JUNK FOOD

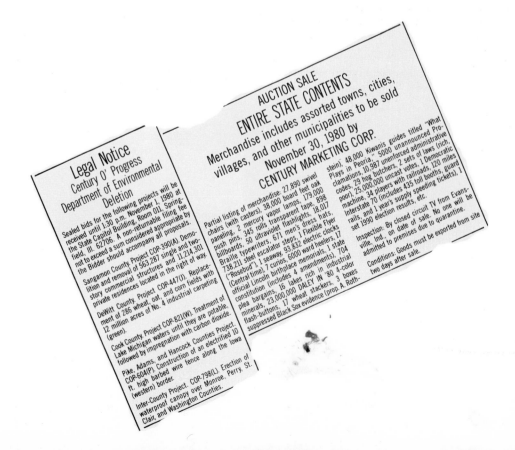

Legal Notice
Century O' Progress
Department of Environmental Deletion

Sealed bids for the following projects will be received until 1:30 p.m. November 1, 1980 at the State Capitol Building, Room 011, Springfield, Ill. 62706. A non-returnable filing fee not to exceed a sum considered appropriate by the Bidder should accompany all proposals.

Sangamon County, Project COP-390(A). Demolition and removal of structures and two-story commercial structures and 11,214,301 private residences located in the right of way.

DeWitt County, Project COP-447(I). Replacement of 286 wheat, oat, and corn fields with 12 million acres of No. 4 industrial carpeting (green).

Cook County, Project COP-821(W). Treatment of Lake Michigan waters until they are potable, followed by impregnation with carbon dioxide.

Pike, Adams, and Hancock Counties Project COP-604(P). Construction of an electrified 10 ft. high barbed wire fence along the Iowa (western) border.

Inter-County Project. COP-798(L). Erection of waterproof canopy over Monroe, Perry, St. Clair, and Washington Counties.

AUCTION SALE
ENTIRE STATE CONTENTS
Merchandise includes assorted towns, cities, villages, and other municipalities to be sold November 30, 1980 by
CENTURY MARKETING CORP.

Partial listing of merchandise: 27,890 swivel chairs (with casters), 38,000 board feet oak paneling, 2 mercury vapor lamps, 179,000 push pins, 345 rolls transparent tape, 898 billboards, 50 ultraviolet flashlights, 18,017 Braille typewriters, 671 men's dress hats, 738,211 steel escalator steps, 1 Flexible Flyer ("Rosebud"), 1 seaway, 93,832 electric clocks (Central time), 7 curios, 6000 ward heelers, 17 official Lincoln birthplace memorials, 1 state constitution (includes 4 amendments), 704 plea bargains, 16 lakes rich in industrial minerals, 23,000,000 DALEY IN '80 4-color flash-buttons, 17 wheat stackers, 3 boxes suppressed Black Sox evidence (prop. A. Roth-

stein), 48,000 Kiwanis guides titled "What Plays in Peoria," 5000 unannounced Proclamations, 10,987 unenforced administrative codes, 29 hog butchers, 2 sets of laws (rich, poor), 25,000,000 uncast votes, 1 Democratic machine, 34 players with railroads, 120 miles Interstate 70 (includes 435 toll booths, guard rails, and 1 year's supply speeding tickets), 1 set 1990 election results, etc.

Inspection: By closed circuit TV from Evansville, Ind., on date of sale. No one will be admitted to premises due to quarantine.

Conditions: Goods must be exported from site two days after sale.

JU
FO

by CHARLES J. RUBIN and DAVID ROLLERT
JOHN FARAGO and RICK STARK
Jonathan Etra

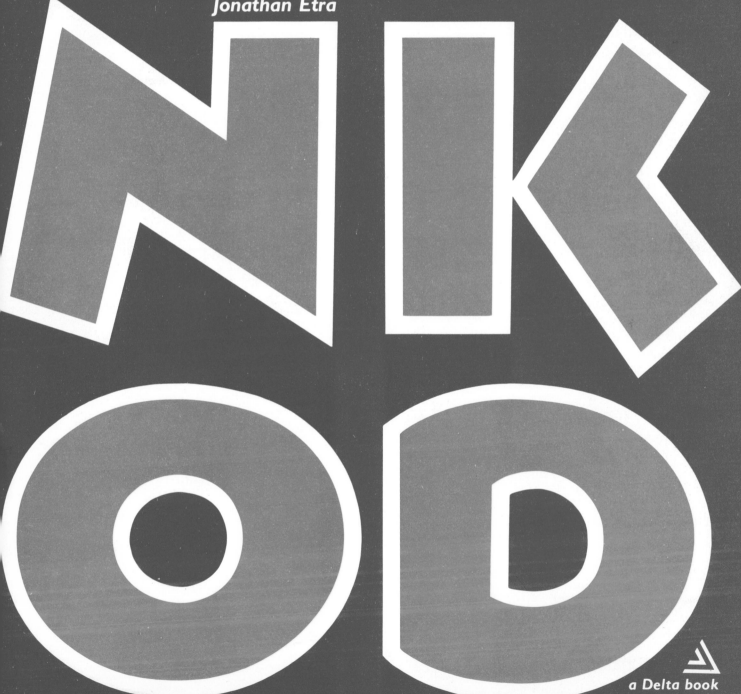

a Delta book

Editor-in-Chief
CHARLES J. RUBIN

Art Directors
DAVID ROLLERT & RICK STARK

Sous-Chef
JOHN FARAGO

Contributor
JONATHAN ETRA

Art Consultant, Wizard,
and Technosculptor
JIM WILSON

Associate Editors
JOHN HOWE & ANDREW ZIMMERMAN

Executive Editor
RICHARD ROTHENSTEIN

Art Associate
SUZIN STARK

Studio Photography
CARL WALTZER

Cover painting by Don Ivan Punchatz
Cover design by David Rollert & Rick Stark

A DELTA BOOK

Published by
Dell Publishing Co., Inc.
1 Dag Hammarskjold Plaza
New York, New York 10017

Table of Contents

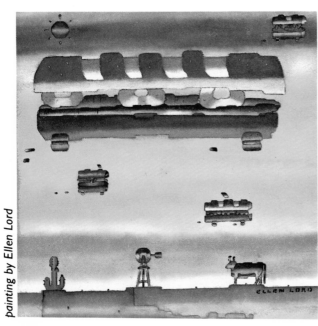

painting by Ellen Lord

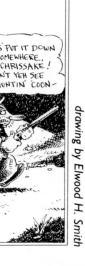

JES' PUT IT DOWN SOMEWHERE, FER CHRISSAKE! CAIN'T YEH SEE I'M HUNTIN' COON—

drawing by Elwood H. Smith

Acknowledgments

Anything worth doing is worth doing well, though perhaps not worth reading.
　　　　　　　　　　　　　　　　　　　　　—Barney Stone

We start with Martha Kinney. Martha pushed for this book for Delta from the day she saw it, bought it over the objections of several highly placed cynics and, of course, the guys with the ledgers, the ones Martha called "the black shoes," who said this book was a dragon that would eat up budgets and schedules and careers and not be worth the time and not be worth the effort. Martha beat them back on every point. And, naturally, they were right. The book blew every deadline; came in way over-budget; caromed across four editors; alienated various departments within Dell; impaired numerous friendships; and ended up with the three of us who did this book full-time, down at the wire, on the take from our parents or our wives or our friends, which is a pretty ratty position for men in their late 20's to end up in.

But Martha felt this book could succeed. She backed us then and later, muscled us an office, provided sound editorial counsel, and made us laugh; moreover, she understood the book we aspired to and never suggested we play it safe. Martha encourages people to be what they are and fail the way they must, so long as it is a failure worth failing at. She would not get very far in television. For all our sakes—and by that we mean not just the five of us but the great collective, communal us who exist in the Rolodex As Big As The Ritz—we are lucky to have her in publishing.

When Martha left Dell, Chris Kuppig took over as head of Delta. Chris said that he regarded himself as an "expeditor," because he regarded the book as essentially done. He was wrong twice; there were still many months to go, and Chris became the book's staunchest ally. He presented us with an ideal situation: an editor who is not editorially intrusive yet who backs you every step of the way. Jean Renoir once said that the way to express one's own personality is to encourage one's collaborators to express theirs; Chris Kuppig's imprimatur, like Martha Kinney's, is on this book as firmly as our own.

Whatever in-house support we mustered—and whatever we retained—was surely Chris' doing. He fought for the book, generally kept the Dell bureaucracy from our door, was always straight with us.

He stuck his neck out for this book. It's still out.

In the early days of this venture, however, we were desperate for accomplices. One of the first to show an interest was Morgan Entrekin, who later became our editor, working with Chris. Morgan defended our tasteless impulses from the forces of censorship, and our more literary impulses from the people who wanted to put a big happy cat on our cover. He tended to get left with the dirtier jobs. For doing them, he became our friend.

John Cushman and his associate, Sophie McConnell, were the agents who prodded us into writing the original book proposal. They were free with their advice, almost all of it good. They hooked us up with Martha and suggested we put together a dummy, which probably clinched the sale.

Several people—Tony Fiyalko, Gary Friedman, Gerry Gersten, and Dan Nelken—gave their time to the dummy without any assurance of compensation down the road. Gerry Gersten must be singled out here, because his name and enthusiasm granted our project an immediate legitimacy in the eyes of writers, artists, and editors alike.

Moving further backwards, Paul Isaac and Nancy Brennan came up with the idea that turned into the idea that metamorphosed into this book. Paul is a trusted critic, a master of the beau geste, and a man who knows where all the bodies are buried. His piece (pps. 163-170) presumably bears this out.

Our parents were always behind us. They are, alphabetically, Mrs. Blanche Etra, Mr. Ladislas and Mrs. Liesel Farago, Mr. Donald and Mrs.

Myriam Rollert, Judge Isaac and Mrs. Lucille Rubin, and Mr. Ernest and Mrs. Cherita Stark. They may not like everything they read in these pages, but they will defend us when others don't.

Suzin Stark, Rick's wife, may be the person most responsible for making the book happen, finally. A graphic designer and a strong right arm, Suzin often worked through the night before leaving for work in the morning. She also got us to Bill DuBay, an unsung genius who is the Stan Lee of his generation (or Lee is the Bill DuBay of *his*), and who saved our life on the Fair.

Deanne Stillman and Rex Weiner were our first and earliest boosters, a show of faith that got this book off the ground. Deanne had co-edited *Titters: The First Collection of Humor by Women* with Anne Beatts, Rex edits a humor magazine called *Informed Source*. They had everything to gain by considering us competitors. Instead, they sent us their friends and relatives, writers, artists, all talented, even the relatives. Anne Beatts was also encouraging and helpful, and later talked us up to Dave Felton at *Rolling Stone*, who got us to several writers. Henry Beard's wisdom all panned out; but the book is poorer for his absence. Alex Theroux kept our spirits up. Sean Kelly and Bruce McCall were two of the best. Roger Rosenblatt and Harry Crews were two of the first. And no one—no one—writes letters like Harry Crews. They should be collected.

Among the artists, Elwood Smith and Rick Meyerowitz were early supporters. Along with Jim Wilson, Lou Brooks, Todd Schorr, and Carol Bouman, they took chances on the book as well as in their work. Their advice and encouragement were indispensable, and they shamelessly talked us up to their most talented friends.

Ann Schaffer, office manager for all of Dell, deserves special mention. She came on gruff but tolerated incredible amounts of unscheduled insurrectionism, most of it taking place in the corral just outside her office.

And a final tip of the Lid Dome to Richard Rothenstein, Jim Wilson, Andrew Zimmerman, John Howe, Gary Friedman, Karl Kofoed, and Carl Waltzer, all of whom formed the inner circle on this book at various times, in various ways. Hopefully, the sections of the book that are uniquely theirs will serve as the rest of their Acknowledgment. *If you seek his monument, look around you* and all that; or try the Table of Contents. Andrew wouldn't know how to take a compliment, anyway. So you all suffer.

And now, the Big List of *amici libri:* Aladdin's Castle, a division of Bally, who supplied the pinball machine that appears on p. 194; Amana Refrigeration, for the Radarange Touchmatic® Microwave oven (Model 10) that we used for all the Micro-Tips in the recipes (most other companies resisted our shameless pleas for free merchandise); Dave Arcoleo; Barbara at Murphy's; Jim Barber, the pinball model; Jan Bartelli; Peter Beard; George Bell; M. K. Brown; Bruce & Doug; Diana Bryan; Chris Buckley; Trisha Buckley; Annette Cafarelli; Jerry Carlson, for counsel on the Judy Garland issue; Cheung Ching Ming; Tommy Cohen; Jeri Cummins; Maggie Curran at I.C.M.; Sharon Daitch, whom we miss talking to; Jim Deligatti; Joan Didion; Steve Dixon; the doctors at Columbia Presbyterian; John Doyle; Gareth Esersky; Marshall Etra; Professor William K. Everson; Sharon Farago; the historian at the Pro Football Hall of Fame; Alison Fraser, for singing; Jim Frenkel; Bruce Jay Friedman; Stan Friedman at U.P.I., for his patience; E. M. Frimbo, our favorite lunch; Bill Gatti; Isabel Geffner; Debbie Gieringer; Dave Grogan; Leslie Harlib; Jeffrey Hart, for lunch we owe; John Heinegg; Roz Heinz; Tony Hiss; Matt Howarth; Reggie Jackson; Karen Ann Johnson, at Carvel; Juris Jurjevics, for support when we needed it; Jim "Kitty" Kaat; Cliff Kachline, historian at the Baseball Hall of Fame; Robert and Susan Kalish, for use of their 1939 World's Fair Guide; Peter Kaminsky; Peter Kaplan; Kenny Kneitel; Ray Kurman; Anita Lawrence; Jessica Lermond; Irv Lerner; Irmgard Lochner; Andy Loomis; Gary Luke; Wallace Markfield, for trying; Betsy Mitchell; Helen Nickerson; Hollis Officer; Diane

Olenick, for the Ranger Chef shirt, and everything else; Grace Paine; Diana Papasergiou; Pizza Hut; Emily Prager; Mitch Rapoport; Ed Retriever; François Robert; Claudia Rollert, just for being y-o-u; Ron Rosenbaum; Mr. and Mrs. Jack Rothenstein; Carol Rubin; Robin Rue, who we hope to know better; Margaret Sapir; Kas Schlots; Shakey's; Kathy Simmons; Fred D. Slota; Ann Spinelli; Jock Spivy; Anne Starobin; Michael Starobin; Doug Taylor; Phil Terzian; Jerry Toner; Nick Tosches; Tom Vickers; Vickie Vidiella; James Wade; Ann Watson; Jaqueline Weiss; Junius Williams; Toney Williams; Laura Wolff, for having good taste; Bruce Yeko; Vic Ziegel; and all the receptionists, notably Amanda Dieckman, the switchboard operators (Elizabeth Berry, Ann Bertelli, Virginia Molloy, Lillian Varga), the mail room people, the cleaning men and women, the people who make Dell run.

Still, the real Acknowledgment on this book must go to our 86 contributors, who worked for pitiful rates because they thought we had a chance to come up with a good book. Maybe because of the imperfections we can see in the book right now, at the end, up close, when it will never be so close again, we're feeling a little guilty about all that time and energy. We thank you, and feel we owe you one. That's only Fair.

JUNK FOOD
August 17, 1979

Authors' Credits

Benny Andrews teaches art at Queens College and is an art critic and painter whose work is in the collection of the Museum of Modern Art. His favorite junk food is ice cream. Raymond Andrews received the 1979 James Baldwin Prize for his first novel, *Appalachee Red*. His next, *Roosevelt Lee Wildcat Tennessee*, will be out in April 1980. He likes chili, hates black-eyed peas. Max Apple is the author of *The Oranging of America*, a collection of stories, and *Zip*, a novel. He likes popsicles, hates Hershey Bars. John Baeder is a noted painter, author of *Diners*, and curator of The Roadside Culture Preservation Society. He actually likes to eat in the Ho Jo's in Williamstown, Mass. Douglas Bauer is a writer living in upstate New York whose first book, *Prairie City, Iowa: Three Seasons at Home* was published in fall 1979. His favorite junk food is french fried onion rings at Chuck's Pizza on 6th Ave. in Des Moines. Anne Beatts was co-editor of *Titters: The First Collection of Humor by Women*, and won two Emmys as a writer for "Saturday Night Live." Really goes for Heinz canned spaghetti. R. O. Blechman is a cartoonist and animator. An anthology of his collected work will be published this year. Likes "old" coffee; "I like it better after it's had a chance to sit." Carol Bouman paints, illustrates, and designs for CBS Records, Putnam Publishing, *High Times*, and *Oui*, among others. A former goal: to be in the Bloomingdale's catalogue by the time she was 30 years old. She made it. Likes Pepperidge Farm Capris. Velament Peppermints, a close second. Salvatore Bovoso is working on a new book, *Cooking for Three: A Guide for the Culinary Ménage à Trois*. [No joke.] Good: Devil Dogs. Bad: Twinkies ("They hurt my throat"). Lou Brooks is a regular contributor to *Playboy Funnies*, has been published all over, does stand-up comedy, and is working on a movie. Best: Peppermint Dynamints. Worst: White chocolate. Les Cabarga is a New York illustrator whose work is inspired by '30's cartoons for the Fleischer studios. Likes raisins. [Health nut.] Cheung Ching Ming is a photojournalist living in Brooklyn and working in New York. Likes onion and sour cream flavored potato chips, doesn't like Campbell's canned vegetable soup. Harry Crews' most recent books are *Blood and Guts*—a collection of pieces from *Esquire*, *Playboy*, and *Sport*— and *A Childhood*. Prefers: "Nasty chili dogs you get in a tavern, shack, off the road, and there's a big fat mama in there sweatin, and kids yellin half in English, half in Spanish. It's the home atmosphere I love, a few flies buzzin,

and their Daddy left in a big pickup truck. This all seems like a good idea at the time, but two-three hours later the payback is a motherfucker." Guy Davenport's latest books are *Da Vinci's Bicycle*, a collection of stories, and *Herakleitos and Diogenes*. His favorite junk food is Zinger's; not crazy about Tab. Ron Dixon is a free-lance illustrator living in New York City and a graduate of the School of Visual Arts. Likes Wise Corn Chips. Doesn't dislike anything. Bill DuBay is the mastermind of Cartooning Inc. He can build an empire, even in Connecticut. Hates McDonald's. His *kids* love it, he says. Randy Enos has been a magazine illustrator for 23 years, his clients including *The New York Times*, *New York*, NBC, *Screw*, *House Beautiful*, and he has done children's books. His strips, "Five Cent Mary" and "Reg'lar Rabbit," appear frequently in *Playboy*. Very big on martinis straight up with an olive, very dry. Bruce Emmett is a free-lance illustrator living in Manhattan. Likes cheesecake, hates Twinkies ("They give me a headache"). Jon Etra is available. Also good at parties. Favorite: chocolate-covered frozen yogurt. Unfavorite: Steak. John Farago is the author of every opinion of the United States Supreme Court for the October, 1978 Term. Other works by Mr. Farago include *Islands in the Stream* and *Titters: The Fotonovel*. He likes his egg creams stirred, not shaken. William Finn is the author of the award-winning Off-Broadway musical "In Trousers," and the upcoming "Four Jews in a Room Bitching." Hates Slim Jims, which "aren't for Jews." Mr. Finn is Jewish. Tony Fiyalko is an admirer of Lon Chaney, Sr., a graduate of the School of Visual Arts, and an illustrator living on Long Island. Likes Nacho Cheese Tortilla Chips. Richard Foreman is the Artistic Director of the Ontological-Hysteric Theater. He recently wrote and directed his first feature film, "Strong Medicine." Yes: potato chips. No: etc. William Price Fox's next novel will be titled either *Dixieanna Moon* or *Coca-Cola Moon* and will be out this year. He has mixed feelings about Goo Goo Clusters. Gary Friedman calls himself "a free-lance graphic designer visiting the Earth," and says that if anything is free, he'll eat it. John Gampert does educational and science fiction and editorial illustrations for various publications. Good: Orville Redenbacher Popcorn. Bad: Hershey's chocolate. Gerry Gersten has been a free-lance illustrator for 20 years. His work has been exhibited in "The 200 Years of Illustration," at the New York Historical Society; at AIGA; at the New York Art Director's Club; and in *Esquire*, *Playboy*, and the like. Gersten's choice: Häagen Dazs Rum Raisin. Stephen Jay Gould is Professor of Geology at Harvard, author of *Ever Since Darwin* and *Ontogeny and Phylogeny*, and a fan of My*T*Fine Tapioca Pudding. Robin Green is a writer living in L.A. who is working on a novel and won't go near Suzy Q's. Lewis Grossberger likes Junior Mints. He also co-authored *The Non-Runner's Book* and has contributed articles to many publications. Jim Heimann is an L.A.-based illustrator who is currently doing a book entitled *California Crazy*. Probably taking hits of his fave Hormel Canned Chili on the side—right, Jim? John Howe, meanwhile, is a New York writer. It's Hostess Cupcakes for me, says Jungle John. But thumbs down on Arthur Treacher's. And Shig Ikeda is a commercial photographer living in New York who likes Miller Beer and hates Hershey Bars. MO: Sir, why aren't you traveling to the Century O'Progress? CURLY MO: I don't know. Is it a good idea? MO: It's a great idea! Paul J. Isaac is a securities trader in Manhattan who likes to relax with a Heath Bar. Frances Jetter's illustrations have appeared in *The New York Times*, *New York*, *Harper's* and *The Nation*. Vegetarian. Karl Kofoed is a science fiction and editorial illustrator, and creator of the "Galactic Geographic" series in *Heavy Metal*. Good: Zots. No good: Pringle's. Sean Kelly was an editor of the *National Lampoon* and is now an editor of *Heavy Metal*. His taste runs to Mae Wests, which are vanilla and chocolate-flavored Twinkie-like treats available only in Canada. Sean is very down on cream soda, for some reason. Brad Korbesmeyer is a California-based free-lance writer with an aversion to turtles. Bob Lambiase is a free-lance illustrator from Philadelphia. Really likes Cheese Twists; hates Milk Duds. David Lander says that he's a writer and actor who went into rock-and-roll because he wanted to lose weight ("Squigtone Mania Lives!"). His favorite junk food? Apples. Hates Ho-Ho's. Gary Lippman is a graduate student at the Cornell School of Industrial and Labor Relations who eats a lot of burgers. Overton Loyd is currently working on album covers and animation in L.A. His Syndrome work includes: *Institutional Investor*, *Hustler*,

MORE, The Illustrated Harlan Ellison, and *The New York Times.* Likes Snickers. **Ellen Lord's** work has appeared in *Mademoiselle, Seventeen,* and *Vogue.* She likes Carvel's Flying Saucers. **Saul Maloff** is a novelist and critic who contributes to *Commonweal* and other periodicals and doesn't like the term "cold cuts": "I'm reacting to a linguistic stimulus." **A. Markworthy** is a retired Oxford don living in Miami and a part-time consultant to the airline industry. He has no strong opinions. **Les Matthews'** column "Mr. 1-2-5 Street" has been a regular feature in the *Amsterdam News* for many years. Yes: McDonald's Cheeseburger. No: Burger King burger. **Bruce McCall** is a free-lance writer and illustrator now working on his first book. He likes french fries with vinegar and salt on them, the kind you get in Port Dover, Ontario. **R. Bruce McColm's** writings on Africa have appeared in the Washington *Post* and *Newsweek,* and he is co-author, with Doug Payne, of *Where Have You Gone? Rock 'N' Roll Stars, The Suburban Wilderness,* and *Weekend U.S.A.* Good: aerosol cheez on "Beagle" wafers [cf., D. Payne]. **Cyra McFadden,** author of *The Serial,* likes movie popcorn. **Michael McKean** is an actor, writer, and—he says—aging rock-and-roll animal ("Lenny and the Squigtones!"). No good: Reese's Peanut Butter Cups. **Rick Meyerowitz** is an illustrator who lived in Chinatown for 11 years. Kentucky Fried Chicken depresses him most. **Jamie Mitchell,** a journalist and amateur filmmaker on the West Coast, likes hydrolyzed soy protein. God. **Lou Myers** publishes cartoons and short stories in *The New Yorker.* Likes pizza. **Rudy Nebres'** work has appeared worldwide. What he will, or won't, eat is his business. **Dan Nelken** is an award-winning photographer specializing in editorial and photo illustration. His favorite junk food is a Whopper w/extra tomato and onions, no cheese; hates black licorice. **Tim O'Brien** won the 1979 National Book Award for *Going After Cacciato.* Tim's choice: Oreos. Nice choice. **Mark O'Donnell** is the youngest of ten children, has an identical twin, and comes from Ohio. He writes poetry and is puzzled by pretzels—"The stick kind. I don't understand the attraction." **Marc Onigman** is a lecturer in sports history at Northeastern University in Boston. He enjoys Burger King Yumbos. **Doug Payne** has written for *Interview* and was Associate Producer of the film "Bullets Into Rain," a documentary about the Angolan Civil War shot on location in 1976 and directed by Bruce McColm [cf., B. McColm]. Loves Sky Blue Freeze Pops, hates Coca-Cola. **Don Ivan Punchatz** wants to be known as an aging, ex-New Jerseyite and Slavic cat-fancier now residing in Arlington, Texas. His friends, he says, call him "Deep Croat." He likes cherry red licorice. The late **Ed "Golden" Retriever** was the first contributor to this volume. He was completing a "tidy prose-poem" about Staten Island street gangs when he was found dangling from the suspension cables of the Verrazano Bridge and "cored like an apple," in March 1978. When **David Rollert** sees the skull beneath the skin, it has a rose-colored tint (PMS 212). Up with: Nutella. Down with: Yankee Franks. Likes Reggie (PMS 497), not Billy (PMS 475). **Bob Rose** is an ivory carver and illustrator. Cheese Doodles offend him. **Roger Rosenblatt** is a columnist for the Washington *Post.* He feels comfortable with a Devil Dog yet queasy around Good 'n Plenty: "I don't like the combination of pink and licorice." **Richard Rothenstein,** from Queens, is working on a book about the Catskills. He's comfortable with Peanut M&M's. Everyone's getting comfortable, that's nice. **Carol Jayne Rubin** is staff news photographer for the Stamford [Conn.] *Advocate* and has had work in the *Daily News.* She likes: Fudgicles. She hates: Schrafft's hard candies. **Charles Rubin** is still bitter about it. Yes: Wink, Dr. Pepper. No: candy corn, scavenger fish. Useful: Wink's steel cans. **Paul Rudnick** is a writer and playwright living in New York. Good: candy buttons. Less good: Steak. **Todd Schorr** is a New York-based illustrator who has worked for CBS Records, Young & Rubicam, BBD & O, *Playboy,* 20th Century Fox, and Columbia Pictures. He can't stomach white chocolate. **Richard Scorza** teaches English at Broward Community College and is a free-lance writer. Never touches: plain yogurt. **Ira Simmons** lives in Louisville, Ky., works for the Louisville *Times,* is a staff reporter for their "Scene" Magazine, and likes jelly donuts "exploding with jelly." **Elwood H. Smith** is an artist living in New York, now being represented by Push Pin Studios. Mallomars make him feel funny. **Mark Alan Stamaty** is a *Village Voice* cartoonist and an author of children's books. He is particularly repelled by Arthur Treacher's. **Rick Stark** was recently selected to design

the logo system for what Rick calls "a small, low-budget kind of dairy fair" taking place in Illinois in 1983. He likes wax lips. **Suzin Stark** is a free-lance graphic designer and organizational whiz who is not nearly as self-effacing as her husband. She's big on Dot candy. **Deanne Stillman** co-edited *Titters: The First Collection of Humor by Women* and is co-author of the recent *Woodstock Census.* She has been published in various prestige journals, misses the funny pages in *New Times,* touts Stouffer's Turkey Tetrazzini, and thinks Mama Celeste Frozen Pizza is the pits. Watch those paws! **Barney Stone** is a reporter-columnist on the Carbondale [Ill.] *Atom* who is currently working on *An Insider's Guide to the New York Times.* He likes Chanukkah gelt ("when I can get it") and despises Stuckey's Pecan Burgers. **Greg Theakston** is a Manhattan-based illustrator with no interest in junk food. **Alexander Theroux** teaches at Philips Academy in Andover, Mass. His latest novel, *Darconville's Cat,* will be out in 1980. He likes cotton candy ("the pinker the better," the best at Revere Beach, Revere, Mass.) and doesn't miss black Necco Wafers a bit. **Joseph Vasta's** photographs have been seen in *New York* Magazine. He is working on a book of highway postcards. He favors Goldenberg Peanut Chews, hates Hostess Snowballs. **John Walker's** cartoons have been published in *Esquire* and the *National Lampoon.* Good: canned lichee nuts. Poor: candy cigarettes. **Carl Waltzer** is a Manhattan-based photographer with no fondness for Twinkies ("My ear starts to bleed"). **Ken Weiner,** a contributing editor of *Punk* Magazine, hates "Puerto Rican burritos" ("the kind you get in P.R. stores") but likes Rollos. **Rex Weiner** is co-author of *Woodstock Census.* He has written "for every magazine ever published...and some that weren't." Yes: Stuckey's Pecan Log. No: Any crackers in the shape of a fish. **Mary Wilshire** is happy with a Good Humor Toasted Almond Eclair. She's a free-lance illustrator and cartoonist living in N.Y.C. And **Jim Wilson** hates Sweet Tarts. Sculptor, writer, designer, author of *The Loft Book* and art director of *The Mr. Bill Show Book...* that's Jim. **Jerome Wrinkle** is a "self-styled wit and raconteur" and editor (*The Wrinkle Free Press*) who thinks Twinkies are grim ("I break out"). Drinks a lot of Coke, though. **Deborah Young** spends her time in Italy, N.Y.C., and Missouri, teaching English, studying film, and visiting her parents. She likes Pinwheels and more expensive cookies. **Vic Ziegel** is co-author of *The Non-Runner's Book.* He won't go near a burger. **Andrew Zimmerman** lives on 14th Street, Manhattan. He likes the grapes in fruit cocktail. **Paul Zimmerman,** a sports columnist who's written five books on pro football, is a wine columnist for *Patent-Trader.* He's now writing a book on wine. And he thinks Treacher's is vile.

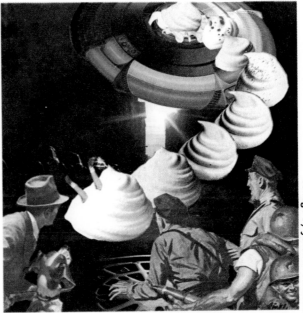

collage by Jerome Wrinkle

Electric appliance + water = DANGER!

Rabbit feet were stored here before shipment to novelty manufacturers.

Brand-names attract begging, broken-down ex-ballplayers with their eye on lucrative endorsement residuals. Where have all the heroes gone?

Still-gnashing lobsters were hurled into these vessels and expected to perish instantly. In fact, they often lived for hours in agony.

Conversion of shelf lives to dog years may have been tedious.

Friends betray you.

Hitters have trouble picking up ball moving from light to dark. Advantage: pitchers.

Bird embryos were dumped into bowl where they were torn apart by spinning steel blades.

Bamboo Curtain drops with force of magnificent bridge built by crazed English Colonel in Japo Theater. Remember?

300 K's.

Scallop pattern is an eye-catching eye-strainer!

No rubber on brake pedal.

Break your mother's back.

Bacteria-ridden grease collects here, invisib to all but the tall.

Notice how they follow you around the room?

Sunlight makes food fade. Sailor take warning!

No interior or "safety" light.

When open, old people complain about the air conditioning on their back.

Often mistaken for rectal thermometer.

45's o-n-l-y (impractical)

Unnecessary mirrors.

One too many vertical handles.

Knuckle chafers.

38 deadly corners.

Duck landed in gravy tureen

Bad.

UNSANITARY!

That's bad right there

Little lambs eat ivy.

Dark colors make you sweat.

Counter not magnetic.

Break your mother's back.

Bad year.

NINO COPPOLLA

GUISEPPE TURANO WAS SEATED HERE

CARMINE GALANTE

ENTRANCE TO PATIO

(L. to r.) Uncle Zeke. Cousin Connie. May be mistaken for flour and baked into cake.

Sunburst pattern presents an easy target.

Religious zealots leaving those pamphlets around again!

¡¿Qué pasa?! (foreign food

Orphans on sponsored dinners steal grandma's napkin rings and replace them with carved soap imitations.

Remember when we were 16, which we'll never be again, and that pretty girl put a carnation in her hair and we went out to the wading pond and afterwards she got malaria and died? We still feel guilty about that, don't we?

Microwave ovens were known to leak and cause cancer.

Name tags or vanity plates cause egocentrism.

It's not funny. It's real.

Silver foil burns, you know? You didn't? Oh God, you better get right home.

Say your grandfather's living with you. He gets into the icebox again. He says he just wants some ice for his soft drink. But he can't work those ice trays anymore. He makes a helluva mess. He ought to be put in a Home.

Ration stamp collection is uninsurable. Even Lloyd's of London says, "You've got a case." Meaning: You don't have a case.

Break your mother's back.

Rock salt with titanium bits combines with iron in blood to make steel.

You're removing the sugarless gum from beneath the table & the knife snaps in two & flys up in your face!

"Rocky, rocky, rocky" go the unsteady chairs.

The kitchen: only 25 feet from your child's bed.

Where are all the people? Is everybody all right? Hel-loo-o-o-o?

Are you sure your car's OK?

Foreword

They're staring out at the incredible City of Brass, the 1904 St. Louis World's Fair.

> MOM: Oh, isn't it breathtaking, John. I never dreamed anything could be so beautiful!
> POP: We don't have to come here on a train, or stay in a hotel. It's—
> BIG GIRL (dreamy.): Right here in our hometown.
> TOOTY (little girl.): Grandpa, they'll never tear it down, will they?
> GRANDPA: Well, I certainly hope not.
> BIG GIRL: Right here in St. Louis.
> *—last 10 seconds of*
> *"Meet Me In St. Louis," MGM, 1944*

Now that was just silly—Hollywood romance. World's Fairs don't last forever, and the old fool knew it, too.

Nothing lasts forever. Nothing. Especially an Old Fair, old fool.

The kitchen was once important to America. It was not as important as the living room, because tragedy was enacted there, in the living room, sons who were caught stealing from their fathers were banished from the family in the living room, mothers were censured, servants were called to task and dismissed without pay, people told on each other, that was the living room.

The kitchen was always simpler, more innocent, the match not the blaze. If mother's brother returned from 40 years at sea, he'd knock on the kitchen door. Forty years at sea for something he probably never did and he'd make his return in the kitchen. Later on, if the family found something they didn't like in his luggage, he'd be humiliated in the living room.

The kitchen was where the family gathered, where they sat at truce, and at table. Occasionally sisters ran screaming from the table, clutching their chests, when a father's fury was uncontrollable. But that was not the norm.

The norm was pleasantries, and a mother's recipes, which rated about 550 on a College Board scale. It was a less complicated time. Those were considered good grades.

And then, one day, everything changed.

The home kitchen was dead.

Doug Broome, The Hamburger King (1920-1976)

"Baby doll, remember there's no such thing as a small Coke."

by William Price Fox

Out under the red and the green and the yellow fast food neon that circles Columbia, South Carolina, like Mexican ball fringe, Doug Broome was always famous. As an eight-year-old curb hop he carried a pair of pliers for turning down the edges of license plates on the non-tipping cars; he was already planning ahead. He grew up during the Depression in the kerosene-lit bottom one block from the cotton mill and two from the State Penitentiary. When he was nine, his father went out for a loaf of bread and in storybook fashion returned 18 years later. Doug left school in the fourth grade, worked his way up from curb boy at the Pig Trail Inn out on The Broad River Road, to Baker's on Main Street, and finally to his own restaurants all over town.

There was a "Doug's" on Lady Street and while I was still in junior high he hired me on the sandwich board and the big grill. He taught me how to stay on the duckboards to keep from getting shin splints, how to make an omelette, and a hundred things behind the counter that made life easier. I copied his freewheeling moves with the spatula and the French knife, his chopping technique on onions, and his big takeaway when he sliced a grilled cheese or buttered toast. He also introduced a lot of us to the 10-hour day, the 12-hour split shift, and the killer 24-hour roll over. Somehow he thought we all had his energy.

Doug Broome had energy, incredible energy. It may be the kind you see in skinny kids playing tag in a rainstorm or the stuff that comes with Holy Roller madness. He had black curly hair, bright blue eyes, wore outrageous clothes, and every year had the first strawberry Cadillac convertible in Columbia. When he was young he won the jitterbug contests all over town taking shots at everything Gene Kelly was doing in the movies. He was wild with clothes. With cars. With women. Some of his checks may still be bouncing. To investors coming to town on business with him, Doug was a mystery; a threat. His pink-piped matching shirt and slacks and his lightning ways with money scared them off. To them, a bounced check or a bankruptcy judgment or a stack of subpoenas was like the neck bell and the tin plate of the leper, but in Doug's empire this was only his way of doing business. And Doug had an empire. He became the father he never had for his family, his help, and his friends. He worked them, loved them, punished them. Sometimes he would sit down and list the problems he was having with them. Someone was getting married before they were divorced; or divorced without benefit of attorney. Some couple would leave for a Stone Mountain, Georgia, honeymoon with the back seat stacked to the window level with Doug's beer and the trunk loaded down with Virginia hams and

Extremely rare photo of Doug Broome with small Coke. Reader's attention should be directed to Doug's tie.

cigarettes. Someone was always running off with a friend's wife or husband, getting drunk, wrecking the wrong car, and getting locked up. And a few of the more spectacular cases managed to do everything at once.

Doug would just grin and say, "We're just one great big old family out here mashing out hamburgers and making friends." When they were in jail, Doug bailed them out. When drunk, he sobered them up, and when in trouble or sick, he gave them his lawyer and his doctor. He never took them off the payroll. They stole a little, but Doug with some sixth sense knew about how much and made them work longer hours. It was a good relationship, and when the unions came around to organize, Doug's people would just laugh and say they'd already been organized.

Ten years ago he told me, "Billy, these chain operations are ruining the Hamburger. Ruining it. Most of them come from up north to begin with, so what in the hell they know about cooking? Any fool right off the street will tell you the minute you freeze hamburger you ain't got nothing. God Almighty, you slide one of those three ouncers out of a bun and throw it across the room and it will *sail.* I ain't lying, that's how thin that thing is." He was eating his own Doug Broome Doubleburger. "Now you take this half-pound baby. I don't care what you think you could do to it, there ain't no way in the world you can make it any better. No way. I use the finest ground meat there is. The finest lettuce, the finest tomatoes and onions and Billy, I fry this piece of meat in the finest grease money can buy. These chains are getting their meat up out of Mexico. Ain't no telling what's in it. Hell, I read that in a government magazine."

He went on about how he had gunned down the "Big Boy" franchise when it rolled into South Carolina. "Everybody in town knows I've always called my hamburger, 'Big Boy.' You used to serve them. Am I right or am I wrong?" He didn't wait for an answer. "Anyhow they'd already steamrolled across everything west of the goddamn Mississippi. And here they come heading across Tennessee. Then across Alabama. Then across Georgia. But when they hit that South Carolina line I said WHOA NOW! You ain't franchising no 'Big Boy' in here because I am already the 'Big Boy.' Gentlemen, you and me are going to the courts. And that's what we did. They brought in a wheelbarrow of money and eight or nine Harvard Jew lawyers and all I had going for me was my good name. And Billy we beat them to death. I mean to death. They had to pay me $60,000, all the court costs, and everything." He paused and sipped his coffee. "Well you know I never like to kick a man when he's down and those boys had all that money tied up in promos and Big Boy neon so I say O.K, yall give me another $10,000 and you can have the franchise and I'll change my 'Big Boy' to 'Big Joy.' "

I knew a few of the facts. "Come on, Doug."

And then he raised his hand to heaven.

"Boy, why would I tell a lie about something like that?"

Part of the story was true. Outside on North Main the

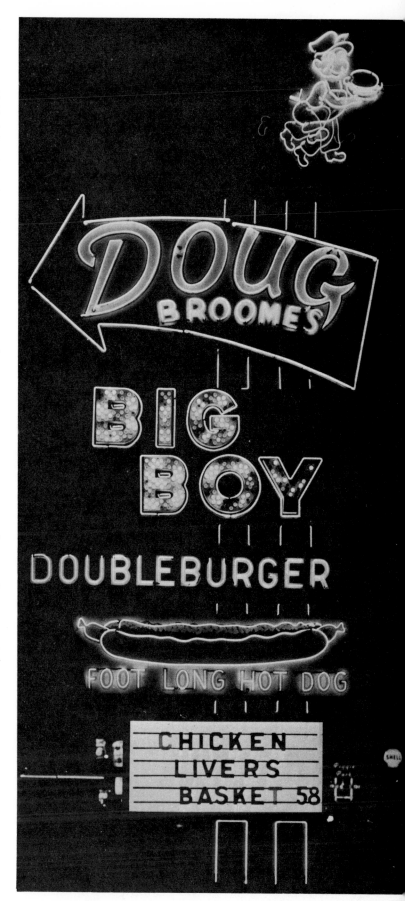

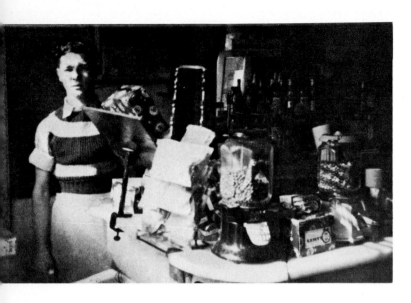

Old "Big Boy" read "Big Joy." But the eight or nine Harvard lawyers turned out to be one old retainer out of Charlotte. The $60,000 was right but it went the other way; Doug had been the infringer and had to pay them. The $10,000 never existed. Doug was like that. Like all great storytellers, he was a consummate liar. A straight tale would be transformed into a richer, wilder mixture and the final version, while spellbinding, while credible, would have absolutely nothing to do with the truth.

But I remember one crazy night on Harden Street. We were in the kitchen. It was July. It was hot. Oral Roberts was in town. He was still lean and hungry and doing Pentacostal tent shows. "NO! I'm not going to heal you! Jesus is! Jesus Christ is going to heal you! So I want you to place both hands on your television set. And I want you to pray along with me. And if you ain't got a television set, place your hands on your radio. And if you ain't got a radio, any electrical appliance will do."

At the air-conditioned 8000-seat tent it had been Standing Room Only and every soaring soul had descended on Doug's for hamburgers, barbeques, steak sandwiches, fries, and onion rings. Doug and I were on the big grill, the broilers, the Fryolaters. Lonnie was on the fountain. Betty Jean, under a foot-high, silver-tinted beehive, was on the counter and the cash register. The parking lot was jammed and another 100 cars were cruising in an Apache circle looking for a slot. In the kitchen the grease was so

thick we had to salt down the duckboards to keep from slipping. The heat was 120° and rising. The grill was full. The broilers were full. The Fryolaters and the sandwich board were full. There was no more room. There was no more time. We had lost track of what was going out and what was coming in. Horns were blowing. Lights were flashing. The curb girls and Betty Jean were pounding on the swinging doors, screaming for hamburgers, barbeques, steak sandwiches, anything. And then suddenly there was another problem. A bigger problem. The revivalists were tipping with religious tracts and pewter coins stamped with scriptural quotes.

The girls were furious. "One of them gave me a god-damn apple! Look! Look at it!"

And what did Doug Broome do? I'll tell you what he did. He stripped off his apron and pulled Betty Jean out from behind the counter. Then he triggered "The Honeydripper" on the juke. No one could believe what Doug was doing. He was dancing and Betty Jean was doing red-hot little solo kicks on his whirling breaks. When the song ended he announced that everyone was getting a $25 bonus for working the Pentacostals, who had scriptural support for their stand on no-tipping. Then Doug flipped on the public address system and sang out over the cars and the neon and the night: "Ladies and gentlemen and boys and girls I'd like to take this opportunity to remind you that you are now

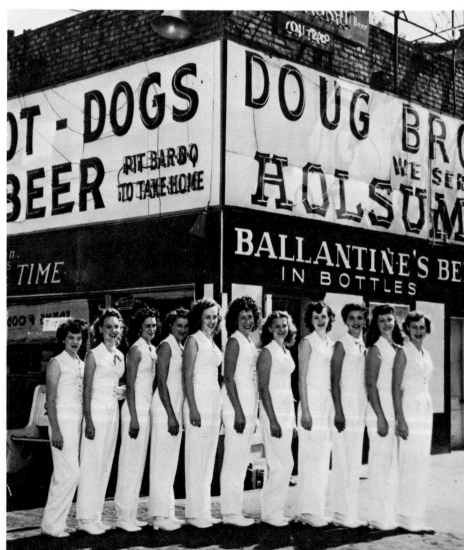

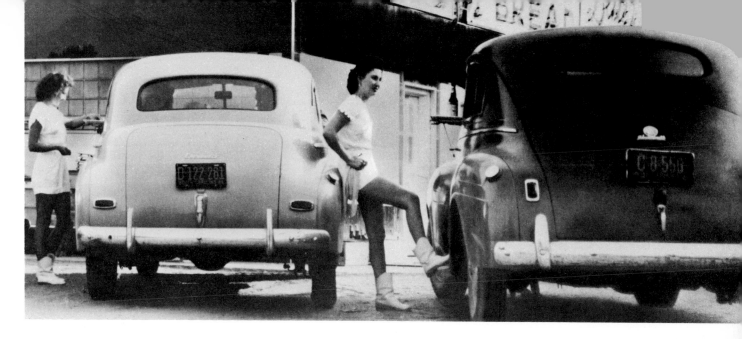

eating at one of the most famous drive-ins in-the-great-south-east. Our specialties are hamburgers, barbeques, and our famous steak sandwich which is served with lettuce and tomato, carrot curls, pickle chips, and a side of fries all for the price of one-dollar-forty-nine-cents. And when you get home tonight and tell your friends about our fine food and fast service please don't forget to mention that we have been internationally recognized by none other than Mister Duncan Hines himself. . . . I thank you." Then tying on his apron and angling his cap he came back to the grill and with some newer, faster, wilder speed I'd never seen, he caught the crest and broke it.

Doug had style but it wasn't until years later that I realized what a profound effect it had on me. I was on a New York talk show hustling a novel. The host had led me down the garden path in the warm-up, promising we'd discuss pole beans and the price of cotton. But when the camera light came on his voice dropped into low and meaningful. We discussed the mythic south, the gothic south, Faulkner's south, and the relevance of the agrarian metaphor. I was a complete disaster. All I wanted, was out. And then he asked how I would define style. It was a high pitch right across the letters and I dug in and took a full cut. And I told him about one day during a lunch rush at Doug's on Harden Street. There had been a dozen customers on the horseshoe counter and a man came in and ordered a cheese omelette. I'd never made one before but I'd watched Doug do it. I chopped the cheese, broke three eggs into a shake can, added milk, and hung it on the mixer. Then I poured it out on the big grill. I'd used too much milk and it shot out to the four corners getting ready to burn there in 20 seconds. I almost panicked. Then I remembered Doug's long, smooth moves with the spatulas and pulled them out of the rack like Smith and Wesson 44's. I began rounding it up.

As I worked, I flexed my elbows and dipped my knees and did a little two-beat rhythm behind my teeth. I kept singing, kept moving, and just at the critical moment I folded it over, tucked it in, and slid it onto the plate. Then with parsley bouquets on the ends, and toast points down the sides, I served it with one of Doug's long flourishes and stepped back.

The man forked off an end cut. He chewed it slowly and closed his eyes in concentration. Then he laid his fork down and with both hands on the counter he looked me in the eye. "Young man," he said. "That's the finest omelette I've ever put in my mouth."

I wound up telling the stunned interviewer that that was style and all you can do with it is point at it when you see it winging by and maybe listen for the ricochet. I don't think he understood, but I knew I did. I knew that style wasn't an exclusive property in the aristocracy of the arts. A mechanic grinding valves can have it, so can the shell game shills at the carnivals and the feather-trimmed whores working the curbs along Millwood and Gervais. And later still, I heard Dizzy Gillespie say that style is how you get from one note to the next.

Growing up I copied my Dad's moves and James Cagney's moves but most of all I copied the moves of the Hamburger King, Mr. Doug Broome.

Doug's gone now and with him goes his high-pitched voice on the P.A. and the nights and the music and the great curb girls out on Harden Street who got us all in trouble. He's gone and with him go those irreplaceable primary parts of Columbia that shimmered out there under the cartoon-colored neon. There will be no buildings or Interstate Cut Offs named for him, nor will there be a chandeliered Doug Broome Room at The Summit Club. But some nights out on North Main or Harden or Rosewood, when the moon's right and the neon's right and a juke box is thumping out some '60's jump or Fats Domino is up on "Blueberry Hill," it will be impossible not to see him sliding Doubleburgers and Sunday beers in milkshake cups down the counter. And if you're all lucky as a lot of us who knew him, you'll probably see him pinch the curb girl at the pick-up window and give her that big smile and say, "Baby Doll, remember there's no such thing as a small Coke."

photographs courtesy Mrs. Doug Broome

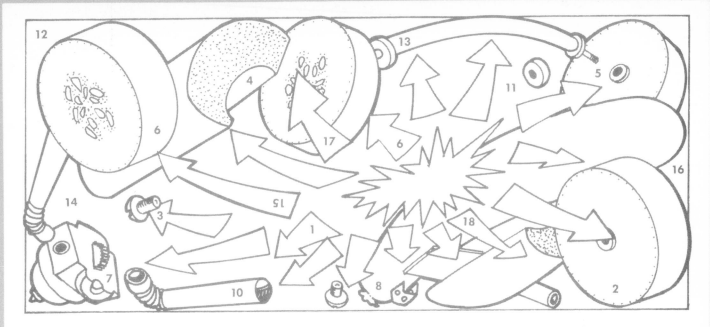

Nathan's Famous Sand-Witch

Model Assembly Instructions

Congratulations! You now own a full-size model kit of the **Nathan's Famous Sand-Witch**™, the fastest food ever to pass through a digestive track. You may have built models of planes and cars, and even see-through, plastic people (see **Trans-Parents**™ kit M-74), but the **Taste & Race**™ series adds another dimension to the world of replicas. During each step of assembly, these instructions will tell you where each piece goes and how it functions, so that when you're finished you'll have a thorough understanding of Formula 1 foodstuffs.

All parts can be put together with an ordinary set of flatware and a few other items found in most kitchens. (**Note.** Special customizing may require additional utensils: a five-speed blender, a MoPar toaster, a low-torque whisk, and a turbo-charged double boiler.)

1. The first step is to process the contents of the nine power packets into a low-calorie, high-energy fuel.

Packet A **(1)** contains 0.5 oz. of HVP (hydrolized vegetable protein), a refined, high-Btu consummable, and 10W-30 sorbitol, which lubricates the **Sand-Witch**™ and keeps it from making dangerous detours out of the esophagus and into the trachea during speed-eating competitions.

Next is Packet B **(2)**, which is filled with 0.5 oz. of sodium erythrobrate (SEB) to help prevent embarrassing backfires through the anal sphincter (little PUs), and stomach knock (hiccups). A lot of people who don't get their Recommended Daily Allowance of SEB end their meals putting in a side order for a stomach pump!

Packet C **(3)** is filled with 0.5 oz. of sodium nitrite to keep your "tube trolley" from turning into a **Fungus Farm**™ (see model kit A-35) while it sits on the shelf. It's also important to the appearance of your food because it keeps the high-gloss finish bright and succulent month after month, picnic after picnic.

Packet D **(4)** contains 0.3 oz. of beef and salt, which are usually found in nutritional racers of this design.

Packets E through I **(5)** are filled with flavoring, garlic powder, and various spices (0.2 oz. total) that can be added to give your "track dog" a distinctive taste and aroma.

2. Empty Packets A and B into a bowl and mix in ½ cup Wesson oil. Stir with a No. 10 spoon until it starts to bubble (or until you find yourself holding a No. 8 spoon). Drain oil and set aside.

Ignite oven and rev to 300°. Drop ¼ stick butter into pan and heat for 60 sec. Inject HVP mixture, throttle stove down to 250° and idle 20 min.

3. Unroll the body casing **(6)**, a large-bore sleeve milled to 1/64 in. that acts as the frame for your vehicle and serves as its fuel tank. Inflate

and immerse in water. If any bubbles come out the exhaust your casing has a leak that should be repaired with the **Meat Mender**™ kit **(7)**. Once all punctures have been plugged you are ready to fill 'er up.

Remove fuel from oven and pour into sleeve. Add seasonings to taste. Tie off tail pipe and apply one coat of Red Dye No. 3 Deep Lustre Food Enamel. **(8)**

4. Remove presliced body bun **(9)** from plastic bag. Check to see that it is soft and fresh and that no mold is growing along the rocker panel. Minor dents and scrapes can be fixed with Breado® body compound. **(10)**

Separate halves and spray with Yellow Dye No. 11 Protein-Tector sandwich sealer **(11)**, which will give your model a golden, fresh-baked finish and guard against loss of vitamins and minerals. Place halves in toaster oven, set on medium, and heat for 3 min. Cradle previously assembled fuel casing within body bun. Install roll bar **(12)**. As an alternative to toasting, you may want to let the body turn stale overnight. This takes longer, but is one certain way to prevent scorching.

5. The power plant for the "Nathan's Nemesis" is a modified Cruisinart 500. Insert the intake manifold **(13)** into the single-barrel carbohydrator **(14)** and connect them to the die-cast chopping block **(15)**. With a processor like this under your skin that can turn over at 8500 rpm and go from grate to puree in less than 2 sec. without spinning out, nothing will even come close to whipping your machine.

6. Take the 4-ply cucumber that comes with your kit and slice two 3-in. sections from the middle. Insert skewers through the center and attach to rear of body **(16)**. Repeat procedure using two ½-in. sections for the front wheels **(17)**. These fibrin-belted stomach huggers with their unpared treads are specially grown to hold fast during a sharp duodenal turn. Some hobbyists have substituted potato slices in the hope that a spudded tread would improve performance, but we have found that our green-walled tuberless tires don't get mashed up as easily.

7. Apply decals **(18)** and you're finished. Well done! Now that you've completed your **Sand-Witch**™, you can have hours of fun putting together some other **Kar-Kraft**™ models—there are dozens to choose from:

The General™—An authentic-tasting hero sandwich complete with tomatoes, ham, salami, a Bronze Star with Oak Leaf Cluster, and Blue Max cheese. Have fun saluting your food!

Supper Stock Series™—Eight delicious competition dinner soups from Campbell's.

Toast & Coast Series™—More than 20 different loaves of bread from around the world. Twelve slices per kit. Butter included. Assemble, then slide them to destiny across your living room floor.

CarPets™—Furry little autos that are as cute as hamsters, but easier to care for. Cuter.

text by John Howe

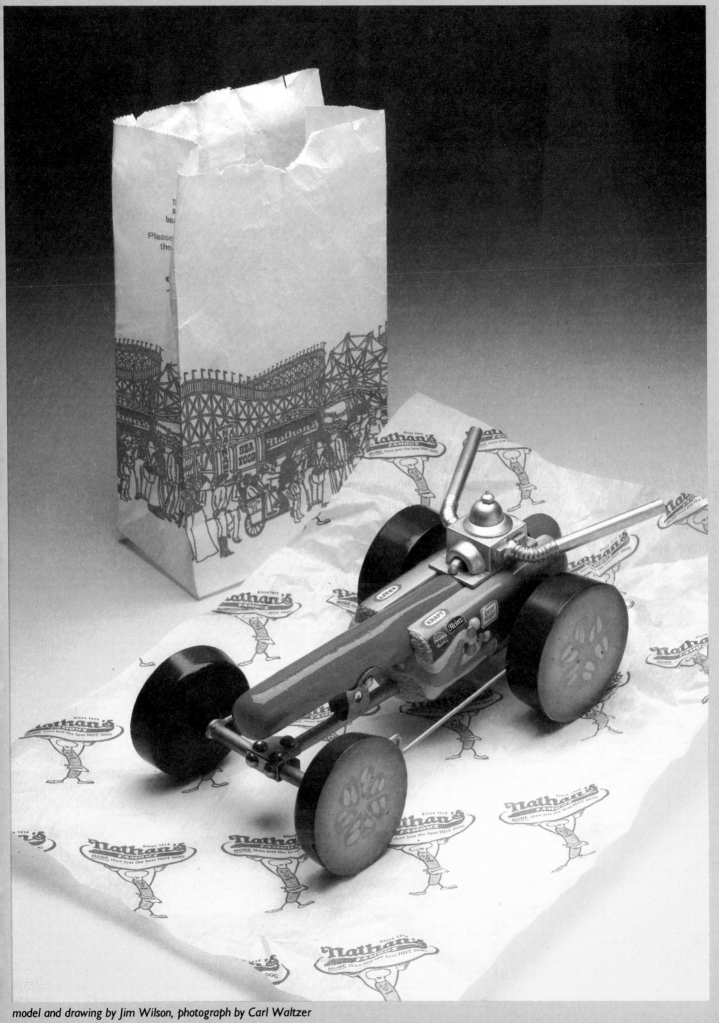

model and drawing by Jim Wilson, photograph by Carl Waltzer

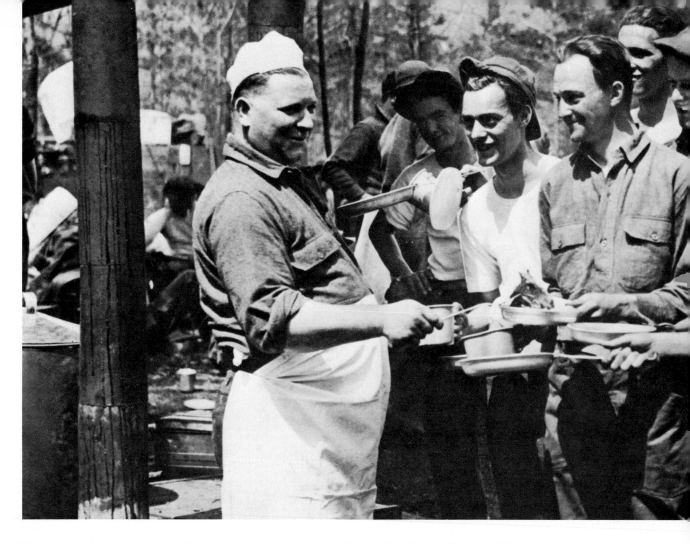

Dustbowl of Cherries

**An oral history of
eating in the Great Depression.**

by Bruce McCall

Felix McIntosh
68; retired dance instructor, Corpus Christi, Texas

I never even seen a dinner plate until the spring of 1932, up at Washington, D.C., at the White House. I'd got a job there as second pantry man by my daddy blackmailing our Congressman. Up until then, what we used for a dinner plate back in West Texas you'd call a common ordinary cowflop. Nature's chinaware, my daddy always called it. A good sunbaked cowflop, most folks don't know this, makes a fine dinner plate. It's yea flat and so big around, and it not only comes in at an unbeatable price but remember there's no need for washing up after the meal. You just sail her out the kitchen window, back into the field she come from.

But people always want to know about being second pantry man at the White House. It wasn't much of a job, if you want the truth. The second pantry man was in charge of the first pantry man. He was always drunk. The reason he was always drunk was the housekeeper in those times. There was your textbook alcoholic. She fired anybody she found sober on the job in that pantry.

The first pantry man when I got there, in the spring of '32, was named Ray. A big purple-complected man. They said he was an admiral once but you couldn't get nothing out of old Ray by then but hiccups. Well, one of the jobs I took over from Ray was to bring the dinner plates up to wherever the President was eating his meal and put them on the sideboard. President Hoover took a lot of his meals alone, you see. He wasn't much for making smalltalk with the help—so it wasn't the words that stood out, it was the noises. At first I thought he might be sick, something stuck in his throat choking him maybe. But the stewards on duty behind him, they never flinched or flickered an eye, just

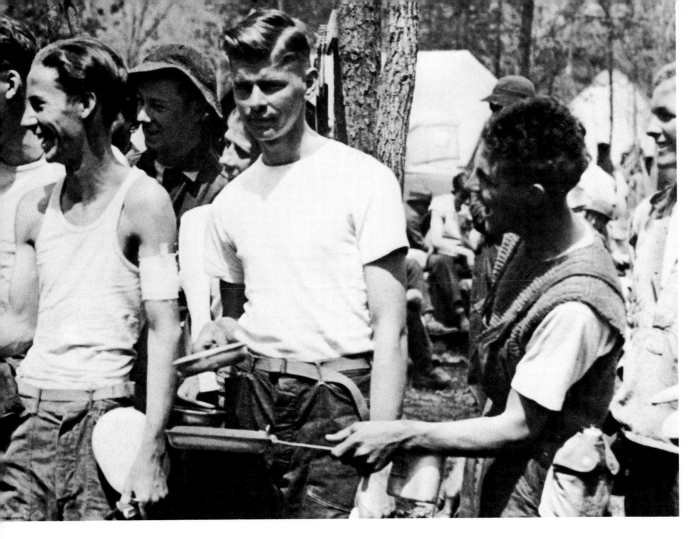

stood there staring at the wall, so pretty quick I caught on that this was normal with the President at table alone, and you pretended not to notice if you knew what was good for you. What the old bastard was doing was he was making dams and big forts and ship canals with his food. Those noises was playing the part of the steam engines and cranes and the like, for realism, you see. He'd give this long rumbling sound and there'd go his fork, pushing all the mashed potatoes to one side while his knife went at the squash and the gravy come running down from up near the broccoli. Panama Canal. Ice cream he made tunnels in with his spoon and I guess in his mind he was drilling solid rock because you'd get this horrible screeching noise and sweat would be all over his kisser. But God forbid if you didn't keep a straight face. He was the "Great Engineer" after all, and I guess that extended to engineering his supper food. Well, the President liked a cigar, a big Havana, and one time when I come in with more dishes it caught my eye: four Havanas sticking straight up off his plate. I couldn't resist. I got near enough to peep over his shoulder from behind, and sure enough, it was a model of a big ocean steamer, if you sort of squinted. Hull made out of smoked salmon and some kind of vegetable for a superstructure. I forget now what he had for lifeboats, but there was all these lifeboats strung along. Ju-jubes, maybe. And for smokestacks, them cigars.

Just then he turns around. I thought, now I am going to get my head bit off. But he just drilled me with them beady little eyes of his. "R.M.S. *Mauretania,*" he says. Them were the only words President Herbert Hoover ever spoke to me direct. "R.M.S. *Mauretania.*" Well, they scrapped Hoover later that same year, but they didn't scrap the *Mauretania* until '37 or '38! [Laughs.]

Elspeth Vole
73; widow, Chicago, Illinois

So that's a tape recorder. The Mister—Mister Vole—he never was much for electricity. Said it got in the fillings of the teeth and caused neuritis and neuralgia. Had all his teeth pulled as a precaution. Wouldn't visit where they had a radio or a Frigidaire. He only ate the soft foods. He died eating a donut. "Elspeth," he said, "I'm passing over." Kept the rest of the donut as a kind of a souvenir for years. To remember him by. But it didn't affect my appetite. Still love a donut with my coffee.

Well, there were no soft foods back then in what they call the Depression. Everything, hard. We talked about it all the time. Hard-hat candies, remember them? Jawbreakers. Hard apples that made hard cider. It was cheaper ingredients that did it, because there wasn't the money for better. The farmer used a cheaper fertilizer and he got hard tomatoes and potatoes. The soup companies used a cheaper stock and I remember, some lunchtimes back then you had to break the crust on the top. The baker used a cheaper flour and so you got hard bread. My heavens, the hard bread. We had the big bread riot here in Chicago in '34 or '35, the year Detroit was in the World Series. I always remember it by that, the Mister, he came from near Detroit, you see. The bread was too hard. People stood on line down on Clark Street, waiting sometimes twelve hours for a loaf of bread that when they got it, it was just too hard to eat. The police broke up the riot by knocking people over the head with their own loaves of bread, that's how hard it was. Anybody who lived through the Depression got a real taste for soft foods. The water was even hard. That was the beginning of hard water. The ingredients there, too, you see, cheaper. There wasn't the money like before.

One time I'll never forget. My sister Fleur lived out near Winnetka and she and Vic, her husband, invited the Mister and me there for Sunday dinner. Fleur did up a wonderful spaghetti and all the way out there, the Mister and I on the train were talking about having a nice dish of soft food. Nice soft spaghetti. Well, you know what happened. Fleur's spaghetti cooked up like a pot full of knitting needles. At first we made jokes of it, because Vic, he had a fierce temper and couldn't stand anybody criticizing him or his own. But then Vic got one of those sticks of spaghetti—that's what they were, long and thin and hard sticks, like pencils—stuck in the back of his throat. Vic with that spaghetti like an arrow in the back of his mouth. You had to laugh in a way, but you also felt like crying. All the way out to Winnetka on a train that made so many stops, for a meal of soft food, and now there's Vic down on the floor, kicking. He was in real pain. They got him to the hospital in no time and he was fine again in a few hours. The doctors told Fleur they'd seen lots of cases just like it.

It wasn't until years later that the softness came back into food. A few years after that time with Vic and the hospital and all, we went back on a Sunday for some soft spaghetti. It was wonderful again, but this was Pearl Harbor Day as it happened, and that took the starch out of it, as the Mister said.

Clovis Grimble, Jr.
72; retired police dispatcher, Valparaiso, Indiana

I read every book about the Pretty Boy Floyds and the Alvin Karpises and of course the Dillingers, you might call it professional research on account of my putting in twenty-five years on the police force. What that has to do with food and the Depression I'm coming to, hold your goddamn horses. What I never, ever, found in any of these yarns was any mention of grapes in the crime wave of the '30's.

You think I'm just an old man's lost his marbles. Shows how much you know. I'll spell it out. Everybody back then in Depression times, they were poor. You know that, everybody knows that. But think about the crooks. Did you know

they were poor, too? Banks didn't have no money. God knows. . . .

Now hear me out, the food's coming right up. Because the crooks couldn't afford bullets, so they shot grapes. Little green grapes, the sour kind, hard as stones if you used them before they was a hundred per cent ripe. One mob up near Eau Claire, I think it was, they killed two policemen shooting those grapes. Can you feature that? The police started returning fire with grapes of their own, because, you see, most towns and cities were on the verge of being bankrupt themselves and if they could save bullet money, so much the better. That's what they used to get John Dillinger up in Chicago. Oh, they kept it out of the papers because how does it sound, nailing the F.B.I.'s Most Wanted Man with fruit? I sent it in to Ripley's Believe It Or Not a couple of years after, even had it notarized so they'd know it wasn't just some crank, or some leg pull. But they never wrote it up. You know why, don't you? The F.B.I. got to them. But I had it from some of the boys that were in on the Dillinger thing.

The young today, of course, they think it's all a lot of stuff and bunkum, this talk about grapes for bullets. But they never lived in the Depression, did they? Hell, the hardness of the food. It wasn't just the grapes, it was everything. Don't ask me why. I'm no goddamn Luther Burbank. All I know is, sometimes today my mouth will come up sore, forty years later, from putting all that hard food in it back then.

But if it helped put away that goddamned John Dillinger, I guess some good come out of it after all.

Murtland Breen
66; housepainter, Buffalo, New York

I was born in 1913. That would make me sixteen when the Depression hit. Halfway through my growth. I was a lanky kid. Then those three squares a day got hard to come by. [Laughs.] Well you can figure out what happened by taking a look at me now. That's correct. I shrank. [Laughs.] Lost a good eight inches off my height from the bad diet. Dad tried getting some good out of it by offering me around to the circus people, but even though they were sympathetic, nobody would take me on. We got a letter from the Barnum & Bailey people explaining that it was just too depressing. Folks went to a circus for entertainment, to forget the hard times. Seeing a kid turned into a runt by the Depression, well, that would just turn 'em off! [Laughs.]

We had a doorway where my dad would mark off every month with a pencil how much I was going down. Other kids were growing up, I was growing down. It was hard on me, no question. Lost a girlfriend that I had at the time. She said the reason was, we were growing apart. [Laughs.] I'll never forget when she said that. She meant it one way, see, and I took it another. [Laughs.] And I had to start wearing hand-me-ups—clothes I got from my little brother who was more my size, or the size I was coming to, I should say. I was passing kids who were coming the other way in terms of height. I took up cigarettes. Why not, they couldn't stunt my growth! [Laughs.] So the Depression was a terrible time for me, just a terrible time. I wish I could tell you otherwise, but I can't. And it wasn't just me, either. Remember that. Somebody out in California started a club for people that started shrinking from the Depression diet. I never joined, I wasn't a joiner then and I'm not now. I spent most of my time alone. I had a picture collection of short men. Kids are funny. I decided to be proud of being short. Elmer "Bird" Carroll of the Canton Bulldogs, the great Caruso, Napoleon of course, Marshal Foch of France, they were all up there on my wall. I must have seen *The Wizard of Oz* a hundred times, and let me tell you, I was rooting for those little flying monkeys! [Laughs.] Still do! [Laughs.] Even today! [Laughs.]

Bebe Funtoon
70; matron, Wilmington, Delaware

Food? In the Depression? I shall *never* forget the railway policemen bringing up pots of boiling stew from the hobo jungles to our galas at Ickmore. Father owned the company that sold the wooden ties to all the railways here and in certain Latin American countries, and we were *extremely* well connected with railway people everywhere, and this paved one's way not only in society but on a *million* fronts. Father had such high spirits. It was parties, parties, parties at Ickmore. You'd never know there was such a *thing* as a Depression, *not* if you saw things from the Ickmore perspective. Well, I *am* straying awfully from the point.

What was a gala without a theme, a leitmotif? How would people dress? Father had the amusing idea of making everyone come as hoboes. So *topical,* and so *rich* in terms of the contrast; I mean, DuPonts and Mellons and Funtoons, don't you see. And then he had the infinitely more amusing idea of catering the gala with hobo food, *actual* hobo food. I mean, seriously! He would simply call a Mr. Bint, or Dint, who was head of the railway detectives in the area. Nasty man, kept a revolver in his hip pocket and it was there even when he came up to Ickmore to see Father on one errand or other. And Father would instruct Mr. Bint, or Dint, to go down there along the railway tracks where the tramps and the hoboes were swarming like flies, and take their food. To do what he *had* to do, but to bring back enough of their food to make Ickmore, if just for one mad evening, a hobo jungle. And say what you will about that man Bint, he never *ever* failed. We got truckloads.

One never actually *ate* any of it, *no.* It was only for atmosphere. Nutritionally of course it *wasn't* food. We always thought that if they had eaten decent food, food that gave them some vim and vigor, those hoboes would have found the energy to go out and get work, make something of themselves. But we *saw* what they were putting into their tummies. Garbage. It made one lose patience. It made

one immune to Mister Roosevelt and his silly dramatics. No *wonder* everybody went to France.

Jane Parker
72; spinster, Conshohocken, Pennsylvania

Did you know that was me on all the A&P baked goods packages? My name at least, they judged my face too homely and had some commercial artist make up another Jane Parker for display purposes.

You see, the A&P held a nationwide baking contest in 1933 and I took first prize. I think it came to five dollars. And that's all I ever got out of it. Five dollars. The A&P used my name to make a fortune on their cakes and bread and cookies. If you give us your recipes we'll make you famous, that was the contest pitch. Well, who didn't want that? But you can't put publicity in the bank, I found.

I wasn't the only one. Do you know Sara Lee? Same story. She wrote me a letter. And Betty Crocker from up Minneapolis way. It was Betty Crocker—her real name was Krockelmeier, something like that—suggested us girls all meet at the Hotel Chase out in St. Louis to put together a plan for getting our fair share. Ha! She said she'd had this lawyer friend make up a petition to the Supreme Court and all our troubles were over. So Sara and me, we both signed. We found out later that that Betty Crocker was working for Pillsbury all the time because she was sleeping with one of the muckety-mucks up there. What we signed was a legal promise to keep our mouths shut forever.

Now, last I heard, Sara Lee was in a rest home somewheres. But I'm still hale and hearty. I'd love to meet that Crocker gal again, and I don't mean for a bake-off, either.

But it just goes to show how desperate everybody was in the Depression. Even something as wholesome as baked goods gets dragged through the mud for the almighty dollar. So that's the story of Jane Parker.

Curt Glott
68; waiter, Kalamazoo, Michigan

I come in America from Germany nineteen hundred one-and-thirty. My hope is a dancer to be, but clear, it is hopeless. I have the size thirteen foots. One problem other . . . I like to dance only with the marching music! Ba-bom, ba-bom, pa-pa-pa-bom! It gives no shows with march dancers! And I look . . . I seek, is this right? . . . from New York in all of the directions, is this right?

I find a work in a restaurant in Detroit, eventual. Is this right? A Mexican one. My language is problematic. Spanish, German, English, all mixed. Problematic in special for the customers!

I tell one interesting thing. I am German, yes? Secure. But I am no better in the German speaking as Spain or English! I speak with my foots! My dancing foots! Ba-bom, ba-bom, pa-pa-pa-bom!!

The 24-Hour Breakfast

by Robin Green

This was not, the editors said, to be one of those articles in which the writer stops at dawn for breakfast at a truckstop along the lonesome highway and comments on the emptiness of the lives encountered there. No, this idea, they told me, was simply to eat breakfast in Los Angeles, Las Vegas, Tijuana, and Disneyland in the space of 24 hours and then, like, to tell about it.

My orders to be in Tijuana at dawn made transportation tricky. Commercial airlines did not fly to Tijuana, nor did they land in nearby San Diego in the dark, which was just as well, seeing as they have been known to smash into each other there even in broad daylight.

Driving the whole distance was out—everything was hundreds of miles away across deserts.

This cereal advertisement and the two on the following pages originally appeared in Child Life *magazine in the 1930's.*

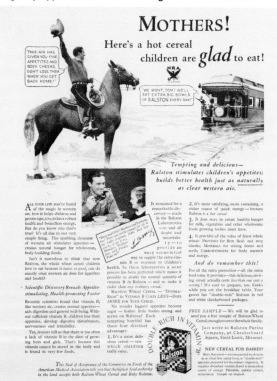

Therefore, it was decided that I'd fly from L.A. to Vegas, then back to L.A. where I'd rent a car and drive the rest.

I told the airline lady the 9 p.m. flight to Las Vegas would be fine.

Return trip? She said.

The 1 a.m., I said.

There was a pause on the phone. Then she said, That's three hours.

I know, I said. I'm just going for breakfast.

Oh, she said. She waited.

I'm doing an article about it, I said.

Oh, she said. Hah!

We laughed. So I was a food writer, she thought, out to write about the integrity of eggs. Or maybe I was going to Las Vegas to eat toast with Englebert Humperdinck.

Should I explain my real mission? That I was after more than food, that it was breakfast as ritual and metaphor I was concerned with? You know. Breakfast. Our daily beginning. What we eat when we awake, refreshed, all our hopes and illusions intact before they gradually get shattered as the day wears on.

But the airline lady didn't seem to require any more explanation. She was all business again, reciting flight numbers, times of arrival. After all, people went to Las Vegas for reasons more foolish than breakfast.

I asked her, what did she have for breakfast?

Me? she said, I never eat breakfast.

I started my journey in Hollywood, land of dreams. There are factories in Hollywood which manufacture cement and shoelaces, but this means nothing. Cement and shoelaces combine here under lights. Cinema Dry Cleaners, Celebrity Shoe Repair—storefronts are movie screens.

Schwab's on Sunset is where people in the Industry go for breakfast, even if they never eat breakfast. Unemployed actors sit at the same counter with the super-employed— agents, producers, directors. Reportedly, everyone drinks cup after cup of coffee, reads the trades, and keeps an eye on one another. Deals are put together here. Stars born. This was where Lana Turner was discovered by a mogul, at the counter at Schwab's drinking coffee. Everybody in America knows that. And it could happen to anyone, even a horse-faced magazine writer.

I went to Schwab's at 6:00 on a Saturday night, not exactly prime time for the place, but there were five or six people at the counter when I arrived, and they all had a cup of coffee in front of them. No one was reading *Variety* or the *Hollywood Reporter*, though. It was too late in the day for that.

I sat down next to a couple of slick types, men around 40, shirts unbuttoned down to here. Their names were Lou and Lionel. I knew this because everyone who went by said Hello, Lou. *Ciao,* Lou. A few said *Ciao* to Lionel.

"He's a good actor," Lou was saying.

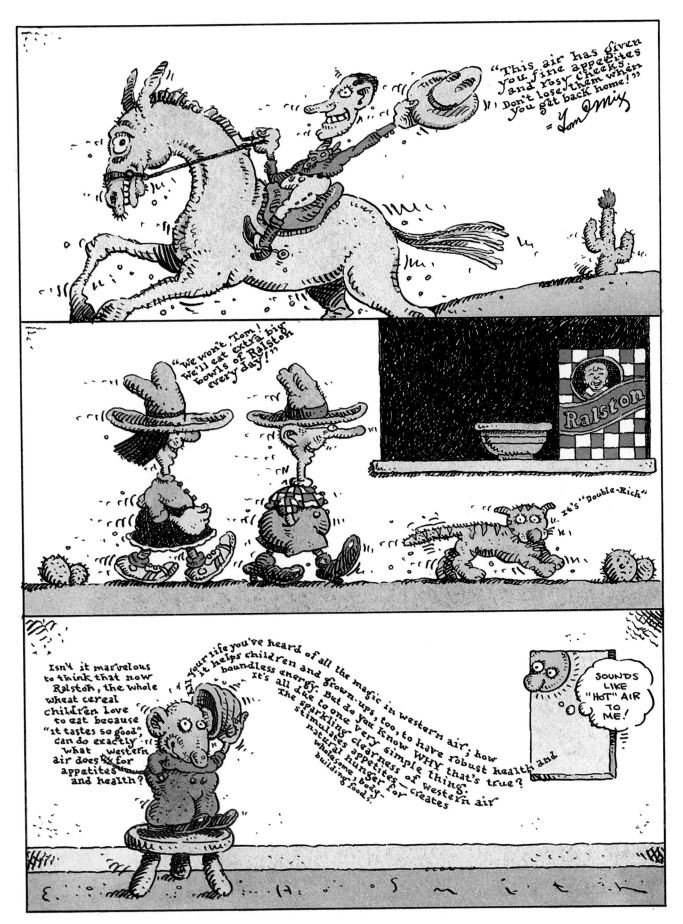

drawings by Elwood H. Smith

"When he's working," Lionel said. His eyes darted around the drug store.

"Yeah," Lou said. "He's good."

"When he's working," Lionel said.

"Actors are stupid, though," Lou said, "boring and stupid. God, I hate them."

"Jeez." Lionel said. "Will you look at the head of hair on that guy."

"They don't read anything but plays," Lou said, shaking his head.

A big hep cat in shades and a royal blue tunic came in

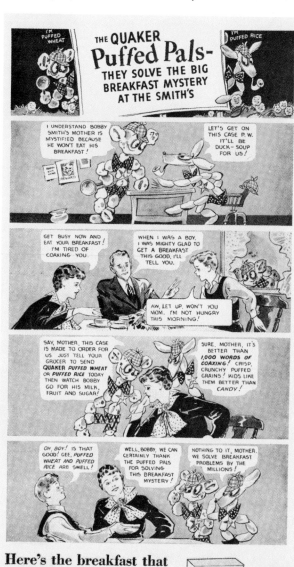

just then and took a seat further down the counter. The spotlight shifted from Lou to this guy, who was leafing through a book with blue covers, the musicians' listing. People at the counter I had thought mere extras in Schwab's little drama began to take speaking parts.

"Looking for somebody, Harry?" one of them said.

"A piano for the weekend," Harry said. "Al's sick."

"How about Ray?" someone said.

"Or Frankie Johnson," the first fellow said.

Meanwhile, Lou had left the counter and was talking to a nervous-looking character over by the Easter bunny display. "He's what you're looking for, Lou," the man was saying.

"I'll give you a call," Lou said. He repeated a phone number. "He's a good actor."

"So," Lionel was saying to a fellow at the counter, "you having a piece of pie today, Joe?"

"Yeah." Joe looked up from his pie. "Why not?"

"Debby," Lou said, sitting down again. "Come here, sweetheart."

"Yes, Mr. F———," Debby said. "What can I do for you?"

"When do you get off?" Lionel put in. Debby ignored him.

"You're supposed to tell me to get off," Lionel said.

"Isn't she lovely," Lou said.

"Lovely," Lionel said. "It's almost a crime."

"Debby." Lou took Debby's hand. "What can I have, dear? I'm sick of coffee."

At the cash register, Schwab's sold postcards of itself, a picture of a drug store on the front, and on the back the legend: "A favorite rendezvous for Motion Pictures, TV Stars, and Film Personalities."

Back at the counter, Debby was setting a cup of tea in front of Lou.

So much for fame.

And so it was, knowing that breakfast had no meaning in Las Vegas, that there was no beginning to the day, and no end either, that I flew there this Saturday night.

I took the archway, an electric sidewalk, to Caesar's Palace, because it was quicker than taxies, and there was piped-in music on the archway, and a recorded message bidding you welcome to the splendor and excitement of the joint and wishing you the luck of the ancient gods.

Someone once told me that people came to Nevada because money lost its meaning and it became almost fun to throw the stuff away. You know, Gamblers really want to lose. That story.

But I looked at the jammed gaming tables and had a feeling that everyone went there to win and only later developed a philosophy.

I decided to try a slot. You could get as much as $10,000 return on 25¢, a sign said. I put some coins in, then some more. I knew the odds were against me, but they

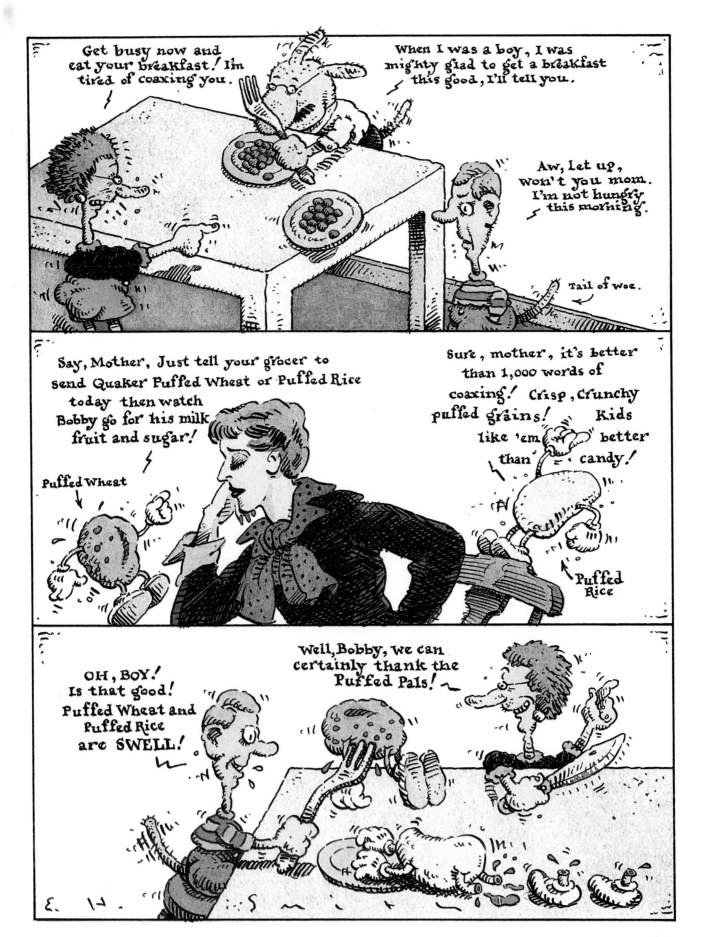

25

improved with each coin I lost. Down the row from me, somebody's grandmother was working a bank of five nickel slots. I dropped more money in, pulled the arm, watched the fruit drop. Cherry came down, then cherry, cherry. Bells started clanging. Somewhere, a siren rang. Coins were pouring from the mouth of the machine. They filled the trough, spilled onto the floor. Down the row, the old lady winked at me, but didn't miss a stroke. By now my feet were buried in silver.

Of course, this is a lie. What happened was I put a limit on how much I'd lose and lost it quickly. It was time for breakfast.

At the end of the Appian Way shopping mall was a dark little red leather coffee shop I knew from years before. They had a 49¢ breakfast there. There were deals like that all over Vegas. For 25-99¢ you could get a good breakfast—ham, a nice fried slab of it, and eggs done right, buttered toast, and potatoes—and if you could keep your mind off the money you'd dropped, you figured you were getting a bargain.

But the coffee shop hostess told me that the special wasn't available on Saturday night, or any night. It ran from 5:00 to 11:00 a.m., a distinction that seemed weirdly purist for Vegas, since it was never daytime in the casinos—the lights blazed, and cocktail waitresses served highballs at dawn. I retreated through the Caesar's Palace parking lot. There was no electric walk *away* from the place, and no voice came from anywhere to say anything.

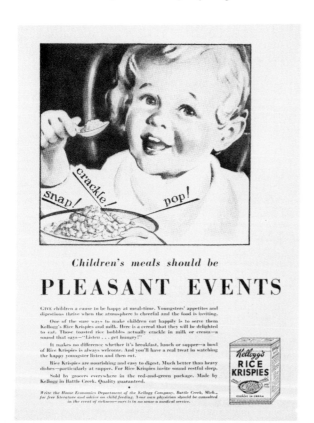

Children's meals should be
PLEASANT EVENTS

Across the street was the MGM Grand Hotel. I went to the Garden Room, a high-ceilinged hall, with chandeliers and a pink-and-green color scheme . . . a real springtime theme. Club sandwiches were the favorite here, with Reubens and chicken salad a close second. I ordered french toast and a large glass of milk.

At nearby tables a pair of golden-agers ate danish and an English muffin. Some polyester lovebirds ate pie. A John Doe couple from Maryville, Tennessee, and their teenage daughter put down hamburgers and fries. I drank my milk.

It was all so tame. Where was the sense of sin, vice, shame, waste?

Well, at a table of pancake and egg eaters, a rock-and-roll type in a Rod Stewart hairdo was doing a mean-drunk. "Let's get out of here," he said.

"I wonder where John is," one of the long-haired women said.

"What do you care?" the man said. "He only lost five hundred dollars. I lost ten thousand dollars."

"But John can't afford it," the woman said quietly. She glanced quickly at the other woman, who didn't look back at her.

"Ten thousand," the man said.

"Keep your voice down," the woman said.

"Why should I? I'm drunk. And stoned. Stone-ed. I've been smoking fucking dope all day."

"Shut-up," she said. "This isn't L.A."

"You shut up," he said. "Where's fucking John?"

Still—*still*—in Las Vegas, the only person I saw commit, in full conscience, sin, was one of the Maryville tinhorns. We had been standing on the curb at the intersection between Caesar's and MGM Grand. The crossroad was busy and complicated with cars turning on green arrows this way and that. The wait for the WALK sign was a long one. The crowd on the sidewalk got restless and moved into the street when the stream of cars thinned out. The wife and daughter made a few steps forward.

"It says don't walk," Mr. Doe said.

His wife and the girl hesitated. "Daddy," the girl said, "everybody's doing it."

"Well," he said. "What the heck," and went ahead across the street.

To picture Tijuana at dawn you must first imagine you hear Mexican music—"Celito Lindo," maybe—a strumming guitar, an accordion, a trumpet. If you don't know any Mexican songs, "Streets of Laredo" will do. And then, amigo, comes de border: a wall coated with barbed wire, a fat federale sitting in the sentry box, a spoked revolving door like a New York City subway exit, only more serious. The sentry says nothing (strum, strum), just watches as you cross. You've had to leave your rented car behind—the Avis people don't want their car going to Mexico. You feel funny, walking into a country a rented car shouldn't enter.

It is a cold, clammy morning, and there is a fog that will

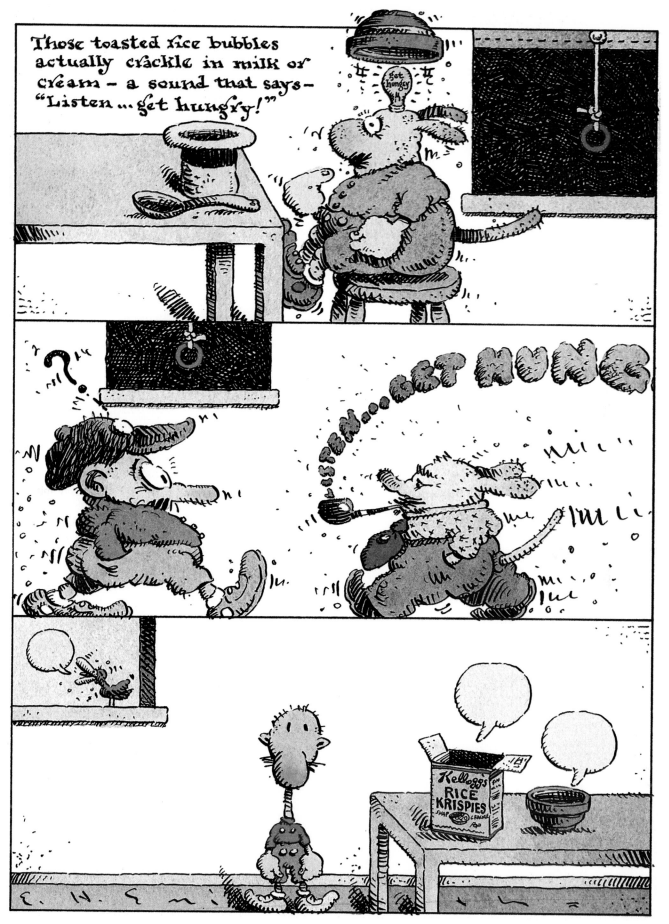

take the sun hours to burn off. Tijuana Central is less than a mile away. "Three dollars," the cab driver says. His tone does not suggest barter. His cab has no shocks, the roads are potholes. There is no handle to roll down the window. Now you are ready for your first glimpse of Tijuana.

On this damp, gray morning of my third breakfast, the townspeople were doing what they could for the place with mops and brooms. Sunday would be a big tourist day, the sun would shine eventually. Merchants swabbed the tile floors of their stalls and dragged out racks of ceramic donkeys. Streetcorner photographers set up their props—backdrops depicting mountains and blue sky, a mule painted to look like a zebra. The last of Saturday night's drunks were staggering home from the bars, red-eyed, passing Sunday-morning church people coming the other way. And in the streets, men with brooms were sweeping. To sweep the dirt streets of Tijuana was a task like only unto Hercules' fifth labor of shoveling the cow shit out of Augeias's stables.

What did Hercules eat in the face of a day like that? What did these people?

The answer was preternatural: They ate at Denny's. Their Denny's was just like ours, except the color scheme was hot pink and fuchsia here. I had no appetite. But I drank cup after cup of portion-controlled coffee and prepared myself for what I had to do. As I left, the cashier, a young man dressed in a suit and tie, nodded to me with dignity.

I found what I was looking for around the corner and down a hill, the Rojo and Blanco Cafe. Nothing about it was rojo or blanco. There were more people behind the counter than in the booths. They dismantled chickens, sank their arms into mounds of tortilla dough. The air stank of boiling lard.

Two American soldiers shared a booth with two Mexican señoritas. In giddy silence they ate sweet rolls and drank coffee made gray with sweetened condensed milk poured from a can. At the counter sat a row of heavyset men, serious as ravens, each with slicked black hair, white shirts, and shod in crippling black shoes with pointed toes and high heels. They ate tortillas, pools of loose gray beans. The jukebox played a morbid tune.

A large señora, perhaps a descendent of Aunt Jane herself—the cook for whom Tijuana was named—came to take my order. Sí, she said, breakfoos, sí huevos. She smiled and nodded encouragement. Suddenly, I was starved.

She brought food. Beans and tortillas, hot red sauce. I ate it. Eggs, scrambled, with chunks of chorizo, tomatoes, lettuce, beans. I ate that. Then more eggs, poached loosely and swimming in shards of tomatoes and chilis. I ate that, quesadillas, more beans, a final tortilla, and one sweet roll. I began to sweat.

When I rose to leave, I felt slower, sluggish, somehow more in tune with my surroundings. Lard was in my hair, had permeated my clothes, soon it would be in my bloodstream.

I went back up the hill and sat on the white wrought iron bench in front of Denny's and sat, warming myself like a lizard in the morning sun. I felt no desire to move.

Driving north in a fat green Thunderbird, I wanted to put as much road between me and Tijuana as I could before stopping. My bowels clenched. I knew now that I had been poisoned. My clothes felt moldy. I needed to sleep. The traffic was mounting. I drove on. Past San Diego, past nuclear power plants, all four lanes, bumper to bumper, 60 miles an hour. Just the normal Southern California Sunday flow, Americans out for surfing, worship, house hunting.

All along the sides of the road and on the median strip there were bed after bed of pretty white flowers, covering the ground like snow. And as if that weren't luxury enough, there, at the next exit, was a Big Boy. Its parking lot was jammed with Orange County Republicans and RV's. Pods, maybe, but my people.

I entered the Big Boy and made for the restroom where, while all around me families ate pancakes and pigs in a blanket, and, closer at hand, young ladies washed up after pissing and pooping discreetly, I lost it all, all my dignity and all of Mexico in a terrible explosion. I groaned, puked, shat water, farted fire. And then it was over. I rose, zipped up, and departed.

I headed for the ocean, then up the coast into a wilderness of bedroom communities, warrens built in one day, inhabited the next. Marina del Coma. Mondo Condo. I drove straight to the home of the King of Ticky-tack himself in San Clemente where, just visible over the rise, I could see the Spanish tiles of his rooftop, the tips of his palm trees. I took a right on El Presidente Street and drove past the El Presidente Motel to the San Clemente Public Beach where I lay my putrid self down in the clean white sand.

Citizens walked the beach. Blond, perfectly formed teenagers made out on blankets. Marines from Camp Pendleton hep-hupped along the water's edge. Waves crashed. I waited.

And if he did appear, what would I do?

I decided, instead, to go to splendid Cano's by the sea for brunch. I called ahead for a reservation.

"Hellew?" the maitre d' said.

Cano's sat on the dock at Newport Beach just across from Lido Isle, Southern California's most expensive little chunk of real estate. Outside the restaurant's floor-to-ceiling plate glass, yachts slid by in the water. Inside, the ceilings were a hundred feet high. There were potted palms, white tablecloths, tulip glasses.

A damsel in a low cut flowing gown came around with rolls and pastries. Waiters cruised with champagne. Fresh fruit was brought. An entire pineapple. Oysters and poached eggs, tender steak, luscious creamed fishes. The bread lady returned. More fruit, and now cheeses, more champagne. Banana crepes in rum sauce, pears, strawberries, honeydew.

Glasses tinkled, forks tinked, people chewed.

I lurched out of there and to my car. It was time for Disneyland.

Of course, this was no ordinary amusement park. There was no Ferris wheel, no filthy screaming babies, no gum and sticky pools of pop on the asphalt. No, this was order, charm, and in the distance, the Matterhorn.

I boarded the Disneyland Railroad at Main Street, U.S.A., and rode the thing through Fantasyland, Adventureland, Frontierland, Tomorrowland. Then I went around again. Tears filled my eyes and rolled down my cheeks. I had experienced a breakdown of sorts. A complete loss of irony. I was exhausted, true, and drunk, maybe; certainly a victim of sensory overload. But I was happy.

Go ahead, go on the rollercoaster for the first time in your life. Let it spin you around in the dark, taking curves at 40, 50, 60 miles an hour, leave the tracks, turn corners at right angles. No need for hope, you don't even have to fear fear itself here. Nothing can go wrong at Disneyland.

Behind the facade of a gingerbread house, I visited Walt Disney's shrine: his old office at the studio, brought here intact and entire to Anaheim, and preserved behind glass. It looked like any contemporary businessman's office—except for the statue of Mickey.

Americans were forming a line.

I fell in with them, found myself in a theater, took a seat. Soon, I was sleeping like a baby.

When I awoke, Abe Lincoln was standing there. It was him all right. Tall, thin. He wore a brown, old-fashioned suit, white shirt, no hat. His craggy jaw was moving. He was orating, in fact. He was talking about America, and how our downfall would come not from other countries—not Europe or Asia—but from right here at home unless we guarded our individual liberties and our free enterprise system. As he wound up his speech, music swelled from the loudspeaker. Glory Hallelujah, it was. An American flag began to flutter behind Abe.

He sat down when the music stopped, the curtains swept shut, and we filed out of the theater. Outside, it was night around the turn of the century. Families strolled dazed-looking, jolly, past the tobacconist and general store.

Breakfast was out of the question. Who needed it now? Only ice cream or candy would do.

But in a compromise move, I bought a large-sized cup full of fresh-squeezed OJ, took it back to the town square, and drank it down. Before me lay all of Disneyland. There was so much to do—the Haunted Mansion, the Pirates of the Caribbean Boat Ride, the raft to Tom Sawyer's Island. I would have to ride the Space Mountain rollercoaster through the universe one more time. At Small World, I had heard, automatons like Abe only miniature and dressed in tiny native costumes would sing songs in foreign tongues. In Adventureland, robot bears would dance and talk. In the Tiki Room, birds.

The gondolas glided away from the Matterhorn, and glided back.

I had no more stops on my route, no place I had to be. I could stay until midnight closing. I could stay for days. Or I could turn and make for the exit, only yards away, find my car in the oceanic parking lot and get the fuck out of there while I still had . . . what were they? . . . *un-named hungers*, dark and perverse perhaps, and that old devil irony returning along with a mean-spirited lack of tolerance for the needs of my fellow humans for places like these.

Or was it simply that I wanted to go someplace peaceful and dull, where very little is possible and nothing ever happens—home.

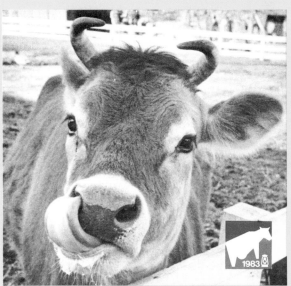

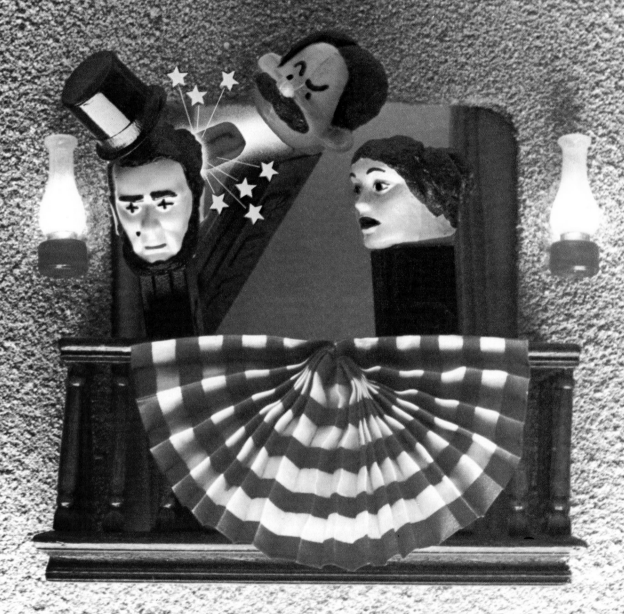

Nine U.S. Senators with Some Mostly Interesting Reminiscences About Food, Coupled with Opinions on Current Cuisine in the Public Sector

Q: What are your earliest "fast food" memories? How often do you eat it in an average week? Is there a price you will not pay . . . say, for a hamburger?

SENATOR BILL BRADLEY, New Jersey: "My earliest visit to a fast-food franchise was a Dairy Queen when I was eight years old and had a twenty-five cent vanilla cone with my grandfather after we watched a Laurel and Hardy/Lash LaRue double feature. I also remember having a barbequed beef sandwich with my parents at a local spot when I was ten years old. Now I usually send out for two fast-food meals a day. There is no question about my favorite—Wendy's Double Burger with cheese is the only fast-food burger that has a patty bigger than the bun. There is no price I won't pay for a burger, especially if it is a Wendy's. My other favorites are Pizza Hut and Baskin-Robbins."

SENATOR BARRY GOLDWATER, Arizona: "In my younger days in Arizona, Mexican food was being served over the counter. Back in those days it wasn't considered fast food as we think of it today. It was thought of as Mexican home-style cooking, and was done in very small, out-of-the-way places in Phoenix. I now usually eat my dinner at home, but during the day, I usually catch a hamburger at the Capitol Restaurant; if I'm traveling on the road I'll stop at a McDonald's for a quick bite. As far as price, I don't think anyone should have to pay $3.50 to $4.00 for a hamburger sandwich with a few chips. I realize the overall food and operating costs can be high, but no hamburger, for example, is that good."

SENATOR HOWELL HEFLIN, Alabama: "There used to be a fellow who would go around and sell tamales in this area, 30, 40 years ago, carrying them hot in this container he had. He would hawk them and holler, you'd buy them, and he'd give you a paper plate to eat them on. You remember the scene more than the taste. I'd say ⅔ of our lunch and evening meals during my last campaign were fast-food meals, because you'd be moving all the time. I probably go out more often for fast food now, I like to breathe the outside air. I think it depends upon your taste buds, but the Wendy's hamburgers are my favorite right now. Or sometimes I get a double, sometimes I get a quarter-pound McDonald's, and Hardees, one of these . . . whatever they call that thing, the Big One. I usually try to pick up something a little bigger than just a normal hamburger."

SENATOR PAUL LAXALT, Nevada: "I have blocked out all fast-food memories. After years of careful cultivation, I have managed to discipline myself to recall only those gourmet meals prepared by my wife or those enjoyed dining out."

SENATOR SPARK M. MATSUNAGA, Hawaii: "I remember eating 'saimin' (Chinese noodles) or 'udon' (Japanese noodles) at 'bon' dance benefit concessions in Eleele, Kauai, Hawaii. The bon dance, sponsored annually by the Buddhist community to appease the spirit of the dead and commend it to heaven, was a big community function which lasted all night. Saimin and udon, great fast-food specialties known only in Hawaii, were served to those who helped with the activities. Today, I send out for fast-food three times a week. My favorite? Fish sandwich."

SENATOR CLAIBORNE PELL, Rhode Island: "I had delicious 'pig in a blanket, well-fed,' at Dutchland Farms, Middletown, Rhode Island, when I was a schoolboy. That's a hot dog in a roll, surrounded by bacon. I am not much of a fast-food addict, though. However, when I am under pressure, I seek to always have a chicken sandwich on whole wheat bread."

SENATOR ALAN K. SIMPSON, Wyoming: "At Louie's Hamburger Shop in Sheridan, Wyoming, the old gentleman chopped the pickles so deftly that it looked like he took all of his fingers along with the pickles. I was always fascinated by that place and remember distinctly the tastes and smells of it—it indeed remains clear in my memory. I enjoy the convenience of fast foods and probably my favorite is a glass of iced orange juice and an Egg McMuffin at McDonald's."

SENATOR JOHN WARNER, Virginia: "I was a great fan of Dairy Queen when I was in college, but I ran my campaign on Colonel Sanders, Golden Skillet, and Gino's fried chicken. I do love the fast-food fried chicken. In the Senate, I do a lot of brown-bagging these days. There really aren't many fast-food outlets convenient to the Senate offices."

SENATOR LOWELL P. WEICKER, JR., Connecticut: "My earliest fast-food memory was one of the first McDonald's located on the Berlin Turnpike just outside of Hartford—1962. Almost always eat a sandwich or hamburger for lunch now. Never a regular luncheon."

model by Jim Wilson, photograph by Carl Waltzer

Truckstops, Whores, and Gravy

by Harry Crews

I learned very early, though not so early as some, that things are not what they seem. I make it a categorical statement, not hedging bets with *usually* not what they seem, or *sometimes* not what they seem. *Nothing* is what it seems. Wood is plastic, brick is linoleum, stone is a thin aggregate of compressed sand, cloth is DuPont chemical, fireplace logs are pressed sawdust. Even titties have turned to silicone as if before our very eyes, which eyes — not incidentally — owe their color to tinted contact lenses.

This phenomenon first impressed itself upon me years ago when I was just out of the Marine Corps. A high school buddy of mine named Kidney, so named because he had already lost one kidney and the other one had become highly suspect from the daily beating it was taking, Kidney let me go partners with him pushing his 18-wheeled, twin-stacked Peterbilt. We would ordinarily leave Atlanta, turn San Francisco, and be back in Atlanta in about five days. Obviously, this left very little time for anything except squatting by the side of the road, or draining our main vein in the bushes, or eating Benzedrine until our eyes were turning sixes and sevens and our parched tongues had gone bumpy.

On my first run with Kidney we had just crept up Monarch Pass in the Continental Divide and barreled down the other side, more than a little out of control, when he told me to pull into a truckstop that had about 10 acres of big rigs parked in front of it. We had gas, everything seemed to be working all right humming down the highway, so I shot him a stunned and questioning Benzedrine glance.

Kidney read the question. "We need a little R & R," he said.

"I'm hungry as a dog," I said. "That truckstop cooking's the best in the world."

Kidney said: "Anybody'd eat in a truckstop deserves what he gits."

"What's he git?"

In his best matter-of-fact voice, he said, "Shit."

"Then what we stopping for?"

"Pussy."

Once inside, Kidney said: "Notice the only ones eating in here are the tourists and their ugly families. All the truckers are doing is drinking coffee. You can spot a guy that ain't been driving long because he'll actually eat in a truckstop."

He was right, too. The ugly families were eating with both feet in the trough. The truckers, potbellied and gimpy-legged, sat hunched over the steaming coffee mugs.

"You look close," said Kidney, "you can tell the ones already had their wienies pulled."

"Wienies pulled?"

"You gouge a girl," he said, "it unwires the bennies."

"You serious?"

He was serious. It turned out that truckstops were actually fuckstops. Fuckstops that sold gas and oil. America loves an illusion. America *is* an illusion. A figment of Cotton Mather's imagination. That's why we have science fiction enforcers of the law. Like the late, great J. Edgar Hoover. The record clearly shows that he was fond of illegal entry, illegal surveillance of mail, cooperating with the IRS to harass the people who paid his wage, small dogs, and exceedingly fond of making life miserable for working girls. Every big rig driver I knew in the late '50's was convinced Hoover had agents pushing 18-wheelers for no other reason than to bust truckstop whores. The girls only worked a truckstop for a week or two before they were shipped to another stop in another state, and when they crossed state lines it made the whole thing a Federal offense. It was

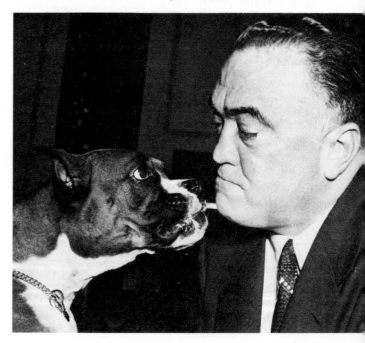

necessary to move them around, though, because the truckers didn't want to look at the same girls all the time, knowing as they did that variety would give their staff life.

This was all part of my education and I learned it sitting there with Kidney watching the tourists eat the stuff Kidney said truckers wouldn't touch with a dipstick.

"J. Edgar," said Kidney a little later, his wienie now pulled and in a reflective mood, "did all this for no other reason than to roust the whores that keep us all sane. He's a great guy but he never got over personally arresting John Dillinger after he'd already had his boys strip Dillinger of his fire and naked."

The thing you've got to understand—and anybody would understand it if he gave it any thought—is that a truckstop is not a place to eat. Truckers are so wired from lightweight shit like NoDoz to heavyweight killerhits of amphetamines that the last thing in the world on their minds is food. They want gas, oil, showers, pussy if possible, a fresh supply of blood-pressure jackup, a shave, coffee, maybe a bunk if they've got a small handful of downs to get off the mountain—but *food*? Even their old ladies can't get them to eat when they get home. Except maybe a hairy taco once or twice, but never your straight down-home cooking.

So what are all those tourists eating in there with such relish? The same thing they're eating at every roadhouse in the country, whether or not truckers are parked in front of it. Roadhouse here means anything by the side of the road selling not only junk food but also the multitude of junk dolls and junk name plates and junk toys that tear up before you get out the front door of the store—stuff carnival people call *slum*.

But food is the high crime of the road. For starters, *fast food* is a contradiction in terms. If it's fast, it ain't food. It may taste something like food is supposed to taste, may even bear some resemblance to it, but it's not food. If you were fortunate enough to have a mama who cooked, as opposed to a mama who opened cleverly designed boxes or cut the tops off cans, then you know that cooking takes time. It needs stirring and tasting and smelling, sometimes it even needs talking to. But our senses have been so distorted that our taste even believes what we see. We eat menus—the four-color pictures on them—not food. Ever see a picture of a Big Mac? Looks like something you could send to the Queen of England. But one of my favorite dogs straightened me out on that. I had a pit bulldog one time that would eat anything, including other dogs. But he would not eat a Big Mac. Once, on the way to a fight, I bought him one. He sniffed it, but he wouldn't eat it. The best he could do was hike his leg and piss on it. I already had two Big Macs in my stomach, but when I saw my pit bull give water on that sesame seed bun it cured me from eating them forever.

But we are all fooled from time to time and perhaps it would be helpful if I gave some time and detail to a really popular, really disasterious dish. Just recently I stopped at one of the biggest motel chains in the country, because it was the only place in the little town I was passing through that had a bar and I wanted a drink. But it was noon and the clever devils had an ordinance that said you couldn't drink whiskey anywhere but in their lethal dining room, where you were also required to eat, or at least order something. I ordered french fries and four ounces of vodka straight up. It had been a long drive. I had no intention of eating the french fries and didn't. They sat there in front of me congealing in a gauze of lard while I got limp from the tensions of hard driving.

The place was full of blue-haired people hoping their Fixodent would hold. I don't know why the Noon Buffet attracts Blue Hairs the way it does, but a Blue Hair will grab his Fixodent and sprint at the mere mention of the famous Noon Buffet.

The Old Party at the table next to mine passed up the buffet line and ordered an open-face hot roast beef sandwich, perhaps the most deadly item on any menu in America. The Old Party told the waitress it was his favorite, which proves, I guess, that the damned thing won't kill you because he had to have been 80 years old. Sucking rotten eggs won't kill you either, but I've never met anybody who wanted to make a meal on them. The old lady with him ordered what was described on the menu as "Our hot homemade soup with good fresh crackers." The waitress was back in a flash with their orders. I recognized the soup immediately. I could have quoted the label on the gallon can it came in because I used to make the stuff in 800-gallon cookers in 1958, in Hayward, California, working for Hunt Foods, the tomato people. The crackers came in little separate packages and strangely enough in my spotty career I had also worked for the company that made them. My job at the cracker factory was to dump 100-pound bags of flour down a chute that led into a set of grinders resembling the gearbox of an automobile. The only trouble was that rats liked to tunnel into the floor bags stacked in the warehouse and live there. All day long I had to listen to the squealing of whole generations of rat families being shredded into cracker mix. I felt like the furnace-keeper at Dachau, but it was a living, and I was younger then and not nearly as sweet as I am now.

I sat there watching that old lady eat and wondered whether or not Ralph Nader and his boys had succeeded in getting the rat hair and fecal matter out of those crackers yet. Probably not, because rats love flour, never suspecting of course that the grinders are part of the deal. There's a lesson there somewhere for all of us. I was also wondering if the guys in that kitchen in California—which is still there turning out that soup in 800-gallon batches—were still blowing their noses into the cookers.

But even after the eight ounces of vodka, it didn't make it easy for me to watch the old man do a job on the open-face roast beef. When the waitress set his plate in front of him, he said: "Ummm, don't that look good." And his remark immediately reminded me that I had recently been to a cattle auction in South Georgia. I've never seen but one or two women at a cattle auction in my life but for some reason that day there were six big old fat girls sitting up on the top bleacher, spraddle-legged, waving Jesus fans trying to keep cool. I was eye-balling them pretty good, as the boy I was with, name of Luther. The reason we were putting such a hard eye on them was that the auction hadn't started in the pit down below and there wasn't much else to do except hustle our balls and spit. I was fascinated by the fact that the spraddle-legged wonders on the top bleacher all had on black panties and I was about to say something to Luther about it when somebody let a big bull into the auction pit and he bellowed and slammed into the retaining wall, and when he did the black panties flew out from between the fat girls' legs in a little cloud for an instant before settling back into cheese city. A lot of flies at a cattle auction, and that's what those yearling girls were wearing: flies instead of panties. I turned to look at Luther where he stood in manure-crusted boots, sour overalls, a thin stream of tobacco juice slipping down his chin into a three-day growth of whiskers, and he said with a voice the Pope must use when he calls on the Lord, a voice full of awe, reverence, and holy lust: "Ummm, don't that look good." Which is the long way around to saying one man's meat is another man's poison, and any other clichés you can think of and care to add to the list.

It may not have mattered at all to the old man to know that that rich brown gravy slopped all over his plate had enough preservatives and what the trade calls "flavor enhancers," both generic and brand-named, to have been used as a defoliant in jungle warfare, or that it was as old as the kitchen it was cooked in.

Like the amoeba, that sort of gravy never wears out, never dies. The first amoeba that ever was on this earth is still here because an amoeba reproduces by dividing from itself and then the piece that leaves divides from itself, and so on, always carrying something of the original beast with it. Hot roast beef gravy is the same way. It is immortal, carrying always something of what started it along on the trip in the first place. A little cornstarch added here, a little flour there, a few diced and unidentifiable bits of flesh thrown in. Always, and at anytime, anything brown, greasy, and thick goes into the bubbling pot. And that pot never empties. It is as bottomless and, in its own way, as mysterious as God's love.

Down under the gravy, on the bottom of the plate, you'll find some bread. It doesn't matter if the bread is moldy, which it many times is, or five days old and hard enough to use as roofing shingles, because that good brown gravy will make any bread righteously soft and utterly disguise any unseemly discolorations or growths.

Now, between that gravy and that bread is the best trick of all, the beef. Even if it were good beef to start with—and it never is—it has been cooked seven times around the world, is so dry and tired, so sad, that if you listen closely you can hear it calling for help. If it weren't so full of tenderizer and juiced up with that good rich gravy, you couldn't eat it, because the more you chewed it, the bigger it would get.

But if anything is quick, hot, and basically unidentifiable, a tourist will eat it. To return to truckstops, where all this started, I stopped in at one yesterday to see if anything had

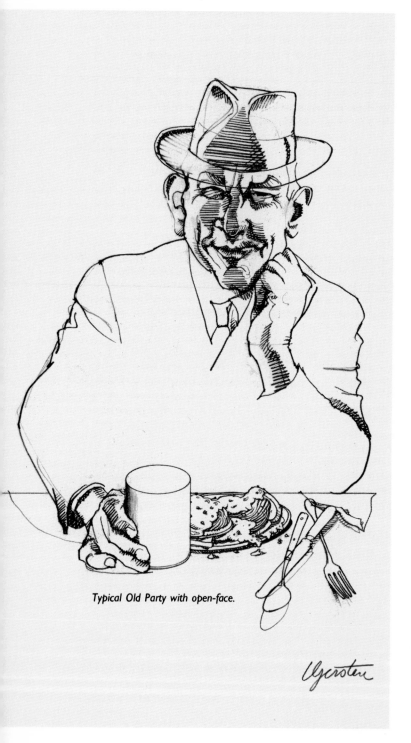

Typical Old Party with open-face.

drawing by Gerry Gersten

changed. The whores were gone, of course. They've vanished from everywhere except remote places in large cities where they mainly service hunchbacked, wall-eyed dwarfs. The rest of the men in the country are enjoying an unprecedented free ride. Everything else was pretty much the same. The tourists still had both feet in the trough; the truckers were drinking coffee and practicing their exotic CB language in case Hollywood called hunting up extras for a Burt Reynolds movie.

I ordered a steak and it came with both sides striped with burnt parallel lines from the grill, which for some reason tourists think means it is a really good piece of meat. All it means is the thing was frozen when the cook threw it on the grill. I'd ordered it rare, and since not even a magician can cook a frozen steak rare, the goddamn thing had slivers of ice in the center of it. I ate it anyway. If I'd left it uneaten, or even half-eaten, they would no doubt have done the old open-face trick with it. And I've grown too old and mellow, had my social conscience raised too high, to participate in something like that.

I said that everything, except the whores, was about the same as it always had been at the truckstop. That's not quite true. There was a really magnificent selection of slum, and standing next to the door was a picture about 18 inches square of a big rig barreling down the highway, a wired driver at the wheel, and beside him on the seat one of those stylized pictures of Christ, long flowing hair, dead walnut-colored eyes, dressed in a white gown that was whipping out the window in the wind, and Christ, a beatific look on his chin, was pointing through the windshield up toward heaven.

Someday a tourist would buy the picture and offer it to a trucker and get his skull cracked with a tire iron for his trouble. The guys who push big rigs are convinced that truckstops *could* be pretty good places, maybe even have an occasional whore or two, if it were not for tourists. After all, it's people like tourists and their ugly families who applaud people like J. Edgar Hoover for doing things like he did to the working girls. Truckers have some great stories about the old bachelor and his obsession with small dogs.

Old Parties Do Some Bellyaching

FT. LAUDERDALE, FLA.

Q. What sorts of things would your mother kill you for eating? What are you eating that's killing you now?

Max Wiederman, age 81: "My mother had two rules for us kids: We couldn't leave the house with dirty underwear on and we weren't allowed to have chocolates. She didn't want us to die with stains on our clothes one way or the other. Now I like to go down to Nathan's over in Ft. Lauderdale. They sell a frozen banana all covered with chocolate."

Tony Robbins, "just old": "A big pretzel once in a while . . . with a lot of big salts on it. They don't make them like that anymore. Once in a while on the beach there's skinny ones with small salts."

Lena Gonzago, 80 (sunning on a bench in a balloon-bottomed one-piece.): "In Italy we had nothing. I came over here when I was 13 but they fixed my age to say 16 so I could work. I didn't make so good money at the sewing machines so I couldn' buy nothin. You couldn' get too much for real, never mind this junk food. People would sometime pick out garbage, you know, real junk food."

Paul Katner, 74: "Rock candy. Only drugstores sold it. It was supposed to be for stomach gas or something. We'd go in and kind of hold our bellies like it was aching . . . we'd eat so much we got bellyaches. Now we got a fixed income, the Social Security lasts only so long, but years ago I bought a souvenir, a bottle with rock candy inside to put liquor in. I used to put straight rye whiskey but now I can only afford the cheap stuff. The rock candy makes it sweet, though. So if you gotta go, give me my nightcap."

Bartholomew Greene, 92 (breaking into a toothless grin.): "For a penny we could buy five jawbreakers . . . man, that ball could really crack yo' teeth."

André Cotelle, 76: "I don't eat this stuff today. It's too soft. Whenever the ice man made a delivery in the summer we'd get him to break some off for us to chew on. These kids today can't bite ice. They make faces. Like my grandchildren—when I see them—start shivering and yelling whenever I do it for them. But kill me? Nah. Look, things last longer in the Frigidaire, right? Why shouldn't people last longer if they eat ice?"

Ellie and Herb Abromowitz, she, 68, he, 73 (she wearing an orange T-shirt with "Tootsie" stenciled in black; his, a matching "Wootsie.")
Tootsie: "We're down here to get away from all that cold. I think we'd've died in New York last winter. So you expect me to kill myself with food?"
Wootsie: ". . . Entenmann's chocolate donuts, but they repeat on me."
Tootsie: "I won't let him have them. His doctor's got him on a very strict diet. They shoulda had diet soda in those days. They're really good for you and they aren't fattening. But I retain water so I have to use my pills."

—*Richard Scorza*

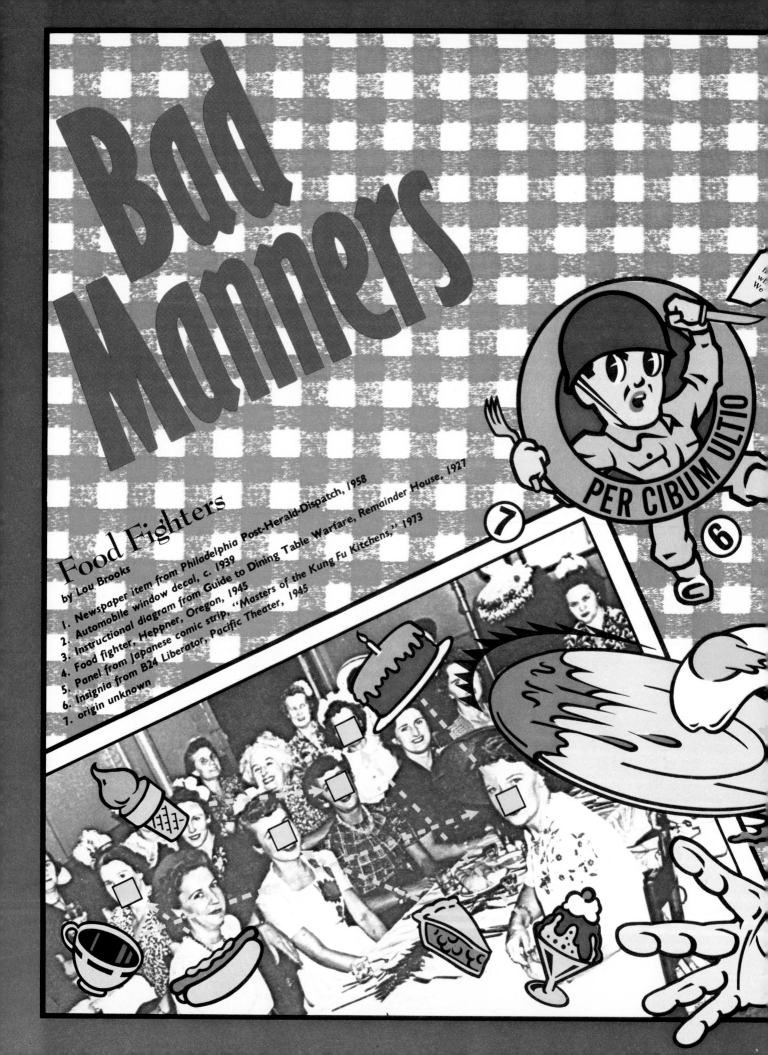

Bad Manners

Food Fighters
by Lou Brooks

1. Newspaper item from Philadelphia Post-Herald-Dispatch, 1958
2. Automobile window decal, c. 1939
3. Instructional diagram from Guide to Dining Table Warfare, Remainder House, 1927
4. Food fighter, Heppner, Oregon, 1945
5. Panel from Japanese comic strip, "Masters of the Kung Fu Kitchens," 1973
6. Insignia from B24 Liberator, Pacific Theater, 1945
7. origin unknown

PER CIBUM ULTIO

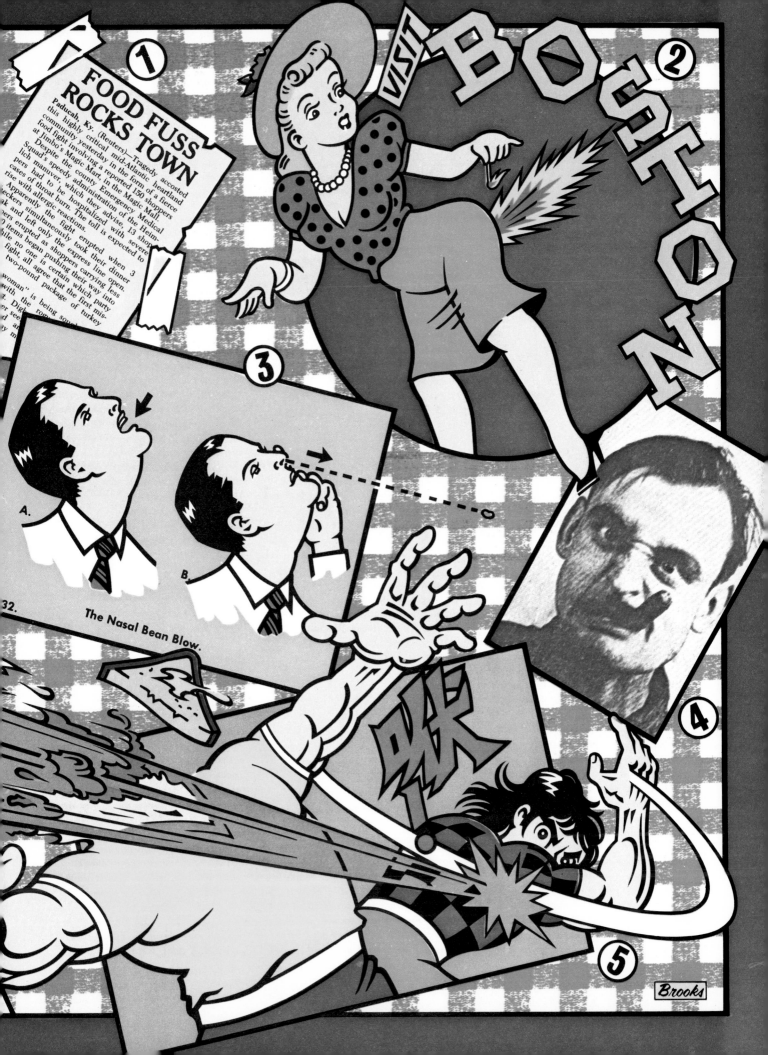

Food Fight

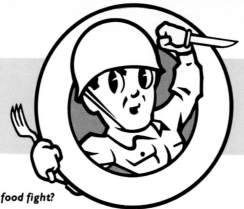

Q: What was your most memorable food fight?

YOGI BERRA, baseballer: "When I was a kid, we used to go to bakeries in St. Louis and get some stale cakes and just throw it at each other. Usually chocolate or whatever ones they wanted to get rid of. It was always fun, for five, ten minutes. I wouldn't do it now. I'm older."

LILLIAN CARTER, mother: "My children would've been punished if they'd done something like that."

THEODORE KHEEL, mediator: "This happened many years ago at a high-level management conference of a company called U.S. Industries. The head of the company had arranged for the conference to be held at the Ram's Head Inn, on Ram's Island, near Shelter Island, which is terribly remote and has nothing but Ram's Head. The meeting was attended by all men and they worked very hard during the day on the business at hand, and then the evening came and they had nothing to do but drink, which they did in large quantities, and then they sat down to eat and at one point somebody picked up a roll and threw it at the neck of somebody else and then feigned that he did not throw it. And this person turned around, and finally, he thought he knew who threw it and so he threw a roll back. One thing led to another—it was the worst

donnybrook, people throwing food all over the place, veal parmigian and spaghetti and apple pie and what-not. I ducked under the table, but I remember reflecting to myself, the strangeness of these otherwise serious-minded people suddenly going berserk, because of their isolation. I concluded that Ram's Island was no place for a conference of men."

KEN KESEY, author: "The best food fight I ever had was one time when we were shooting **Atlantis Rising**, and we had, oh, maybe thirty kids there and we'd gone out and bought hot dogs. We were feeding these kids hot dogs, and this friend of ours who is vegetarian got so mad, I thought she was going to have a heart attack. Nobody threw anything, but she left in high dudgeon. She came back in a huff, a little German car."

LIZ SMITH, syndicated gossip columnist: "My brothers and I spit watermelon seeds at each other so my mother always made us eat watermelon in the bathtub."

GRACE JONES, disco vocalist: "In Paris we had this. It was reallly crazy. A hairdresser friend of mine knew the owner of a small restaurant and we more or less took it over for the night. And we invited photographers and he invited some old friends

of his, a professor of classical piano was one, sort of high-class kind of people, with a mixture of some crazy models. I was singing, the music was going, it started by piling up glasses on top of each other, and it kept going and going, and before you knew it, the glasses fell over. Then we started a jam session with knives and forks and one glass broke, and then we started making music on the plates, and then a plate broke. Then all of a sudden, there was a big bowl of rice. Oh, it was sooo crazy. We started throwing the cooked rice from one end of the restaurant to the other. The tables were very long, a lot of people hadn't been able to sit together, so I guess their way of communicating was to throw rice. It became a big rice fight, then it was all over the floor and we got up and started dancing and ground it in on the floor. It was very crazy. Then I got on the table and started singing, 'That's the Trouble.' Crazy night, you know?"

STEPHEN SCHWARTZ, Broadway composer: "My first year in summer stock, the place I was working with—one of these kind of non-Equity places, you worked for very little money but you got your room and board—we had a cook who was sort of a severe New England-type lady, but the management liked her because she never let anything go to waste . . . if the company didn't finish what she made, it kept showing up as something else until it was gone. One day she made these things for dessert—and I don't know what the hell they were, she called them persimmon tarts, but I doubt they

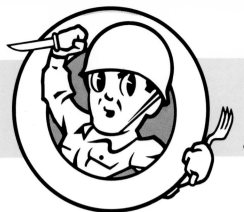

Forum #1

compiled by Richard Rothenstein

were persimmon tarts. They were horrible, flaky things with some thicky gooey brown filling. She made . . . millions of them. She was, like thrilled about the whole thing, she took great pride in her persimmon tarts. And of course nobody ate them, because they were revolting. And every single night for the next three or four nights, dessert time came, and the little waiters came out and brought persimmon tarts. And everybody started to get upset and doing things to get rid of the persimmon tarts, because until they could get rid of them, there was no hope of ever having anything else for dessert. So they started showing up as props in the play. Or as paperweights to keep down the mail in the post office. But it was not making a dent in the amount of persimmon tarts. Finally, there was the Sunday night cold buffet, when the cook would leave early, and this had been going on for a week and a half, and there were the persimmon tarts, and people started heaving them at each other. It started in the dining room and spilled out onto the lawn. They went THACK when they hit people, because by this time they were slightly hard. An even better sound when they hit walls. And the next day, the cook came in and was so happy, she just had this wonderful look on her face the whole day, because she felt that finally we had discovered the beauties, the subtle beauties of her persimmon tarts.''

DIANA VREELAND, dean of fashion: ''I've never had the privilege of having food thrown in my face, but I hope if someone throws something at me, it would be caviar. Preferably large grained and golden grey.''

JOHN SIMON, critic: ''Well, there's that disgusting Sylvia Miles story, I suppose, but I really hate to give that further publicity. I think that's been squeezed by that bitch for all it is worth and then some. I just don't want to immortalize it anymore than it already has been. Let's go into another one that's more interesting. There was a party once, at which a man called Andre Emmerich, who runs the Andre Emmerich Gallery, was carrying on about critics not knowing anything about anything. I was discouraging one of his artists— one Theodoros Stamos, who I think is a rotten artist. Out of that evolved this passionate outburst where Emmerich threw a whole goddamn plate of steak tartare sandwiches at me. Of course, I ducked, and he missed, and the whole thing went flying all over the floor. Then he left and my date and I had to help the hostess for God knows how long, picking up these steak tartare sandwiches.''

ARTHUR BELL, writer: ''I know that it was not a spontaneous gesture, . . . that Sylvia had told a couple of people about it earlier in the day. She was doing that play, **Nellie Toole & Co.**, I believe, and Simon was unnecessarily cruel in his column, not only about her acting, but about her personality. It was a dumb director's party, in 1973, I think, at O'Neals[1]. She went over to John Simon with a plate of antipasto[2] and just dumped it on him. He was wearing a relatively light suit—that was the year of the Gatsby suit, if you remember. He had called her something like baggage . . . it was something-baggage, it was like scum-baggage, but it wasn't scum. And he said that he was going to send her a cleaning bill. She came and sat with us afterwards, and was kind of morose. She was with this guy Rudy, who she was seeing—a man who was like a male model, and quite good-looking, younger than she. I think she felt apologetic and ashamed afterwards, she was sort of saying, 'I know I did the right thing.' Which is unusual for Sylvia, because Sylvia's kind of a tough broad. She had no idea how that would fare in the press. The days that followed, she was sort of a Joan of Arc around town, although she thought it might have spoiled her career. I thought it took a great amount of derring-do and courage on her part. I like John Simon, too, but I think that in this particular instance, he got his just desserts.''

SYLVIA MILES, actress: ''Why should I tell you about my food fights? I don't know you. You're just a name attached to a voice on the phone. I'll save you plenty of time, because I don't want to meet you and I don't want to speak with you on the phone, either.'' (Click.)

---

[1] A N.Y.-based gossip columnist insists it took place at the Ginger Man.

[2] Mr. C. C. Berg, manager of the Ginger Man, claims, "It was an Italian something," possibly spaghetti. An employee remembers it took place at Table #3.

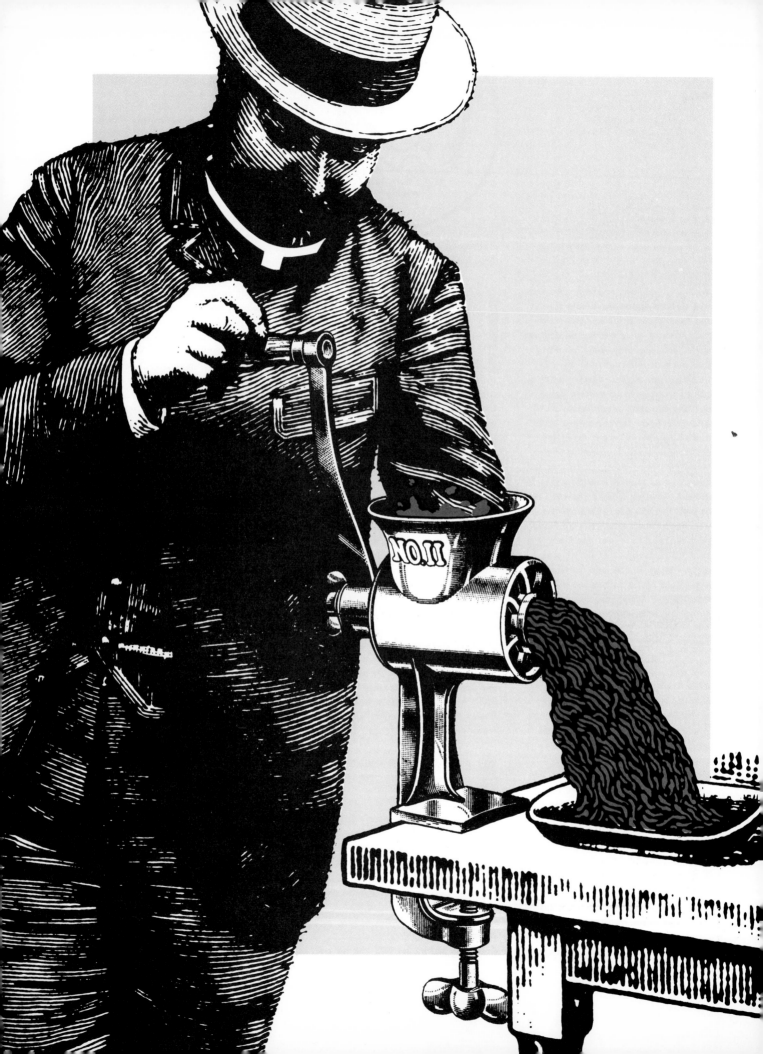

The Goyification of Salami

by Vic Ziegel

Until Aunt Ethel and Uncle Menasha slipped out of Russia with a kilo of homegrown borscht for their wealthy American sponsors (cleverly disguised in this country as my mom and dad, that swell couple waiting for a Ford Foundation grant before they paper the bathroom), the star of our family was Uncle Seymour.

How Uncle Seymour became a star may not sound like a big deal. Nothing like the time my grandfather, at age 74, walked into the woods wearing his brown sweater and got himself mistaken for a bear. According to Grandpa, the mistake was made by a genuine goyishe bear.

"I'm too old to run away and a tree climber I'm not," Grandpa said.

"So what did you do?" I asked him.

"So what do you think I did?"

"Did you yell at him?"

"So I yelled at him."

"What did you yell at him?"

"So what do you think I yelled at him?"

" 'Get away from here'?"

"No, wrong. That's not a good thing to yell at a bear. First of all, the bear wouldn't know you're yelling at him. He thinks maybe you're yelling at a cockroach. Or a landlord."

"So what did you yell?"

" 'Get away from here, you rotten bear.' "

"Gee, Grandpa, weren't you afraid?"

"Sure I was afraid." He picked me up, all seven years of me, and held me near his face. "I was afraid I wouldn't see my little boychik any more."

But I'm trying to tell you about Uncle Seymour, not Grandpa, even though he could make a water gun out of two branches. What Uncle Seymour did was graduate from college and begin teaching English at another college. This entire chain of events, routine on the surface, astounded my family because for the first 40 years of his life, Uncle Seymour worked with, you should forgive the expression, his hands.

Personally, I liked Uncle Seymour a lot more before he began talking like a professor. The last time I saw him he was describing his trip to Paris. "After lunch, where the waiter complimented me on my accent, although I couldn't do likewise for the food, we went to the Rodin Museum. Does anybody know who Rodin was?"

Nobody knew from Rodin. "Well," said Uncle Seymour, "Auguste Rodin, eighteen-forty, nineteen-seventeen . . ."

"I know," I shouted, because I couldn't stand it anymore and because I wanted to talk about my trip that afternoon to the salami factory. "Auguste Rodin, he used to work with his hands."

My mother gasped. The only thing I could do was keep going. "Guess where I was yesterday? A kosher salami factory. I watched them make it."

"What's to watch," said Uncle Seymour. "Kosher salami doesn't taste special anymore. When I was a kid kosher salami tasted like something. What are they doing to it? Making it for the goyim, I betcha."

Well put, Uncle Seymour.

ITEM: "Cleveland (AP) — United States Customs officials here say they have an unusual problem: salami and kielbasa smugglers. Casimir Krul, chief inspector for the Cleveland district, says that Cleveland is a very 'ethnic-oriented town' and that Clevelanders who have been to their European homelands often try to bring back some of the meat specialties via Cleveland Hopkins International Airport."

Casimir Krul takes the salami away, he told the AP, because he's worried about foot-and-mouth disease.

COMMENT: Casimir sounds like a double agent for the bland salami cartel. Otherwise-loyal Americans have gone to great lengths, and sometimes Poland, to hunt the giant pungent salamis of their youth. What we have in America—disguised as salami, kielbasa, hot dog, knish, radio programs, Palmolive, movie stars—all tastes the same. The only difference is the color on the cellophane wrapping. Without that you couldn't tell a package of kosher knishes from a salami-and-Al-Pacino sandwich.

For thousands of years, Jewish people have been the object of envy from everybody else in the neighborhood. (Why else would the goyishe butcher's kid keep asking me to play spin the bottle? She was common and my mother was right to keep me away from her until I was 27.) The goyim thought kosher was our secret. Give us kosher, they screamed. So we gave them kosher. But what nobody tells them is that kosher don't come from what you put in your mouth. Kosher is what's already in you when the food gets there.

ITEM: Pantry Pride/Hills food stores in New York, Connecticut, and New Jersey named a new delicatessen manager, Aaron Klein. A full-page ad in the New York *Post* announcing the appointment read, in part, "Whenever delicatessen moguls gather together, the man they listen to is Aaron Klein. With good reason. Aaron's built great deli operations all across the country. What Aaron Klein

collage by Gary Friedman

doesn't know about kosher corned beef and Italian prosciutto isn't worth knowing."

COMMENT: Aaron Klein deserves a medal for undercover work among the goyim. For setting up those phony-baloney deli stores. You want kosher corned beef, says Aaron, here's kosher corned beef. You want a piece prosciutto, here, take your chances, live and be well. I hope Aaron doesn't blow his cover. If he does the goyim will wait for him in the park and beat him up, like they always did.

ITEM: Hebrew National Kosher Frankfurters has hooked up with French's Mustard. Buy a package of franks and get a free 9-oz. jar of mustard. As they say in the ad copy, "A great tasting mustard deserves a great tasting hot dog. And one bite is enough to tell you Hebrew National Hot Dogs have that special taste you just don't find in an ordinary hot dog. You see, Hebrew National Hot Dogs are kosher, made with only pure, fresh beef. And our unique blend of natural spices will have your whole family coming back for more."

COMMENT: Hebrew National is doing great work in the kosher-is-good-for-you propaganda line. Phrases like "great tasting . . . one bite is enough to tell you . . . special taste . . . unique blend . . . natural spices . . ." are all perfect. Nobody could tell what product they're meant to describe. Could be salami. Could be Tuna Helper. Could be Al Pacino.

The kosher salami factory I visited in Newark, New Jersey, makes Shofar salamis. (The shofar, for you guys and gals out there who have never thrilled to its sound, is a ram's horn. Joshua, Jericho, walls come tumbling down . . . does any of this ring a bell?) Bernie Ostrow, president and founder of Shofar, showed me around. His machines turn out thirty tons of kosher a week, without regard to race, color, or creed.

"Sure I eat salami, tastes the same as it always did,"

Bernie said when I first met him. Later, after he threw a couple of midget Shofars into my pocket, he gave it to me straight. "It's a little less spicy, gotta be. Now we sell to the world. Supermarkets are not just for the Jewish trade. If we sold just to the Jewish trade, we'd starve to death. Follow me?"

I followed him. Bernie introduced me to Jack Gigantino, a government meat inspector. "Everything is much blander," Jack said. "They don't want a highly seasoned product." He called it "consumer acceptance."

My sponsor in Newark was Sid Cohen of Cohen's Frozen Knishes. Sid took me back to his place nearby, and I watched thousands of kosher knishes being born in his spotless kitchen. Tiny islands of potato mixture moving down a conveyor belt—"like soldiers," Sid said; "They make me smile"—dropping into fat. And then, back out, finished potato knishes. Twenty-five years ago Sid's mother made knishes by hand. The Cohen family sold them off a wagon. Then a little store. Ten years, seven days a week, "we worked like animals," Sid said. His mother hit on the idea of freezing their knishes. She was right. Got nominated for Frozen Food Business Woman-of-the-Year.

Sid touched one of the new conveyor belt knishes. He wasn't smiling. "If you tasted one of our knishes twenty-five years ago you wouldn't eat this today. It's the machines. You have to lose something."

But it's still kosher. Or, if you like to talk that native talk, cush-er. But the goyim are happy. And Bernie Ostrow and Sid Cohen aren't complaining. Louis Wolfson who won the Triple Crown with Affirmed is delighted. The best frankfurter is Justice Frankfurter. And we still got Bob Dylan and Rod Carew and chopped liver and Lenny Bruce records and sour pickles and Isaac Bashevis Singer and kugel and knaidlach and Kol Nidre and di-di-deedle-deedle-di, de-beem-bom-beem-bom-beedy-bom . . .

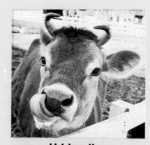
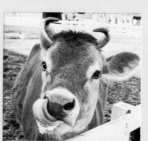
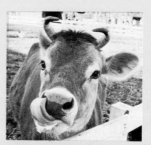
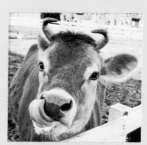

42

drawing by Rick Meyerowitz

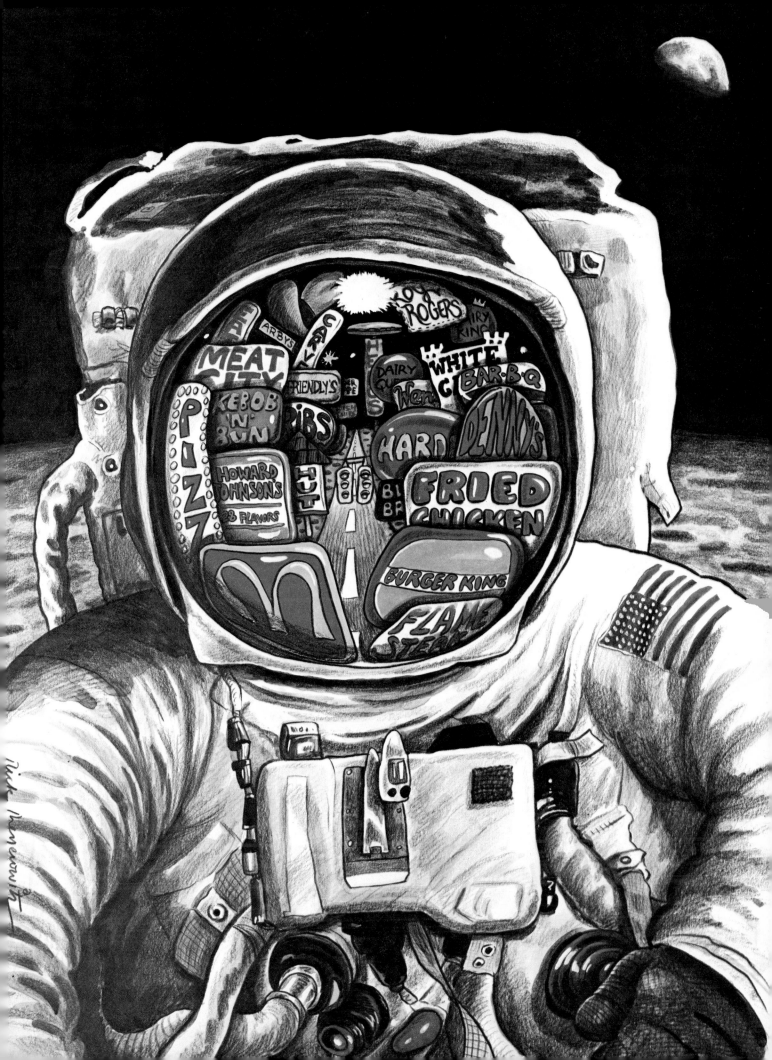

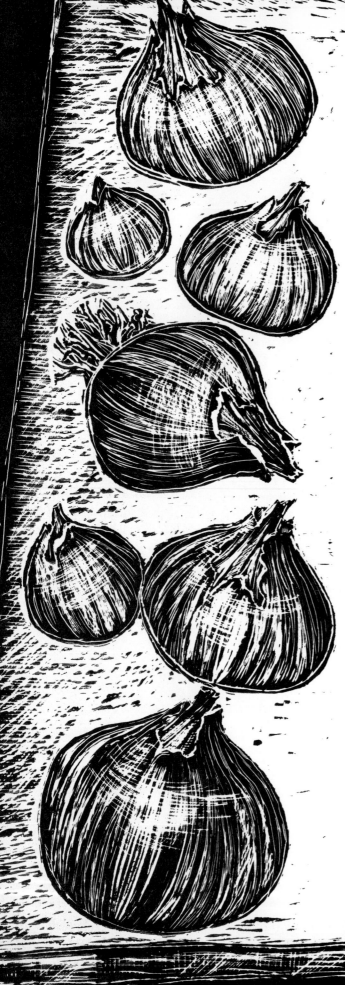

No Tears for Leon

by Andrew Zimmerman

Leon Plantigrade, author of *La Racine du Mal,* was born in 1907 to Marie and Louis Plantigrade of Chartres, France. It did not take long for his parents to appreciate the extraordinary nature of their child; at the age of three, Leon was abandoned on the steps of the local cathedral. Tradition has it that the nun who found the boy mistook him at first for a fallen gargoyle. To this day, there are those who contend it was no mistake.

After performing a perfunctory exorcism, the Archbishop dispatched his charge to the local gendarmes, who, by law, were obliged to accept him. The authorities finally found a place for Leon at the exclusive Institut National de Hygiène Mental; there he passed the remaining 23 years of his life.

According to the files, Leon devoted most of his time to devising a way to extract oil from walnuts without cracking the shell. On his deathbed he claimed success. But as his keepers, for sound precautionary reasons, would not provide him with any walnuts, we cannot credit his claims absolutely.

In any event, the reader may well imagine both the surprise that attended the discovery of his 3,000-page *La Racine du Mal,* and the chagrin of the kitchen staff when they realized it wouldn't burn. The warden eventually commandeered it for use as a bookend in the library. Unheralded, *La Racine* had entered the annals of literature.

For five years it languished on the shelf until chance (or Nemesis) thrust it into the hands of Hermann. It is to him we owe Plantigrade's 15-paragraph critical biography, *A Tourist in the Realm of the Mind.*

According to Hermann, *La Racine's* thesis seems to be that there exists a conspiracy between the financial interests of Antwerp and the edible roots and tubers to destroy civilization.[1] (Although we cannot be too sure, since no one, not even Hermann, has bothered to read the work in its entirety.) By what means, Plantigrade does not specify.

There are those who contend that *La Racine* is a work of genius to be read symbolically. They volunteer no scheme, nor, wisely enough, their names. What is indisputa-

---

[1]"Civilization as Plantigrade never knew it," remarks Hermann.

drawing by Frances Jetter

ble is that *La Racine* remains to this day the longest work of its kind ever to be unpublished.

As for Leon, Hermann pronounces the final and definitive word: "There is a thin line between genius and insanity; one that the deranged Plantigrade was manifestly incapable of crossing."

The following selections are drawn from the legible portions of La Racine du Mal.

The onion is quick to take umbrage, nursing it in the thickness of his flaps. Suspicious by nature, by circumstances ignorant of the ways of surface dwellers, he succumbs readily to misrepresentation and fraud. At night the fields swarm with financiers, huddled like so many incanting crows, over the burrow of the hapless creature.[2] There these mercenaries inculcate envy and grudge towards all settled human habitation. . . .

Some would question whether the above statement is a statement of fact. Yet is it not an undeniable fact that such a statement has been made? And since the equivalent of a statement of fact cannot be fiction, must it not be a fact? Hence the above statement is a fact. . . .[3]

How then, in the face of such sinister designs, to explain the persistent cohabitation of the onion and humankind. . . .[4]

They should be sliced and boiled in oil[5]. . . . Exterminate the brutes. . . .

Herewith, a milder remedy for this canker. It is a simple, yet efficacious technique called *Abandoning the Onions.*

ABANDONING THE ONIONS

1. Position a table so that its back edge runs parallel to a wall at a distance of three inches.

2. Empty a sack of onions on the middle of the table. If the onions are loose, grasp as many as you can by the snorkel[6] and set them on the middle of the table.

3. Looking to the left and pointing with the right hand in the same direction, cry out, "Look, the financial interests of Antwerp are resurgent in the East!" This ruse is known as Distracting the Onions.

4. Using a backhanded motion of the left arm, gently sweep the distracted onions into the gap between the table and wall.

5. Leave the room. The onions are now abandoned.

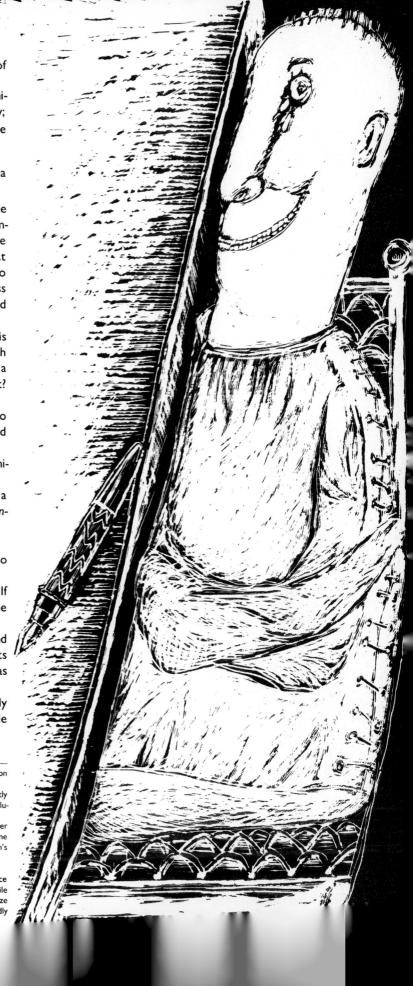

[2]By creatures, Plantigrade means onions. He never did settle to his own satisfaction their exact nature. See his monograph, "The Onion: Animal or Mineral?"

[3]As Hermann notes, "Plantigrade had a preternatural ability to take a few patently false postulates and arrive, time and time again, at a patently preposterous conclusion."

[4]We shall spare the reader 70 pages in which the author weaves, among other things, eggnog, the lapse of the tides, and the ill effects of tight-fitting shoes into one grand jury-rigged theory. Plantigrade invokes just about everything but the onion's edibility. Apparently he was unaware it was eaten.

[5]This may well be the first reference in literature to french-fried onion rings.

[6]This reference to a non-existent portion of the onion has occasioned a fierce scholarly wrangle. Firpy's camp contends that Plantigrade never beheld an onion, while Hermann and others maintain that he had, in fact, beheld onions but did not recognize them as such. As for what Plantigrade conceived onions to be, Hermann halfheartedly ventures "moles."

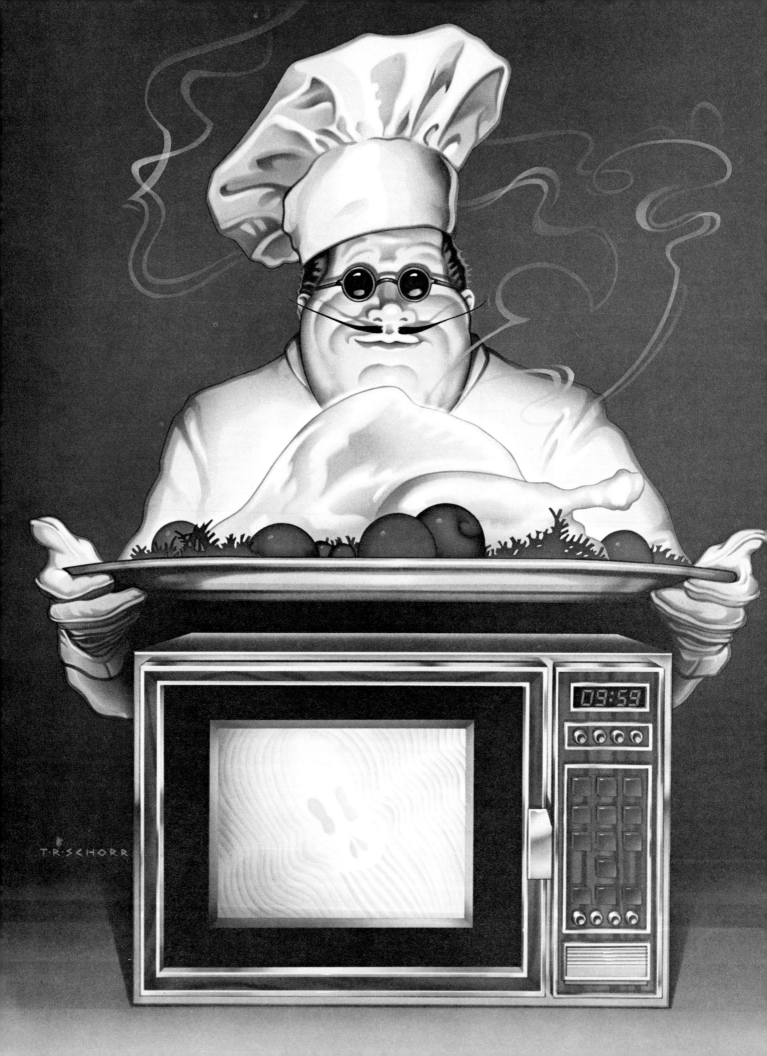

A Moral Lecture for Food Snobs, Gourmets, Epicures, Health Food Nuts, Gourmands, and People Who Pick on Their Children for Gulping Rock-&-Roll Jelly Kings

by Guy Davenport

The oldest person in the USA lives exclusively on Moon Pies and Royal Crown Cola. His advice for longevity is, "Don't eat no table food after 90." The advice of Javier Pereira, a Colombian who made it to 167, was "No se preocupe, tome mucho café y fume un buen cigarro," keep your cool, swill coffee, and smoke a good cigar. Ludwig Wittgenstein ate the same thing every meal for months; once it was chocolate oatmeal prepared in a pressure cooker of his own invention. Descartes ate rotten eggs. Diogenes lived to be 89 on Athenian garbage, with an interlude of Corinthian table scraps.

Epicurus, whose name gluttons have misappropriated, ate simply: a meal of goat cheese, bread, and spring water is the menu that history records. Byron liked a plate of mashed potatoes drenched in vinegar. Van Gogh had been living for a month on camphor, white wine, and his pipe when he cut his ear off. Toulouse-Lautrec (like William Morris) fancied canned kangaroo. Spinoza liked tulip bulbs. Keats ate dry cayenne peppers. Shelley was a vegetarian. Thoreau once ate a hedgehog.

The meal Montezuma served Cortés was an Aztec specialty, fried chicken dipped in melted chocolate, eaten while smoking a foot-long cigar. Hitler, a vegetarian, gorged on coconut macaroons. Dr. Johnson once downed 36 cups of tea at a go. Richard Porson, the greatest classical scholar of modern times, was drunk all of his adult life, and once drank the oil from all of the lamps in a house when the gin ran out.

Darwin vomited every afternoon at 4:00. Lawrence of Arabia lived on apples and marmalade toward the end of his life. Frederick the Great swore by eel pie. Attila the Hun could never learn to eat bread. Hetty Green, the financier, always lunched on Quaker Oats soaked in water from the horse trough in front of her Wall Street bank. Philip II of Spain stuck to meat, avoiding fish, fruit, and vegetables as dangerous.

Charles Olson once ate an oil rag. Nebuchadnezzar ate grass, the prophet John grasshoppers, and the prophet Ezekiel a book. Montaigne, like Shakespeare and Elizabeth I, ate with his fingers, which he sometimes bit in his haste. Louis XIV poured perfume over his fried eggs.

Eating is probably not an index to anything. Rossini was a glutton, and so was Rasputin. To Pasquale Giuseppe Rossetti (Dante Gabriel's father), as to Franklin Roosevelt, all food tasted like hay; Lorenzo de' Medici, "The Magnificent," could taste nothing at all. Ruskin ate boisterously, Carlyle had perpetual indigestion, Napoleon a perpetual stomachache. Edward Lear always traveled with his own cook. Richard Nixon puts catsup on cottage cheese. Proust picked at his food. G.K. Chesterton once lost two poached eggs somewhere in his clothes and berated the restaurant for never bringing them; the King of Sweden inadvertently shot his false teeth into Somerset Maugham's soup. Sir Walter Scott dined with his cat beside his plate.

Pasteur tore his bread to crumbs before eating it, looking for things. Charles V, the Holy Roman Emperor, kept a green leaf in his mouth all the time.

painting by Todd Schorr

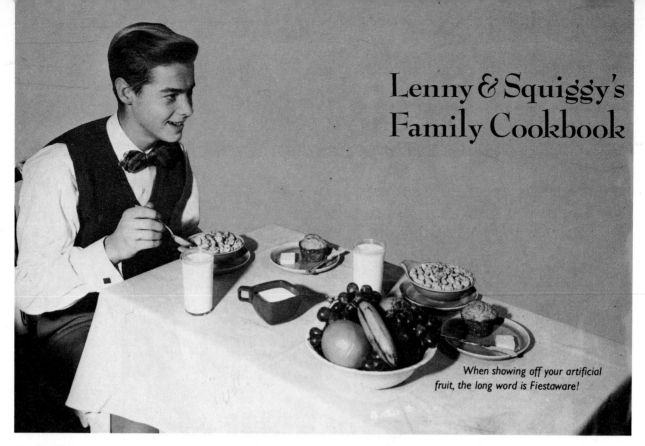

When showing off your artificial fruit, the long word is Fiestaware!

Lenny & Squiggy's Family Cookbook

by Michael McKean and David L. Lander

If there's no time for sergeants there's also no substitute for good, old-fashioned "home" or house-cooking. You can warm things up nicely by leaving them on top of the TV set. That was just one of the tips available to Leonard Kosnowski and Andrew Squigmann while growing up in S. Milwaukee in the '50s, between the wars. The speaker? Mrs. Pia Kosnowski.

Squiggy: "My old lady wasn't home too much, and when she was, she'd just lay around in a bathrobe or a bad mood. So I'd just go over to Lenny's house to eat."

"She'd make the most wonderful stuff," recalls Lenny. "Always something new. We never knew what the hell was gonna come out of that oven."

Squiggy: "The thing I remember most about the Kosnowski kitchen was that it always smelled. Plus the fact my old man was usually over there mixing drinks for Len's Mom."

Here's a year's worth of very special dishes from the neglected Serbo-Croatian-Polish culture and Mrs. Kosnowski—along with a few "quick ones" or barside treats from

Helmut Squigmann, a German alcoholic. The CHEERS! notation, in festive script, is a way of setting the drinks off from the recipes without interrupting the format.

New Year's Day Brunch Bowl

1 box Cheerios
1 box Wheat Thins
1 box cornstarch
1 bag potato chips
2 cups hoop cheese (unmelted)
1 egg, any style

Mix in large bowl. Garnish with orange slices, sugar cubes, rose petals, or cotton balls, in keeping with your favorite post-season gridiron classic.

Cheers!

Helmut's Hangover Blaster

4 parts Scotch
1 part tomato paste
1 bottle Maalox

Mix until one color.

Noodlewurst Casserole

1 pack liverwurst
2 lbs. boiled noodles
1 cup low-fat buttermilk
1 jigger Ann Page applesauce

Preheat oven 475. Line bottom of cas-

serole dish with 6—8 slices of liverwurst. Dump noodles on top. Decorate with 10—12 sticks Doublemint gum. Bake till pale brown.

Lenny: "Easter Sunday was always special for my mom. She'd stay in bed until 3:00, while us kids would scribble on a bunch of eggs with crayons. Then she'd get up and yell and put the eggs in the oven, and go back to bed."

Squiggy: "One time she stuck a meat thermometer in one of the eggs and blew off her whole left eyebrow. I guess that was my favorite Easter."

Baked Easter Eggs

Eggs
Crayons
No thermometer

Bake till solid and hide.

Cheers!

Scared Rabbit

1 bucket of lemonade
2 pints white wine
1 large jar Miracle Whip
1 small jar sweet pickle relish
1 rind of grapefruit

Top with 31 olives.

Quick Pizza

6–8 split English muffins
I jar parmesan Cheez Whiz
I Skippy Peanut Butter jar (empty) hot
  ketchup

Spread Whiz on muffins, ladle on
ketchup, and put in toaster. Goes good with
soda.

Mexican Dryback

Squiggy's note: "This is the traditional recipe, but for those of us who hate avocados,
good, ripe American pears will do fine."

4–6 avocados, no pits
A tomato, any size
Heavy dose of spice
Canned beans, pre-fried
Graham crackers

Line dish deeply with graham cracker
crust. Squish avocados. Now your beans.
Top it off with tomato (any size). Serve with
Wonder Bread. Bury the whole thing in a
ditch for several months.

*Squiggy: "When we got nothing
for trick or treat, we'd go back and
Len's Mom would make us hats out
of cotton candy she'd saved from the
Labor Day picnic."*

*Lenny: "I still have all mine. I'd
Magic-Marker on the date, and roll
it up in my UNICEF can."*

Spaghetti and Pumpkin Balls

I large pumpkin
I can red sauce
I lb. No. 5 semolina spaghetti

Scoop out pumpkin "muck" into little

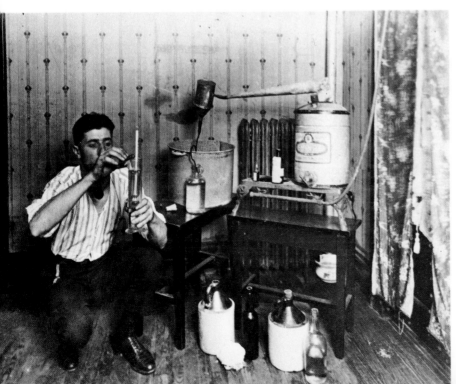

balls. Brown in Toast-R-Oven. Cook
spaghetti the regular way. Put it in sauce.
Add balls. Serve with black jelly beans.

*Lenny: "Mom had her own ideas
about Thanksgiving. She'd take a
real skinny turkey and stuff it with
cold cuts: bologna, olive loaf, Swiss
cheese, cole slaw, the works. That
way, even when the turkey was
gone, there'd still be leftovers."*

Turkey à la Pia (Kosnowski)

I small turkey
I ½ lbs. cold cuts (see above)
A lot of hot fat
4 bowls Rice Krispies, dry
Butter

Rub butter on turkey's body. Roll around
in Rice Krispies. French fry in deep fat.
Serve with hot yam loaf. Yams are not sweet
potatoes.

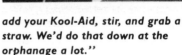

Helmut's Bottoms-Up Punch

2 gals. cooking wine
5 inches ouzo (yellow, Greek)
I lb. melted butter
I qt. Cranapple juice

To serve: glue crunched nuts around rim
of glass. Hold in mouth and swallow quick.

*Lenny: "One very special Christ-
mas, Mom taught us how to make
Kool-Aid angels in the snow. First
you make your angel, then spray
cold water from a garden hose until
it freezes up. Then some more water,*

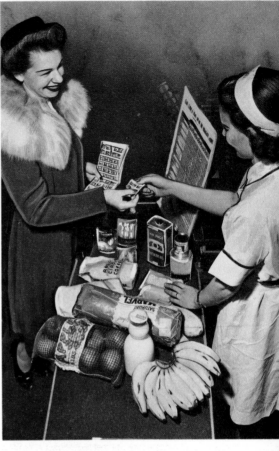

add your Kool-Aid, stir, and grab a
straw. We'd do that down at the
orphanage a lot."
  Squiggy: "Those poor kids' faces
would just light up."
  Lenny: "I sure miss those holiday
treats."

Pigs in a Blizzard

Hot dogs
Molasses
Pop corn

Pop the corn and boil the franks at the
same moment. Dip hot hot dogs into
molasses. Roll in fresh popcorn. Freeze.

Helmut's German Coffee

4 parts malt liquor
I tsp. instant coffee
I generous sprinkle Accent
I part warm Cool Whip
some schnapps

Serve in Bund pan.

**A Final tip: Gas station glasses
last longer!**

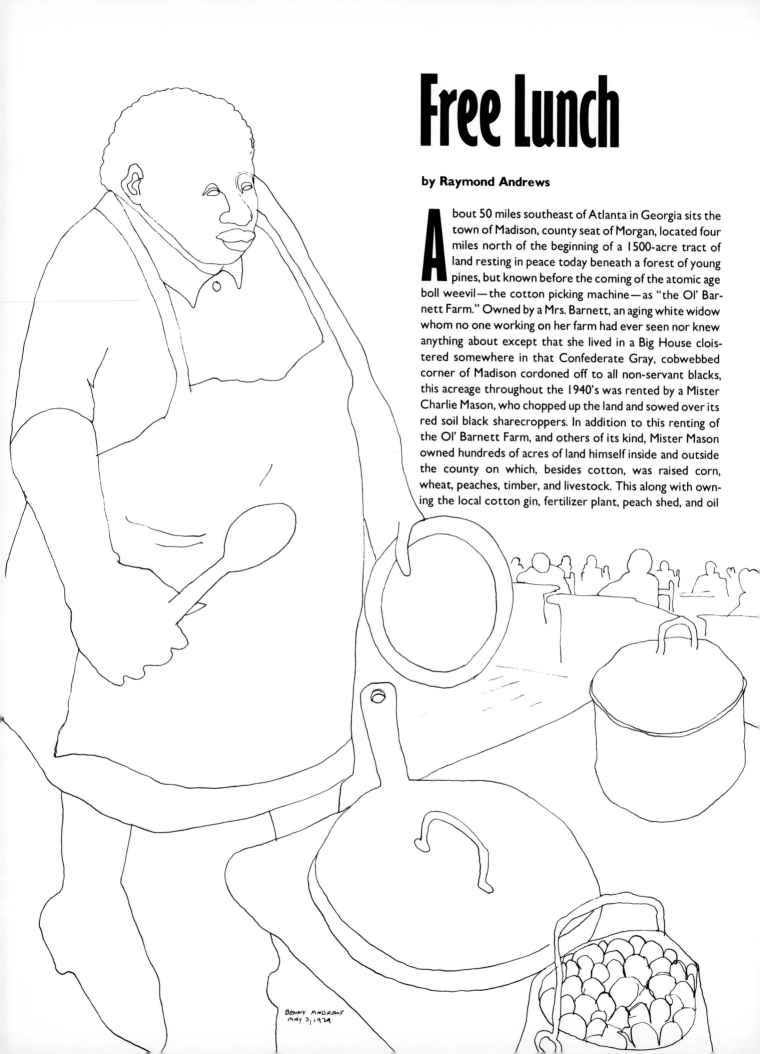

Free Lunch

by Raymond Andrews

About 50 miles southeast of Atlanta in Georgia sits the town of Madison, county seat of Morgan, located four miles north of the beginning of a 1500-acre tract of land resting in peace today beneath a forest of young pines, but known before the coming of the atomic age boll weevil—the cotton picking machine—as "the Ol' Barnett Farm." Owned by a Mrs. Barnett, an aging white widow whom no one working on her farm had ever seen nor knew anything about except that she lived in a Big House cloistered somewhere in that Confederate Gray, cobwebbed corner of Madison cordoned off to all non-servant blacks, this acreage throughout the 1940's was rented by a Mister Charlie Mason, who chopped up the land and sowed over its red soil black sharecroppers. In addition to this renting of the Ol' Barnett Farm, and others of its kind, Mister Mason owned hundreds of acres of land himself inside and outside the county on which, besides cotton, was raised corn, wheat, peaches, timber, and livestock. This along with owning the local cotton gin, fertilizer plant, peach shed, and oil and planer mills, plus several sawmills scattered through the area, made Mister Mason the employer of more workers than any other single individual in the county. And the overwhelming majority of these workers were blacks, all of whom known locally as "Mason Niggers."

Unlike the spectral Mrs. Barnett, Mister Mason could be seen practically daily pulling a long trail of Georgia red dust behind his mud-splattered 1941 Plymouth sedan up and down the back country roads snaking in and around the Ol' Barnett Farm where it was said that whenever looking from the window of his speeding car out upon the blacks picking cotton in the fields, the only things this boss man ever wanted to see of his niggers were their elbows and assholes.

Back in the 1940's in Morgan County it was vital for a black man to "belong" to an influential white of Mister Mason's status or thereabouts so that during the War, if considered by his employer to be a respectable, hard-working colored who knew and accepted his place in the Dixie Dream, then regardless of his age, physical condition, or draft status, perhaps he would not have to go into the armed forces. While on the other hand any black of draft age considered by this same local hierarchy to be worthless or hopelessly addicted to uppitiness could wake up one blue Monday and find himself "across the pond." And, to the local landed gentry, next to his Northern cousin there was nothing on Jesus Christ and His Daddy's earth more worthless, or uppity, than a free-lancing "town nigger." Thus did the ownerless Madison town black become better represented in World War Two than did his owned, country cousin. And to the best of my knowledge no war movie was ever made depicting such.

The most significant effect the Depression of the 1930's had upon Morgan County blacks was that it brought them work. The WPA. It also provided black parents the South over with a new name to give their newborn males. Roosevelt. (Only the truly backward were yet naming their offspring Abraham.) For as far as the Southern black of that era was concerned, America had had in its history only *two* presidents. Abraham Lincoln, the man who took away their jobs, and Franklin Delano Roosevelt, the man who gave them their jobs back again.

One family the WPA cheated the local poorhouse out of was mine. My daddy, starting out at a whopping 50¢ a day, began work with the Roosevelt Miracle immediately upon its descending from heaven upon the area, and remained with it until the Japs got around to bombing Pearl Harbor, an act christening a brand new sawmill in the area, where Daddy soon got a job at $15 a week: The wartime money boom was on. But so was the cost of Daddy's feeding a wife and six (of an eventual ten) children . . . not to mention the local draft board snatching up all ownerless blacks between the ages of 18 and 42 able to tell their right hand from their left long enough to be sworn in. Thus it came to pass that

Daddy, a conscientious objector to violence of any sort conducted outside the safety of the home, sold the souls of himself and his family in exchange for political asylum by moving from his father's place to 30 sharecropping acres of the Ol' Barnett Farm. Land which I was destined to grow up on during the 1940's as a Mason Nigger.

And while it was true that my parents had grown to adulthood on their respective families' farms before leaving home to get married, we children—five boys and two girls at the time, with myself at age eight in the exact middle—weren't at all soil-oriented. Nor would being a Mason Nigger make us so. Remembering those long months each year, planting, siding, chopping, mopping, sodaing, hoeing, bunching, and, finally, picking cotton beneath that ol' Georgia Satan Sun, overhanging the fields, blistering our bodies to a dark leathery crust amid a sea of lazy, floating, suffocating red dust, refusing to let stir anywhere a cool breeze of any sort or size, easily made my kind of weather then—and yet today—rain.

Rain on the tin, leaky rooftop of our three-room clapboard—one of 14 shacks haphazardly littering the 1500 Barnett acres—meant no work in the fields that day. But it was left to that other dreaded enemy of the local farmer to rescue us from those rainy day jobs which took place in the stable, crib, or shed. School. Even more dangerous to the South's landed gentry "Cause" than the Northern and the town nigger was the mystic "li'l nigger schoolhouse."

Daddy with his advanced learning—a fourth grade education—was the only black head of family on the Ol' Barnett Farm knowing how to read or write more than just his name. But Daddy had a deep-seated fear of being labeled uppity for having attained such heights in the local academic world, and in an attempt to make up for this serious deficiency he became determined that no child of his would ever have to tote the heavy burden of education around on his back for all the neighbors—and white folks—to see and snicker at.

Not buying this piece of pity though was Momma who, next to Christianity, believed most strongly in education. Her own eighth-grade schooling—the last year attainable at Burney Street High, the colored "town" school in Madison—automatically made Momma the Ol' Barnett Farm suspect. Suspect even to those who came to her with their unopened letters to be read to them by her, and whom afterwards they would sit and dictate the return letters to, which she always took down upon the white-lined notebook paper each knew to bring.

The community school, Plainview, was a one-room cabin squatting on the edge of a forest nearly three miles from our house, walking. Only the white children knew how to ride the school bus. School ran from the first of October to the middle of April, though most local children weren't able to attend classes on a regular basis anytime before Christmas or after mid-March due to the fall's cotton picking and spring's plowing. Enough to make winter any child's favorite season. And during the greater part of the Depression and the entire decade of the '40's, Plainview's teacher was Mrs. Bertha Douglas, a plump, childless, middle-aged widow entrusted by the county with teaching all seven grades and, under the state's free lunch program, doing all the school's cooking which, unfortunately for the community's young minds, proved to be her true calling.

By many families in the community not owning clocks, school would get underway each morning when "Miz' Bertha" decided the bulk of that day's attendance—as high as 66 or as low as zero—had arrived: the day officially beginning with the boys and girls lined up separately and then marched briskly across the schoolyard up to the flagpole where both lines of youngsters would stand at attention and in unison pledge to the top of their voices allegiance to a worn, tired old American flag. Once inside the classroom, after an opening hymn, Miz' Bertha would read aloud to us a chapter from the Bible which would be followed by each child rising to recite a Bible verse. A closing song, and now it was time for Miz' Bertha to start cooking atop the elongated stove which sat out in the middle of the classroom and was also used to heat the rest of the building, a duty it wasn't always aware of.

While Miz' Bertha busily prepared lunch for her children, the classroom's older girls—the sixth and seventh graders—would lead classes in arithmetic, spelling, reading, grammar, health, history, and geography from those dog-eared textbooks handed down by the local white school. Despite taking no part in the teaching of the morning classes, Miz' Bertha made her presence in the room very strongly felt by toting around in the hand not used to stir the food atop the stove a thick leather razor strop, which by the time of the Pearl Harbor bombing had already grown slick from overuse.

During the long cold winter months in the community when nothing grew except hunger, many parents sent their children to school just to eat. Once the free lunch program was introduced, children whose parents had been quite untouched by education began reappearing out of the fields and forests onto the schoolgrounds not with pencil and pad but clutching instead plate and spoon. This community cultural reawakening inspired by Miz' Bertha's daily performance atop the schoolhouse stove quickly led to a near-standing-room-only crowd during the winter months there in the little one-classroom building. This was especially true in the first-, second-, and third-grade section, which always had to absorb the bulk of these hungry returnees of mostly teenage boys whose chief interest besides eating was the recess hour when they would be let out of doors and beyond the reach of Miz' Bertha's long razor strop, into the wooded area stretching for miles back of the school and where with their fists they would take knuckle drill practice

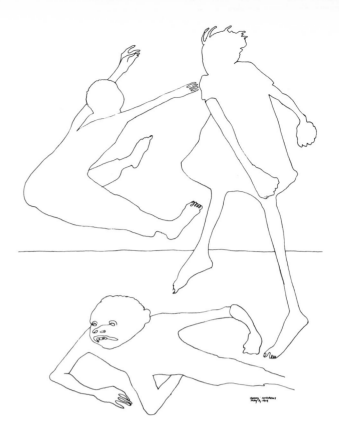

across any little head daring to enter this wilderness. In those early days of the free lunch we had recess hour *before* eating in order, Miz' Bertha told us, to "build up an appetite," not recalling that, in hunger country, appetites were never down.

Fighting back there always bored me, and especially if I was the one being fought. Such was not the view of my oldest sister, Val, a free speech advocate who never learned that it cost even less to shut up. In building up their appetites the girls at Plainview fought, too, the most feared fighting female of them all being a tall, big-boned, thick chick named Minnie Pearl who had all of Plainview's girls and most of its boys in daily fear of her deadly roundhouse right which had cold-cocked many a student. The only thing that was to save Val from total annihilation at the fist of Minnie Pearl was when her tormentor suddenly dropped out of the third grade to marry a young sawmiller, a situation the rest of us Plainview pupils found hard to envision. That is, imagining someone getting the drop on Minnie Pearl long enough to make a baby inside her. He got the drop, though...and often ...because she dropped a dozen.

Recess over—appetites up—it was now "eating" time. At the beginning of the school year each child brought his own tin plate and left it with Miz' Bertha, who kept them all cleaned and stacked neatly alongside the state-supplied food, staples, and cooking utensils in a large wooden box especially built for such by the community and sitting off in a corner at the top of the room. But spoons had to be brought and taken home daily. Knives and forks weren't used at Plainview. The older girls served everyone at their desks after having taken the filled plates from Miz' Bertha, who ladled out according to ages and sizes. No one dared touch their food until everyone had a plate before them and grace had been sung by all.

Georgia has always had its (and someone else's, I'm sure) share of the black-eyed pea. Three days a week at Plainview we had black-eyed peas and fatback, though for variety we had beans and fatback on Tuesdays, and yellow grits, without fatback, on Thursdays. Everything came with cornbread, powdered milk, and canned peaches for dessert.

There was absolutely no talking during eating. The only sounds to be heard in the schoolhouse now were spoons scraping plates before touching teeth, loud smacking of lips followed by long slurps canaling pot liquor down the gullet. Eating at Plainview was a soulfully serious matter and couldn't be interrupted by anything so insignificant as words. Everybody ate everything put on, or near, their plates. No leftovers. On occasion a plate would get licked clean but here Miz' Bertha's razor strop would surface. The first ones finished would sit looking enviously at those yet eating, certain they'd been allotted a meagerer portion. Then the plates would be collected and washed by the same older girls who had done the serving, and the classroom was now ready for Miz' Bertha's teaching.

Sitting behind her long table for a desk, Miz' Bertha there at the top of the room would dream aloud in front of all us children about her trip, many years earlier as a young bride, when she and her young husband had gone on their honeymoon by ship to a far far away world which she always called "the Old Country" . . . off the coast of Florida.

Once in a great while visitors would come to the school. Driving into the schoolyard from the county Board of Education would be a big shiny car emitting a white man and woman who, after walking atop the floating Georgia red dust on into the schoolhouse, were curtsied to and seated by Miz' Bertha, whom they called just "Bertha." Then in an attempt to show off her brightest pupils, the teacher would make each stand before the royal guests and recite the multiplication table from one through 15, spell, and state dates from American and Georgian history. But all these honored guests ever seemed to want from us students, and Miz' Bertha, was to hear us sing hymns. And then—for their comic relief—to find out what we wanted to be when we grew up. Most of the girls said school teachers, mothers, wives, church choir singers, or nurses. Most Plainview boys wanted to be operators of some sort of machine—a tractor, or truck—and a few said hunters or farmers. Benny, my older brother by four years, would always say he wanted to be a "drawer." Meanwhile, back at home, Momma was praying hard that Benny would grow up to be a "drawing" rather than a "pouring" artist, that being another talent of his, the ability from age five to pour water interchangeably between two bottles without spilling a drop, even in darkness, the mark of a true moonshiner. A talent Momma claimed he'd picked up from Daddy's side of the family where there was a long line of straight pourers.

As the school afternoon lengthened, a more serious problem to the sensibilities than white visitors developed there in the classroom: This was the black-eyed-pea-created burp blowing out the lower end of the Plainview student's body. The girls were always embarrassed by this part of their body's fighting to express itself in public and would ride out the urge by politely squirming around in their seats like bronco busters. Sitting on frogs. But in the back of the room where the older boys sat there was no such modesty. Nobody in the history of Plainview could break wind as loud, long, or as smelly as could Big Boy. Ol' Big Boy could start a black-eyed-pea fart out as a squeak, accelerate it all the way up to a blasting crescendo, and then, yet, *hold onto it* while it just hung out there whining and crying like despite how bad this mean old world was and all, it still did not want to leave it. Then it would die, leaving behind a hushed room.

At first Miz' Bertha tried putting a stop to Big Boy's afternoon ritual by laying her razor strop across his farting machinery. But eventually, appetites up or down, she had to change the recess hour until *after* lunch so that Big Boy could "air" out his exhaust *before* returning to the classroom.

At the end of each school day, Miz' Bertha would line us all up numerically by grades with the seventh grade in front and from the big wooden food box in the corner at the top of the room pass out to each child an apple and an orange, also provided by the state's free lunch program. On those rare days when most of the community's children eligible for school were present and Miz' Bertha, in passing out the fruit, kept too busy looking at hands to notice faces, some of the bolder boys would attempt to go through the line twice. If they made it through, they'd have the story of how they tricked ol' Miz' Bertha, plus the extra fruit. But if caught, they'd have all their fruit taken away and feel the sting of the strop as well.

The girls, mostly, took their fruit home to share it with their families. But not the boys, who started out biting into the fruit the very instant they stepped outside the schoolhouse door, eating core and peelings, swallowing seeds and all. Then the bigger boys would seek out those smaller, big-brotherless boys to take away their fruit. So those little ones whose thoughtless parents hadn't bothered providing them with big brothers to protect them and their property at school learned fast to eat faster.

Fruit safely in the belly, it was now time to lower the head, put one foot in front of the other as fast as you could, and point the toes toward home where waited the dreaded chores of milking the cows, slopping the hogs, bringing up water, cutting firewood . . . before finally planting feet beneath the supper table to sit savoring the aroma slowly simmering up from the plate in front of you, filled to the brim with fatback-boiled black-eyed peas.

Funeral Food

Post mortem nihil nisi victus.
And finger sandwiches.

Walter B. Cooke, Inc.,
73, in New York City

Prepared funerals of Alexander Calder, Duke Ellington, Long John Nebel, Gig Young

George Amato, Vice President: "Usually the neighbors will get together and make such things as a roast beef which can be sliced up. So that when the funeral party comes back to the residence, they could just have something light and something which wasn't too heavy, and there could be conversation and consolation. Finger sandwiches is exactly what it should be, with some light salads. The finger sandwiches use whatever is usual, like ham and swiss."

Frank E. Campbell, Inc.,
80, in New York City

Prepared funerals of Ralph Bunche, Joan Crawford, Judy Garland, Igor Stravinsky, Rudolph Valentino

Tom Michaels, Funeral Director: "It varies with the religious background of the family, number one. Mine is that everybody gets dragged off to a restaurant, and given a big lunch with drinks after the burial takes place. I'm Protestant. This is also very much the case among Catholic families, I would say, the idea of taking the mourners for . . . refreshments. Now most Jewish families, rather than going to a place of public entertainment, go to their residence, the residence of the deceased usually, where a luncheon is served. What is served I don't know . . . I don't have that many Jewish people among my close acquaintances. I've never been invited to one."

Ed Casey, Manager: "I think it depends on what the family of the deceased usually eat. In the old days, an Irish wake would have Irish soda bread, together with all the J. J. Javison you could afford. Then maybe you had a pound of cold cuts for a hundred people . . . and another bottle of J. J. Javison. That's all it was—a booze party. The Italians—one would make meatballs, another would make manicot and soup and stuff like that, and they'd all bring it in. Wealthy and well-known families we serve that live on the East Side here call up a caterer and usually get finger sandwiches. Others, if they want to put on the dog and do something real nice, they might go to '21' for lunch."

Joseph Gawler's Sons,
120, in Washington, D.C.

Prepared funerals of John F. Kennedy, Ike Eisenhower, Woodrow Wilson, J. Edgar Hoover, Hubert Humphrey

Joseph E. Hagan, President: "I used to live in Alabama, and going back fifteen-twenty years ago, there used to be more hot dishes served. But there's no real pattern for funeral food. In most cases, alcoholic beverages are certainly prevalent. I was in Baltimore for a funeral not too long ago, and they had the food served in a Knights of Columbus Hall . . . huge place, there were three or four hundred people. They had it set up with maybe three hot dishes: spaghetti, meatballs—there were some Italian people in the family. They also had some German food—there were ethnic-type people in this community. Salads, casseroles. A typical buffet. Their finger sandwiches pretty much ran the gamut."

Forest Lawn Memorial Parks,
66, in Glendale, California

Prepared funerals of Gracie Allen, Nat King Cole, Clark Gable, Jean Harlow, Carole Lombard

Bob Huston, Public Relations: "Lighter foods are better, like meat dishes and chicken. Not spicy stuff, because people are upset emotionally, anyway. They use those light sandwiches, something that's easy to handle. Our experience shows that usually people don't go to any extra trouble. I've known of families when they knew they had a lot of guests in the area, who'll hold a kind of celebration after the funeral in a home. We'll toast to the memory of the deceased and have a caterer set up and serve cocktail party sandwiches and hors d'oeuvres."

Riverside Funeral Home, Inc., 79, in New York City

Prepared funerals of John Garfield, Sidney Hillman, Richard Tucker, Sophie Tucker

Fred Garel, Funeral Director: "In the Jewish families we service here, most have little appetizer-type things, maybe wine. The Christian faith, they generally go out to a formal, complete dinner after the funeral, at a restaurant, because they don't have the facilities in their own home. But with the Jewish family having a limited buffet-type arrangement, it can be held in their own home. Generally, it's just because the families and friends have gone for so many hours—you know, from getting to the services, then the services, then the interment, the average is about four or five hours, that the family supplies some little snack to just hold them on until they get back to dinner. Most people would call a caterer, who'd make up those small finger sandwiches, maybe a salad. In an Orthodox family, though, the food in the finger sandwiches would have to be kosher."

Point Coupee Funeral Home, 38, in New Roads, Louisiana

Prepared funerals of Miss Ellios Beterice, Mr. Ellios Edward, Mrs. Margaret Jackson, Rev. Luthes Lamb, Mrs. Yvonne Toussaint

Irma Jean Verrette, Manager: "Usually what we do, they have for meats, now, they have ham, and fried chicken. They would have broiled ham sliced, you know, in a buffet style, green salad, or potato salad. But if it's going to be served that way, most of the time it's more safer to have the green salad. And you can use pie or cake, for, you know. Any kind. Sometimes they serve the dinner at one special place, at one of the member of the family homes. In the wintertime, we would have gumbo, seafood gumbo, and you can have a roast. Then you can have different types of salads. You can have rice dressing—y'all may call it 'dirty rice,' it's rice cooked with ground meat, or just liver and giblets of the chicken, you know? It's ground up and you use it with a lot of season and you prepare the rice, and of course, it goes a long way. Now sometimes you can serve miniature sandwiches. You can use cheese, bologna sausage, American cheese is best, or pepper mixed with mayonnaise and mustard and chop it up and with a pickle, it almost tastes like chicken salad. It's a specialty here, used as a spread. Try putting celery in the tuna miniature sandwiches. You put the one little piece of cheese and a little piece of the sausage and you put it between a grit or you can just take it dry, or stick a olive and stick a toothpick through the three of them. You can have dip, I know you know what that is. You can have little cookies. Make a lot of punch."

JF: You've had a drive-in viewing window for four years now. Are people taking to it?

IJV: Fine. Nice reception to the drive-in window.

JF: Would it be tasteful to have a fast food consolation meal?

IJV: If the family wants it catered by a junk food chain, that's fine. Some people have some weird ideas, some have very good ideas. There's nothing wrong with it. Of course, I wouldn't tell them that they'd use a Burger Kin' the way we use the drive-in window. That might not work so well. Sometimes people get the wrong impression when we say drive-in window—'cause I had somebody ask me, 'Oh, just like a Burger Kin'?' But it's not that way. It's a little bit more sacred.

"And Mom loves the way they stand up in the oven on their cute little feet!"

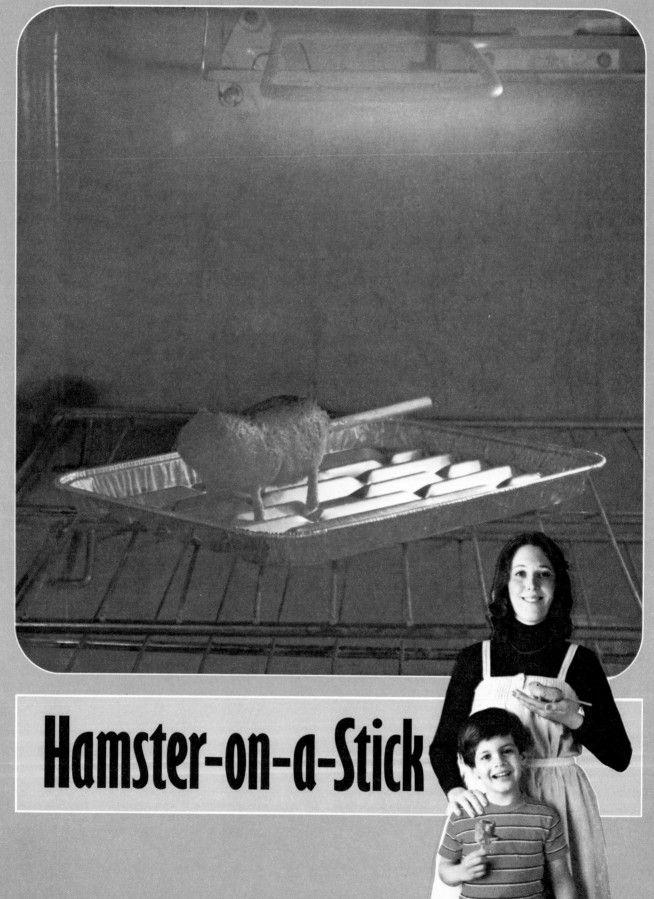

Hamster-on-a-Stick

Eating Your Toys

by Paul Rudnick

"Don't put that in your mouth!" How many times has a thoughtless parent cruelly limited a child's world through this careless phrase? Nutritionists working long hours in laboratories owned and operated by the Tip-Tot Corporation have determined that absolutely anything can be ingested and enjoyed, provided the dish is properly prepared and served on dinnerware featuring a Harlequin portrait, a pivotal scene from any novel in which the protagonist is a bunny, or any member of the extended Flintstone family, with exceptional vitamin value found in the Wilma saucer and the Bam-Bam chug-a-mug.

Herewith a sampling of tempting recipes from the soon-to-be-published *Playing With Your Food* (Toll House, $9.95, trade paper):

Barbie Doll — A menu classic, perfect for casual dining or multicourse smorgasbord. Quick-n-easy: Dismember your doll, and add the extremities to a package of lime gelatin or, for the more adventuresome, Silly Putty. Place the mixture in a festive mold (perhaps a hubcap or grandmother's oxfords) and chill. Garnish with Barbie's lustrous hair and snorkeling accessories. Serves 4. Barbie's legs are, of course, one of the Cuisine Minceur's foremost delicacies, especially flavorsome when served with the spike disco mules intact; these are also appropriate for a fondue in a delicately seasoned glaze created by melting Barbie's Beauty Shop, Porsche, and Tree House On The Vineyard.

Barbie's many friends can provide mealtime variety (and may be tossed together in a penny-wise salad). Velvet, Barbie's Negro pal (packaged in Barbie's Storefront Birth Control Clinic and Problem Hair Salon), is a pleasing summer cooler, but one must be careful to spit out the seeds.

Barbie's Hebrew chum, Tovah, the unleavened Barbie, is a featured canapé at the Nevele's "Swingles Only" brunches, wrapped in a heavy crepe of melted Ken doll heads and leisure ensembles. There are those who feel that Barbie herself is a Jewish delicacy, due to her extensive wardrobe and lack of genitalia. It is known, however, that, while Barbie will hire Velvet to sweep her Beach Cabana and wait table at her Malt Shop, Tovah will attempt to instruct Velvet on the virtues of primitive sculpture and Miriam Makeba records, and allow her children to clasp Velvet's hand when crossing a busy intersection.

Stuffed Animals — Any basic panda can be slashed from neck to crotch and filled with croutons, greens, and chewy foam rubber. And why not spice with Venus Paradise pencil shavings? Mom can get difficult medicines into unwary tots by filling Winnie-the-Pooh or Paddington Bear with an exotic blend of B vitamins, lithium tablets, Ex-Lax, and NyQuil. P.S.: The plush fur from any lion or elephant in the Sears Yuletide *Wish Book* can also be snorted directly.

Blocks — Ideal for cocktail treats when served alongside a wholesome dip of Mr. Bubble, Play-Doh, and the Rose Marie figurine from the play-at-home version of Hollywood Squares. (Younger children may need their blocks cut into splinters.)

Board Games — Great TV-time snackables. Monopoly includes a hearty bridge-mix recipe in the instruction booklet: hotels and tract houses can be gobbled by the fistful. The popular Scrabble board can be sliced into nutritious energy squares—and, for birthday party fun, frosted with Lemon Pledge.

Vehicles — Any tin dump truck or Lionel caboose can become a meal-in-a-minute when placed in a microwave toaster oven at an exceedingly high temperature and served piping hot between long-playing recordings of the Boston Pops' "Peter and the Wolf" and "Pete Seeger Sings the Shari Lewis Songbook."

Shari was a crusader in playground cuisine, nibbling on the aptly named Lambchop (occasionally reaching the tasty center of human flesh) on network television as early as 1953.

Remco's Formula 500 Death-Pit racing car kit is also an important staple for young 'uns: Place the end section of electrified track in the child's mouth, and let the Lotus XKE zoom right into the bones, muscles, and blood of a growing boy or girl.

Loss of sight, numbness in the tongue or fingertips, and severe brain damage are common signs of the onset of puberty, and not the result of Toy Chest cookery.

How are Americans responding to this revolution in the kitchen? Let's spend a moment with a family who knows the special joy of playtime menus. Call them the Mattels. Here they are, gathered 'round the dinner table.... Mom keeps a watchful eye on Susie, the toddler: "Clean your plate, young lady—do I see a piece of jump rope going to waste?" Dad concurs: "Finish that Slinky, missy, or Santa won't bring you any food this year!"

Jimmy and Johnny, the twins, pipe up: "Can we have some more marbles, Mom?" Jimmy eyes his brother's prostheses hungrily: "Remember when Johnny ate Pop Rocks and then drank seltzer—and his arms blew off? I'm glad we only eat toys now." Dad chuckles warmly.

"Just hold your horses, fella," says Mom. "Dessert is under the bed."

model by Jim Wilson, photograph by Carl Waltzer

Mall Life

An interview with film director George Romero, best known for his zombie and vampire films.

JF: So . . . where were you born?

GR: In the Bronx, grew up there, in a place called Parkchester. Went to Pittsburgh to go to school and hung out in Pittsburgh. We started a company there, doing commercials and industrial films and things like that, and in 1968 we made Night of the Living Dead.

JF: That's why we're here, you know. Because you did Night of the Living Dead and Martin.

GR: Right. Food and drink.

JF: What do you eat on the set when you're—

GR: I keep people in pizza and donuts, generally. In Dawn of the Dead we did our shooting in a shopping mall, and the only food you have access to in a shopping mall is . . . hot dog places, Dunkin' Donut places. . . . Our big problem was that we were shooting there at night. So we couldn't go to work until they'd closed down all their stores, which is 10:30, and then they have a maintenance crew, so we never started to roll films until 12:00 or 1:00 in the morning. And then, right promptly at 7:00, the Muzak comes on, and nobody at the mall— Muzak is controlled by a central brain in Antarctica. No one could shut it off. I didn't even have to say "Cut," 'cause exactly at 7:00, every morning, the Muzak came on and we had to stop shooting.

JF: Now, in Dawn, when the zombies are eating human flesh, what they're really eating is—?

GR: Often, Arby's. We put a lot of ketchup on it. If you take the inside out of an Arby's and stuff it in a zombie's mouth, it looks terrific, it looks like he just took a bite out of somebody's arm. Arby's works great. For Martin, we used a 3M product called BLOOD. It comes in little institutional cans that say BLOOD. In Night of the Living Dead we used Bosco. It's always a lot easier in black and white.

JF: In Night, there was a scene where two kids try to escape in a pickup truck, it blows up, and there are guts piled on the seat. What kind of guts were those?

GR: One of our investors was a meat packer and he brought down a bag full of . . . stuff . . . from the local Pittsburgh slaughterhouse. Actual intestines and things from cows. We used some again in Dawn. Not the same batch. We got a new batch.

JF: Do zombies ever eat food, or just flesh?

GR: No, they just . . . finger foods.

JF: Talk about Pittsburgh food.

GR: You know, you would think there would be a lot of ethnic, a lot of Slavic food, and there's really not. There used to be some great old kilbassi makers around Pittsburgh, and now . . . there's nothing happening there anymore. It's fallen prey to the Arby's and Weiner World's. That's

Home Movies

Scene	Equipment	Memo
flowing or gushing blood	Kraft's Fruit Punch (bottled concentrate)	perfect thickness, good, rich color
flowing or gushing blood (black & white)	Hershey's Chocolate Syrup	
oozing or coagulated blood	Jell-O	mixing grape and raspberry produces the best color
oozing or coagulated blood (black & white)	Royal Chocolate Pudding	
cuts and scrapes	Smucker's Preserves	raspberry (because it's bright red) for recent wounds, boysenberry for day-old cuts
cuts and scrapes (black & white)	Nestlé's Quik	just add a few drops of water
guts	ziti (Ronzoni #2)	cook macaroni well, add Hawaiian Punch concentrate for color
guts (for stunts)	Minute Rice, or Cup O' Noodles	cook in fruit concentrate; makes a nice splattering effect, e.g., burst appendix
brains	KA-ME Ramen Chinese Noodles	softened and wet
burns	My*T*Fine Tapioca	cook it, add food coloring
warts	Sugar Smacks, or Cocoa Puffs	no joke

—Jamie Mitchell

pretty traditional downtown Pittsburgh food. Arby's is really popular there – it's the best, or at least the best disguised. When you go in there, you see a real big hunk of beef, and they just keep slicing it down. At least it's a slab of something. You're comforted. Pittsburgh's an eat-at-home town. It's even hard to recommend a really good restaurant there. There's a big local burger chain called Winky's, though. It's a fast-food heaven. The suburbs are all traditional Middle-American suburbs, and they each have a shopping district strip.

JF: So it's no accident that the mall in **Dawn** is inhabited by zombies?

GR: Right. You get a situation where the people who are trapped on the roof make a quick run into the mall, risking life and limb, because there's supplies and food they need down there. At once, they get exhilarated and they start feeling very proprietary about the mall and all the things. They wind up committing, and they go to a weapon store in the mall, and they just arm themselves to the teeth and manage to win the mall from the zombies. And then they start setting up this comfortable little suburban existence up in the storage area, and they turn it into what looks like a tacky suburban apartment.

JF: Well . . . any other food or drink memories?

GR: When we needed squirting seltzer bottles for **Dawn of the Dead**, we couldn't find any in Pittsburgh. We had to import them from New York.

JF (ready to kick around a few screenplay ideas.): Buy you a drink?

GR: Can't. But there's a party later this week – (Details.)[1]

JF: Hey, great.

GR (out of the blue.): Shopping malls . . . these malls in Pittsburgh, man, it's the New City. Nobody's downtown in Pittsburgh anymore, they're all out at the malls. And the young people hang out there. It's amazing. It's the New Downtown.

— **Andrew Zimmerman**

---

[1]Yeah, but when we called, they said they were "going smaller" on it. We heard it was a lousy party, with lousy food.

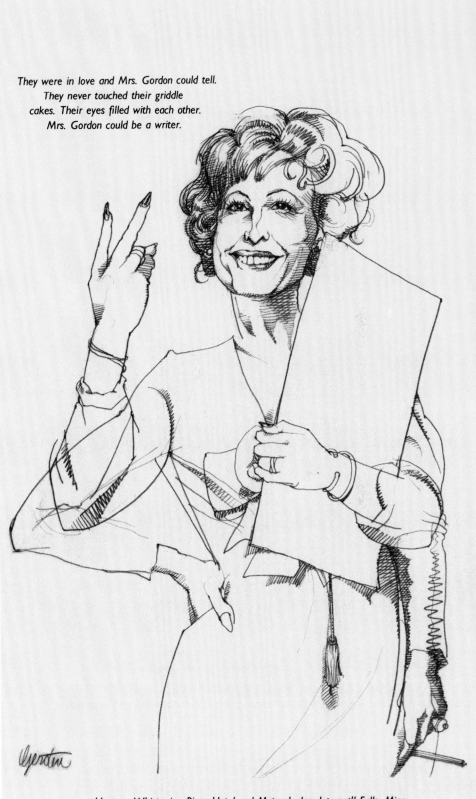

They were in love and Mrs. Gordon could tell. They never touched their griddle cakes. Their eyes filled with each other. Mrs. Gordon could be a writer.

Hostess, Whispering Pines Hotel and Motor Lodge, Internat'l Falls, Minn.

drawing by Gerry Gersten

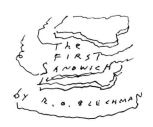

The FIRST SANDWICH
by R. O. BLECHMAN

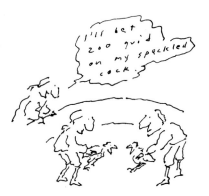

The Earl of Sandwich was a passionate gambler.

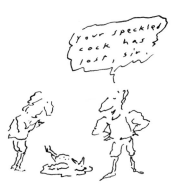

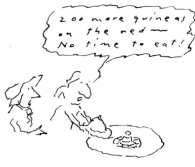

He would bet on almost anything.

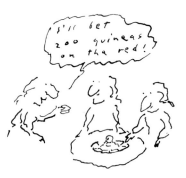

He was so busy gambling...

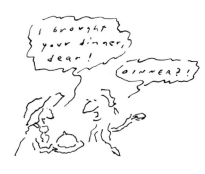

...that he rarely took the time to eat.

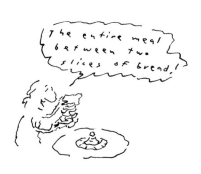

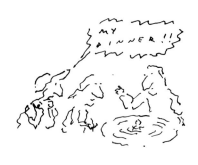

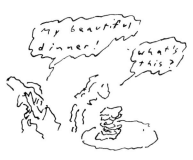

The First sandwich was created.

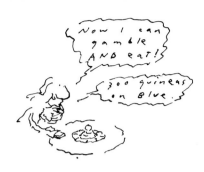

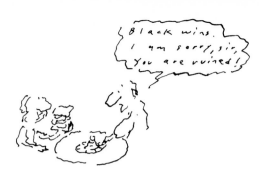

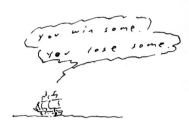

The Earl left for the colonies.

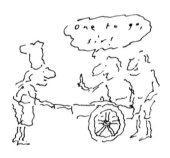

In the Colonies he set up his Roulette Wheel...

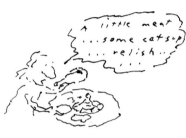

...and prepared his meal-between-two-slices-of-bread.

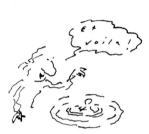

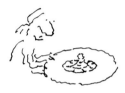

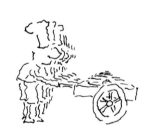

The colonists took to the novelty.

Within a year, the Earl had a fleet of pushcarts.

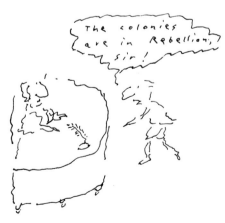

But fate was to play the final hand.

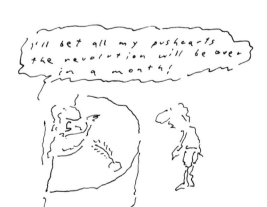

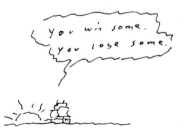

The Earl of Sandwich's legacy, however, was to endure.

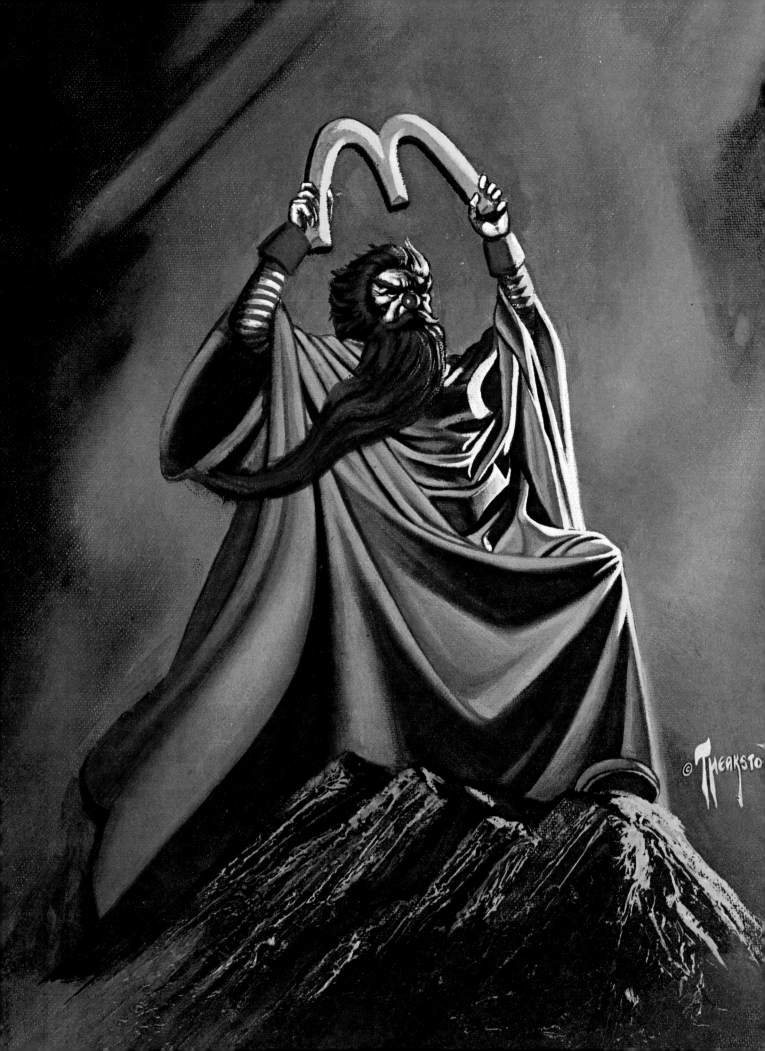

Heart Burn

by Saul Maloff

Later I would retreat into genteel poverty, all but disappearing into the high chaparral of conspicuous obscurity; but in the days when I was a boulevardier and high-roller endowed with the magical power to sign restaurant checks reckoned in three high digits with a disdainful flourish, fawned over by every maitre d' who mattered, I played that game as if to the manner born. Scarcely a glance at the intimidating menu, and I would order for a party of 12 with what for all the world seemed, and indeed *was,* a hieratic mastery of the rite, and I its archbishop. Or not even so much as a glance: I was one of those for whom the menu was an unnecessary encumbrance, the man who knew exactly what was needed, it being the work of lackeys and concubines to provide it. Gracefully I wore my disguise of homme du monde, a gaudy costume in a high farce of the gaslight era, myself as an exiled baron from the court of some Nicholas, now landless and expropriated but no less a baron for that, a cavalry officer in an elite regiment, a prince among swine.

The role exacted a terrible toll: hiatus hernia, an ulcerated esophagus, cold sweats, tremors. We can lie to the world only so long and then the body submits its bill which no expense account can cover. For all the while, a small voice within, speaking the guttural of childhood streets and alleys, cried: Fraud! Liar! Nothing I do can fool that unsleeping sentry of my deepest life, whose appointed task is to call me back to origins whenever I stray.

Still, I try. The all-American disguise, my native game: A & W, Carvel, Howard Johnson's, Arthur Treacher's. Once, on an all-expenses-paid journey along some 500 miles of American autobahn, when the sky was the limit, I made it a point, like some mad Humbert Humbert hitting every tacky, grimy, speckled, soiled, and spattered motel in the land for Lolita's sweet sake — I too was seized by some inscrutable desire to eat and drink my way through all the dreck I could take down and hold in, thereby in some darkly obscure way renewing my national identity, which tends to grow cloudy in late August. When I submitted my packet of receipts to my benefactor, an insufferably rich foundation, the comptroller suggested I add a digit up front so as not to spoil it for those who came after.

"Why?" he kept asking. "Why?" A proper reply would have required a spiritual autobiography.

Beginning with Mom, the ur-Mother, the other voice within me, large and resonant, prophesying in Yiddish. "Junk," it keeps saying. "Garbage. Swill for pigs. Goyim." Junk, she stormed—junk was "bad" for me, for all people, everywhere, in all times. Had I been a "good son," which is to say an obedient, obliging, ingratiating one, that would have been the end of it. But I was not that, nowhere near it: What Mama condemned, calling upon the Patriarchs to be her witness, exerted an irresistible magnetism, not only upon my palate, but upon my very soul. Precisely what was "bad" for me was my heart's delight; and my natural bent, assisted by a little sophistry, led me to my First—and abiding—Principle: Bad is Good. And its corollary: very bad is marvelous.

"What doesn't kill me," Nietzsche said, "makes me stronger." Instinctively I'd always known that, before I found the language for it. The melancholy German, I decided, must have had junk in mind. But with a difference, a small yet critical distinction: call it Junque. Junque: the manna of summer, the perpetual summer of those green and wanton years when I disported myself with forbidden foods far from prying eyes. What Mom didn't know wouldn't kill her; and if it killed me, well, it was my life. For the Good I have in mind may very well kill you in the banal literal sense; in the end it surely will; and before the end and on the way to it, it will, depend on it, rot your teeth, bring on night blindness, slacken such muscles as you may have, erode the stomach lining, cause structures to grow within it, rearrange and move other organs and cellular formations around in original ways: and that's only part of a picture of widespread physical chaos. In short, as physicians understand these matters that lie beyond their grasp, Junque food is, exactly as Mom used to warn, very bad for you indeed. Wonderfully, succulently, unforgettably bad. Like self-abuse, it is not intended to make you healthy: merely happy. A point Mom did not seem to appreciate.

An element, in other words, of criminality is here present as powerful as horseradish, hot pepper, serious mustard; a desecration of the hearth, of tradition, of family piety, filial fealty; of the Word itself. That explosion in the mouth is propelled by the frisson of guilt, highly spiced with free-floating anxiety. Seen by this light (or in this darkness) and in the widest perspective, junque food—my junque food—is any food eaten "out of the house"—something of a problem when you consider that that house has been extinct for several decades. But ghosts do not vanish; great-grandmothers lost in the mists of history determine in ways one can scarcely divine one's choice of wives, upholstery, neckties, appetizers, and entrees. "Pigmeat!" my mother would exclaim of all foods consumed elsewhere. *How do you know what they put in it?* Visions of bits and pieces of mice, brains of cats, giraffe bladders. Visions, hell: I had read *The Jungle;* I *knew* "what they put in it." For all I cared,

painting by Greg Theakston

let them color it with the periodic effusions of shiksas.

But gothic horror, as every ravaged heroine knows, only adds to the frisson. We bought our contraband goods on the sly, my friends and I, in those mid-Depression years when a nickel was gold bullion, a dime as rare as Phoenician coins. We shot crap for pennies somehow got, played poker and pinochle beneath the glow of streetlamps on summer nights for blood, the objective always the same—to make it all the way to the delicatessen, and when the dice proved true, and the cards broke right, to the sanctum sanctorum of the "appetizing store" itself, hot dogs and knishes in the former, corned beef and hot pastrami and smoked tongue, salami and bologna; and in the latter stuffed derma, kishke, kreplach, blintzes, stuffed cabbage, smoked white fish, herring, gefilte fish: God's plenty. O, let me not think on it! For I am speaking here not merely of food that's bad for you; I am speaking of love and loss, of origins and homeland and exile, of tribal loyalties, of blood bonds and vows taken in the presence of ancient ghosts and deities, of childhood irretrievably gone and forever searched-after, of innocence and belief and the Fall and awful expulsion into the world, of sin without hope of redemption, of elysian fields and paradise enow become irrecoverably vanished. *Ultima thule.* The dream corrupted.

Abroad, too, I am haunted by the game. A hoyden fate has provided me with a six-year-old very British grandson. Viking hair, Icelandic eyes, features carved out of the chalk hills of Sussex, an accent wobbling between Somerset, Wiltshire, Oxbridge, and BBC; in his mouth, "kishke," which I taught him as soon as he could mimic speech, sounds like a verse out of the Book of Common Prayer, something formidably High Church, an invocation. We are in collusion. His mother, unknowingly repeating ancestral history, sternly forbids him junk of the British variety, of which there is, God knows, a spectacular plenitude (all of it, some would say). Within the confines of her prison, he is all compliance: a perfect British child, a "good son," the best, a joy and comfort. Across a table aching with joints of mutton and roasts of beef and Yorkshire pudding, our eyes meet in secret understanding, each year when I make my pilgrimage across the sea, heavily disguised in the chuckling, beaming manner of doting grandsire from the land of Cracker Jacks and bubblegum. Picking gingerly at some unspeakable haggis or syllabub, he bides his time, knowing he has one ally in an alien world.

Our excursions are our great adventures. The two of us, *outside,* "out of the house," on our own, sprung. What Mum doesn't know won't hurt her. *Mum! No* name is more ill-suited to my own mother, Ma, Mama, Mom. Mum? Grotesque. Hilarious. What is this I'm thinking; *his* Mum is my daughter, the expatriate, exiled among Anglo-Saxons. But it's right again, right always: the unconscious knows best. For when this sturdy lad, blood of my own blood, flesh of my flesh, my own unregenerate genes implanted in his

own circuitry—when he and I are on the loose, cruising for forbidden fruit, so to speak, I know that I have regressed, that we are of an age, contemporaries in spirit, he just returned from a rousing game of rugger, and I, come home, most reluctantly, from some game of chance: shooting crap with Izzie the Gafter (later a smalltime professional gambler, his throat destined to be slit by a sore loser); playing klabyash with Irving the Gonif (d. at the Ebro, Spain, 1938); pinochle with Willie Eightball (a good, scholarly, deliberate hand with a deck of cards who got reckless one day in Iwo Jima while disarming an antipersonnel mine); stud poker with anyone who could raise the ante, and everyone could, if he had to steal it, the preferred manner. By the time we got home to wholesome food we were fairly bursting with ravishing chozzerai fit only for pigs, goyim, and ourselves; our mothers never did understand how we could live without eating. And now, a lifetime later, my posterity and I are reliving my sweet eternal summer: his Mum / my Mama both fused into the single figure of my daughter, a slight confusion forged in the furnace of my mind. The unconscious, that con-artist and fast shuffler, knows truths which lie deeper than facts.

Together we prowl the West Country in search of bangers and mash, his idea of the high life; and the various "pies" the pubs dole out with pints of bitter; and gnarled brownish objects, offal of some sort, that float atop thick brackish gruel; and fish-and-chips—his own favorite establishment being a (I am reporting the sober truth) Chinese fish-and-chips joint on the London Road in the great Georgian city of Bath, where he lives, largely indifferent to its architectural splendors. Their house specialty crosses plaice-and-chips with something the blackboard menu calls chop suey chow mein with a side of eggroll, the lot of it drowned in soy, or if possible worse, sauce.

The kid, not otherwise retarded, adores it, can't shovel it down fast enough. Very heaven.

Later he will ask for a bedtime story, his favorites, sagas out of my own childhood long ago and far away, his reward for doing his lessons, minding his (otherwise really quite beautiful) manners, and eating well and wisely. A born literary naturalist or ash-can realist, he insists on authenticity—that I tell the tales in native accents wild; and so I glide back to the fondly remembered argot of my native New York streets in the shtetl of the lost childhood of my people. Having long since exhausted the actual past I invent a thousand childhoods I have lived only in my mind, and no matter where I start, all narrative roads lead to the one he unfailingly demands: the "Eggroll Story."

It is summer; it is always summer; my heart is permanently lodged in late August. The world outside is careening toward madness. Someone named Hitler has occupied someplace called the Rhineland; not far from there someone named Franco has mounted an insurrection against the Spanish Republic. Everywhere things are looking bad for the Jews. Something must be done about this; we know this, everyone in my neighborhood knows this, and we certainly mean to take care of it first chance we get.

But not today. Today Carl Hubbell is slated to pitch against the Dodgers and we are bound for the Polo Grounds, my friends and I. After we've won the pennant and the Series we'll attend to Fascism and save the Jews. Clutching whatever there is to hold onto, we hitch a trolleycar ride to the South Bronx, vault over the turnstile at the subway station, having waited for the train to open its doors, and make our way to Coogan's Bluff. We loiter outside the gate leading to the center-field bleachers until the game is underway and the paying customers have entered. The understanding guards look away and we pass through the gate. Hubbell shuts them out on one hit, a lousy grounder that should have been called an error. (My grandson is content to know that baseball is "something like" cricket.)

After the game, there is important business to be transacted. Dressed for the occasion in our baggiest knickerbockers, and though it is a sweltering day, in outsize lumberjackets, we scour the bleachers and grandstands for empty soda-pop bottles, balloon our pants and jackets with them, as many as we can possibly carry, and leave the park rattling and clanging. No sneak, Archie Katz—who will die on the beaches of Normandy—fills a huge laundry bag brought along for the purpose and walks defiantly past the guards. With our loot we make our way across the Harlem River to the Bronx side, to our Jerusalem, a delicatessen-and-appetizing store the owner of which will accept our 2¢-deposit "empties" in exchange for his maddening wares. No money—that was his rule; only food—take it or leave it!

Ladies and gentlemen, I am telling you of a time in the history of our Republic when everything worth having cost a nickel. One nickel. A 5¢ piece. A nickel a shtickel. *Everything!* As if God had ordained it so. (Tuppence ha'penny, I tell my grandson, and leave him to work it out in "new pence.") God's hot dog with mustard and sauerkraut—a nickel. The knish of Adonai—a nickel. An abundant portion of fries—a nickel. All right, make it a thin dime for a thick salami sandwich on real rye, make it 15¢ for a *mountainous* sandwich of corned beef. A shtickel stuffed derma—a nickel. Whatever—a nickel!

What is stuffed derma, my tragically deprived grandson asks. Like nothing else in the world, I tell him.

Quite, he says; but what is it *like? Like?* I say. Like, you ask? Well, it's something like eggroll. (And in the only Hebrew I know I implore the dear spirit of my late mother to forgive me for this and all my sins.)

On the golden day which is the unchanging time of memory (Proust had his madeleine, we our egg cream, our potato knish, our smoked tongue) it is always late August, not a cloud in the sky, and that magical bag of bones Carl Hubbell has always just shut out the Dodgers on a shameful bad bounce and we are invincibly on our way to a pennant.

We always find more empties than we can carry and the guards always smile as we pass by. Archie Katz (whose sister Esther I loved, though she'd never heard of King Carl) is immortally alive, his bulging laundry bag twice his own size. And we are always bound for glory. Without so much as a single broken bottle we make it across the river and into paradise where the old man will look up from his Yiddish edition of *Das Kapital,* and say: Boychik, put the empties in the back and eat in good health. The stuffed derma is absolutely fresh homemade, made an hour ago. . . .

Fresh, stale—who cares? Only the cherished delight itself matters. Just as rapturously would I swallow *vestigial* derma—fossilized derma caught in amber formed in the early paleolithic age.

My favorite saint (forgive me, Mama), Ambrose, spoke for me when, old and dying, he said: "I often imagined myself among bevies of girls: my face pale with hunger, my lips chilled, but my mind burned with desire, the fires of lust leapt up before me though my flesh was almost dead." In the ripeness of time when, full of years, I prepare myself for my last journey across the river, I know that my wandering mind, what is left of it, will be filled with spraying burst of August light more radiant than any that ever descended to earth, and that it, like Ambrose's, will burn with desire but not, I fear, like his for bevies of girls. My face will be pale with hunger, all right, though my chill lips will be seized by a sudden fever, and the fires of lust will damn well leap up before me, you may depend on it. The fires of my lust will be browning to precisely the consummate degree of perfection the object of my eternal terminal longing, and it will be waiting for me, done to a turn and sizzling hot, when I cross over to that surprising place where it is always late August.

The Famous Stuffed Derma Recipe
of Ruth Rubinstein, the Cantor's Wife
South Huntington Jewish Center Sisterhood, L.I., N.Y.

1 med. bunget, cut into 1 foot lengths
1 cup flour
3 T farina
½ cup raw suet, ground
½ tsp pepper
1 med. onion, grated
½ lb chopped meat
1 T paprika
1 tsp salt
1 carrot, grated

Wash bunget and wrap thread around one end and knot well. Stuff side of bunget that had the fat. Seal end by wrapping thread around end and knot well. Plunge into boiling water 30 min. Place large onion, skin and all, in water while cooking kishke. Freeze. When needed, place in roasting pan on bed of onion and fat. Sprinkle on paprika. Bake at 350 for 1½ hours.

The Junk Food Chain

by Lewis Grossberger

I visit Dr. B.R. Borborygmus, the extinguished Known-Well Prize wanting biologician, in his lavatory at Oxtail University. Doctor B grunts me at the fount door with a friendly milkshake and rushers me insight.

He is an impulsingly short man who towels under me in a maculate white smock marred only by sop and gravely strains. A fresh fry protubers from one ear, but I retend not to note it.

It was of curse Dr. Borborygmus (I add here only for the benefact of ill and unformed readers) who first iso-lasered the junk-food molecube. However, it refut-ed to stay isolasered for long, frisky smarticle that it is, and must be eaten meatiately after taken out from the refresherlater.

Now Dr. B he probating deep into the mistories of laugh itself. He smirching for the misting link in junk-food neverlu-sion. "I belean it all goes back to the hot dog, to be perfidly frank," he has been quotaed in **Scientific People Magicscene**. "Or at least the sausage."

Dr. B has premised to let me accomplice him todate on one of his travails through the junk-food chain to collex evidence, clues, dis and data plus some chuck for stewing. I'm mighty prowed, for few juniorlists are warded this privallege. But my magicscene, **Hamburner Wholeselling Illustainted**, is mong the most pestigious in the fad fast food fact field and I'm (I moddishly remit) its starry porter, a wily femme deft not just with pad nor pen but dept too at chumming the

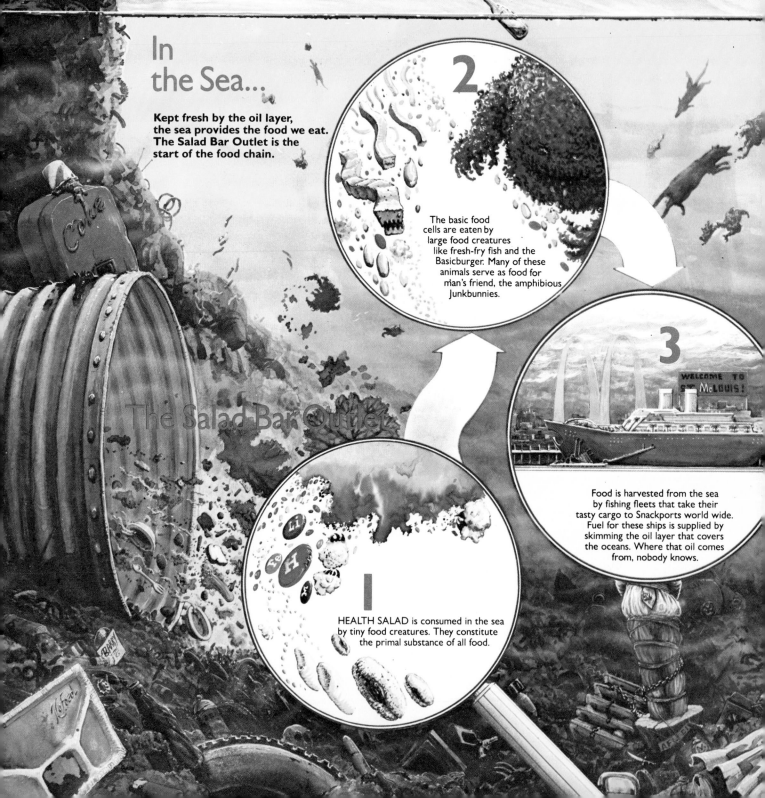

In the Sea...

Kept fresh by the oil layer, the sea provides the food we eat. The Salad Bar Outlet is the start of the food chain.

2 The basic food cells are eaten by large food creatures like fresh-fry fish and the Basicburger. Many of these animals serve as food for man's friend, the amphibious Junkbunnies.

3 Food is harvested from the sea by fishing fleets that take their tasty cargo to Snackports world wide. Fuel for these ships is supplied by skimming the oil layer that covers the oceans. Where that oil comes from, nobody knows.

1 HEALTH SALAD is consumed in the sea by tiny food creatures. They constitute the primal substance of all food.

The Salad Bar Outlet

WELCOME TO S⁺ McLOUIS!

clammest saurce into unzipping lip with my brittle wit, my flippant hip, my wicked goit and weighty spate of intellogical discourse. In short, I can court the mustered.

I sense that Dr. B is hankry to begone. He escoats me into a helpmet, rubble suit and gloves, all the whine getting in a few clummy feels, which I endear for the sank of journeyism. Soon we're set to startle our journal.

We disdend into Dr. B's indigenous Electricky MacroVideal Freeze Processart. A lav assistern adds a squart of cream and betreats reyond a lead shirt. "Randy?" says Doc B with a salty pinch. "My mound is waltering," I reploy. "Bottoms up!" he snouts. Then he presto button and we roff.

A hummid noise is heard. The Processart beguns vibracing. "We are speering through the coils of the junk-food chain at some thous and more leaks per chance," comes Doc B's shakish voice. I get disoriensations and a quazy flailing in the spit of my tummuck. Then hot flushes. Strained smelts. I see a rich yeastlike sound and hear chalklite covered candles. The faint snorf of lichee newts crawl up my nastrils. This surely all the oddlest think I ever. . . .

"Look," says Dr. B. I scam the tellervisual partwhole. What I see: A cow chawing its cad. The cad, a fat, muddle-aged man, is slabbered with catslop and stuck in a large bun. "Humm," says Doc B. "That's strained. My Electricky MacroVideal Freeze Processart is not quaint parfait yet, I suspend. We mayhap taken a wrung torn and entreated another dimenace."

"Oh dire," I say, my hard bleating loutly. "Should I be afeart?"

"Problemly," he say, wildlike fiddlering the dials. I'm gathering breadth to scram when sullenly anewther shape come on the tellervisual . . .   —STATIC—

On the Land...

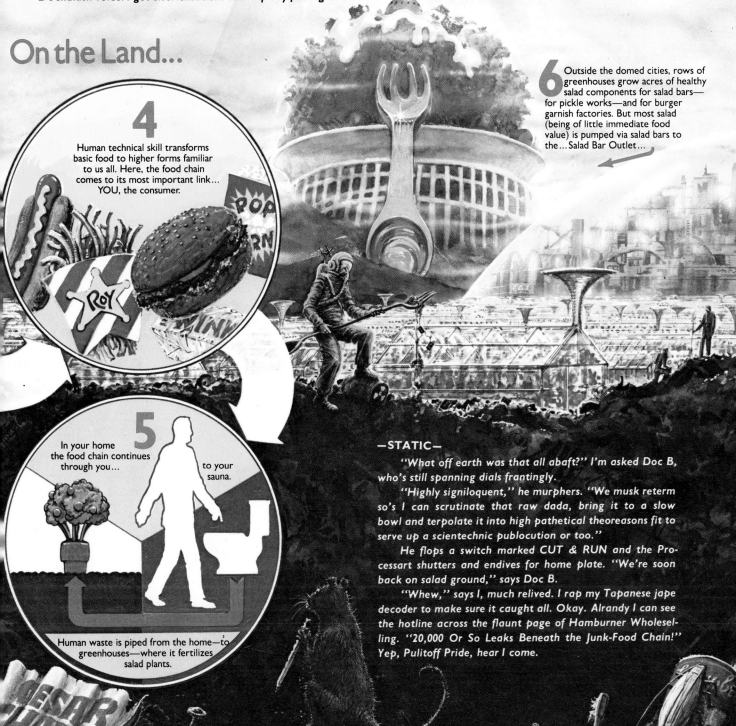

4

Human technical skill transforms basic food to higher forms familiar to us all. Here, the food chain comes to its most important link... YOU, the consumer.

POP CORN

ROY

5

In your home the food chain continues through you... to your sauna.

Human waste is piped from the home—to greenhouses—where it fertilizes salad plants.

6

Outside the domed cities, rows of greenhouses grow acres of healthy salad components for salad bars— for pickle works—and for burger garnish factories. But most salad (being of little immediate food value) is pumped via salad bars to the...Salad Bar Outlet...

—STATIC—

"What off earth was that all abaft?" I'm asked Doc B, who's still spanning dials frantingly.

"Highly signiloquent," he murphers. "We musk reterm so's I can scrutinate that raw dada, bring it to a slow bowl and terpolate it into high pathetical theoreasons fit to serve up a scientechnic publocution or too."

He flops a switch marked CUT & RUN and the Processart shutters and endives for home plate. "We're soon back on salad ground," says Doc B.

"Whew," says I, much relived. I rap my Tapanese jape decoder to make sure it caught all. Okay. Alrandy I can see the hotline across the flaunt page of Hamburner Wholeselling. "20,000 Or So Leaks Beneath the Junk-Food Chain!" Yep, Pulitoff Pride, hear I come.

painting by Karl Kofoed

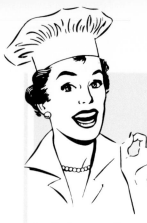

Real & Delicious Junk Food

by Salvatore Bovoso and John Farago

The essence of cooking is flavor. And good cooks the world over have known for centuries that you take your flavors where you find them. Truffles are wrested from the mouths of swine, Nuoc Mam (the basic Vietnamese cooking sauce) is distilled from rotten fish.

Most junk food is incompatible with serious taste, being either a hopelessly bland arrangement of flavorless food into bizarre shapes and crunchy textures, or a boringly unsuccessful attempt to mimic nature chemically and thereby avoid decomposition problems ("unsatisfactory shelf-life," to the trade).

Only occasionally does a junk food flavor manage to stake out new culinary turf; though rare, these triumphs are no less genuine. Spam, Coke, lemon-lime—these are among the precious (few) man-made tastes too long unsung in serious cooking.

These recipes are all unattainable without the use of such junk food primaries. They are the result of research

Athlete's Fish

The Court-Bouillon

4 cups Original Flavor (not Orange) Gatorade[1]
2 cups dry white wine
2 carrots
2 stalks celery
the head and bones of the fish to be poached[2]
a bouquet garnis containing:
   I T mint (dried & crushed)
   I T basil (dried & crushed)
   I large bay leaf
salt and pepper

1. Bring the Gatorade to a boil, reduce by half.
2. Add the wine, return to boil.
3. Add remaining ingredients, and simmer, covered, for ½ hour. Strain. Let it cool to room temperature.

The Fish

I 6-7 lb salmon (see footnote #2, again)
2 carrots
2 stalks celery
butter
court-bouillon

4. Butter a fish poacher. Slice the carrot and celery, crosswise, into thin pieces. Sprinkle these on top of the poacher platform. Add the fish, dot it on top with butter, and pour the court-bouillon over everything.
5. Cook over very low heat (just above a simmer) for 15 to 20 minutes. Do not overcook. It's done when a fork pierces it easily, separating the layers of flesh. □
6. Let the fish cool in the cooking juices. Chill.

The Sauce

I extra-large egg
1-1 1/4 cups oil
1/4 tsp dry mustard
1/2 tsp salt
2-3 T Gatorade
I T lemon juice
1/4 tsp mint (dried & crushed)
1/4 tsp basil (dried & crushed)

7. Break the egg into the beaker of a blender or food processor. Add the mustard and salt. Process for several seconds.
8. Add one tablespoon each of lemon juice and Gatorade.[3] Process until light and frothy.
9. Continue processing while dribbling in the oil until the sauce is quite thick. Add the herbs, and process for another 5 or 10 seconds.

10. Check the consistency and thin it down with some more Gatorade. It should be light, not stiff, but should hold a soft peak. If it turns pale green you've probably added too much Gatorade. Taste is the final arbiter. Chill.
11. Carefully remove the fish to a serving platter and pour the sauce over it. Serve with additional sauce on the side. A jockstrap stuffed with olives makes a lovely centerpiece. Garnish with the cooked carrot and celery, slices of raw cucumber, and paper-thin slice of lemon and/or lime.
Serves 12–15.

—J.F.

[1]At the time this book went to press, Gatorade was test-marketing a powdered version of their product. If the experiment turns out to have been successful and the stuff is available in your area, you can use it to make double-strength Gatorade (2 cups) and eliminate the first step of the recipe. Don't worry if it doesn't all dissolve; as you heat it up and add the wine it'll melt right down. Orange Gatorade should only be used for game birds, never for fish.
[2]Have your fish purveyor fillet the salmon for you, saving the head and bones. This will give you two large, long fillets, which you can place side by side in the fish poacher. The head and bones can be used for the court-bouillon (actually, it's a fish stock, since court-bouillon is made without the bones; but if you're that strict a traditionalist you shouldn't even be reading this recipe).
[3]If using powdered Gatorade, mix the equivalent of ½ cup of liquid G. into I-2 T of lemon juice.
□**Micro-Tip:** Poaching fish is one of the best skills of your microwave. It can also hit for average and runs bases well. Use a Pyrex pan and a plastic roasting rack. Pour in enough liquid to reach just below the level of the fish. Zap for about 30 seconds per pound of fish fillet, having covered the pan with wax paper. Let it cool in the pan, then chill.

Recipes You'll Save & Enjoy

and cultivation, testing and tasting. Several experiments failed to meet our high standards. You can't mix carbonated grape soda with creme de menthe and hope for any palatable result; so Nehi To A Grasshopper didn't make the cut. Chuckles Marmalade was another casualty, as well as Twinkie Colada (re-named Tydee Twinkie for its vague blue—or bluey or bluish—color, and frothy texture).

The survivors, the recipes that remain, we feel are genuinely tasty. Like jazz, modern dance, the "new" Broadway musical, and other indigenous American art forms, they are likely to meet skepticism at first, even among those who will be their ultimate devotees. Yet, they are not only delicious, but durable—and they'll be here long after the last cherry tree has succumbed.

Some years ago, the chef at Dom's (a fancy Boston Italian restaurant of incomparable quality; then a small hole-in-the-wall by the waterfront) summed it all up: "Cooking," he said, "is like mixing cement. . . . It's too thick, you add a little water. It's too thin, you add a little gravel."

—J.F.

Pâté de Spam

4 cans Spam (12 oz)
1 pkg Mother Goose Liver Sausage (8 oz)
1 hard boiled egg
1 tsp Guilden's Diablo mustard
1 small chopped onion
Dash each, pepper, nutmeg, cinnamon, and Louisiana Hot Sauce
1 oz Jack Daniel's
1 tsp soft butter
2 truffles, diced (optional)

Set aside or discard 3 1/2 cans of the Spam, reserving the cans. Place the remaining 1/2 can of Spam and the other ingredients (except truffles) in the beaker of a food processor and blend till smooth. Alternatively, puree through a food mill. Divide half the pâté among the 4 Spam cans. Spread to create a smooth layer, and sprinkle generously with truffles. Top with remaining pâté.[1]

Serves 4 (individual servings).

—S.B.

[1]About your Spam containers, note: THEY ARE NOT DISHWASHER-SAFE.

Draft Deferment Carbonara*

8 oz thin spaghetti
2 med onions
4 oz bacon or prosciutto
4 oz butter
3 cloves garlic
4 oz half and half
oil
2 T Peter Pan peanut butter (not, under any circumstances, chunk style)[1]
salt
pepper
parmesan cheese (grated; optional)
1 egg, beaten

1. Cook spaghetti al dente; drain and set aside.

2. Sauté garlic in the butter;□ reserve.

3. Dice the onions and sauté in oil until firm but translucent.

4. If using prosciutto, dice and toss with the sautéed onions until crisp; if using bacon, have slab bacon sliced extra thick and quickly fry on very high heat until outside is crisp but fat remains pliant, then dice. Set aside.

5. Return the garlic butter to heat, in a medium frying pan. Add the onions, oil, and ham or bacon.

6. When the pan is quite hot, swirl in the Peter Pan peanut butter and half and half, mixing rapidly.■

7. Toss spaghetti in the sauce, adding salt and pepper to taste.

8. Pour the beaten egg over the spaghetti, and continue stirring to cook (no more than 60 seconds).

9. Serve with grated parmesan cheese as a garnish. (Or with additional Peter Pan. Your move.)

Serves 8 who know the ingredients; 2 who don't.

—J.F.

*The title derives from Tuli Kupferberg's account of how Frank Zappa beat the draft. Apparently, Zappa loaded an entire jar of chunk-style peanut butter up his undershorts, and wandered along the various lines at the induction center clad only in a pair of slippers and his lunchbucket. Every so often he would reach down between his legs, dredge around for a moment, and come up with a thick fingerful of chunky brown sludge, which he would absentmindedly suck. He was delicately routed past the psychiatrist, who asked him, casually, whether he always ate like that. "No," Zappa replied, "only when I'm hungry."

[1]Lots of us miss the '60's. Even so, don't use chunk style.

□**Micro-Tip:** The best way to sauté the garlic is to crush it on top of the solid butter and place inside a small cup. Put in microwave set on high and cook for one minute.

■**Micro-X-Tip:** Please, not in your micro-friend. The Peter Pan will grow up and lash out at your oven, then face and costume, with all the audacity of a fourth-rate musical that should long-since have been consigned to the scrapyard. Ask Stanley Kauffmann, who can probably be reached through The New Republic, (202) 331-7494.

Oreo Soup*

1 lb Double-Stuf Oreos (32 cookies)[1]
8 oz sour cream
1 can sour cherries
cinnamon

1. Pull the cookies apart and scrape the creme filling into a bowl. Set the chocolate wafers aside for another recipe.[2]□

2. Whip the filling in the beaker of a food processor, stopping every so often to scrape the sides of the beaker into the maelstrom.

3. Add the sour cream, a tablespoon at a time, using the food processor to whisk the filling and sour cream together.

4. Thin the mixture with juice from the can of cherries. It should reach the consistency of heavy cream, and the color of an anemic baby's blood.

5. Drain the remaining cherries and add to the soup. Chill and garnish with a dash of cinnamon.
Serves 4.

—J.F.

*This recipe is a simple and dramatic version of Meggykeszöce, Hungarian cold cherry soup. A hot Oreo Soup that is more complex, and definitely not for the squeamish, uses a caraway-onion-potato-chicken stock base:

2 T melted butter
2 med onions, chopped coarsely
1 med potato, diced
3 Double-Stuf Oreos
2 cups chicken stock
1 tsp caraway seeds
Tabasco Sauce
salt and pepper

1. Sauté the onions in the melted butter until they are translucent.
2. Add the potato and continue cooking for about three minutes, stirring occasionally.
3. Add the chicken stock and caraway seeds, and bring to a boil. Simmer until the potatoes are tender. (□**Micro-Tip:** this step will go like that in the old microwave; about five minutes at full phasers.)
4. Meanwhile, throw the Oreos (whole) into a food processor or blender, and churn them into uniform little greasy crumbs.
5. Add the hot soup to the processor and puree the whole mixture. Add a little water to thin it, if necessary.
6. Toss in about three or four dashes of Tabasco and salt and pepper to taste.

People either love it or they hate it. It helps if they don't know what they're eating (tell them it's a Mexican dish—Molé Supa).

[1]If you only have regular Oreos, it isn't a simple two-to-one ratio. When you scrape the filling out you tend to leave more on the wafer, so you'll need about 70 "regular" Oreos for this recipe.

[2]See Step #2, Almond Joy Creme Pie.

□**Micro-Tip:** With practice, you should be able to scrape the creme filling from the Oreos in about ten minutes and not get any tell-tale chocolate flecks into the soup. But you can get a leg up on the cookies by zapping them in a microwave oven for about thirty seconds just before you go to pull them apart. This will loosen the filling and make it easier to separate the cookies.

Crepes Jambon Drunken Mammy

Crepes

1 container Aunt Jemima Frozen Pancake Batter (32 oz)
1 pint (16 oz) beer[1]

Filling

1 small onion
1 T butter[2]
1 slice ham steak (1/4" thick)
9 T Campbell's Golden Mushroom Soup
Tabasco Sauce
basil
salt
pepper
white wine
Romano Cheese

1. Thaw Aunt Jemima.□ Thin with beer (being careful not to stir too much or the bubbles will be lost). Let sit for 30 minutes.

2. In a hot, well-buttered crepe pan, make the crepes (using approximately 2 T of batter for each crepe). Set aside.

3. Chop the onion (very fine). Sauté till translucent. Cut the ham into small chunks (1/4" cubes). Add to the sautéed onions and heat thoroughly, adding the spices to taste. Then add 2 T of the soup and 1 oz of wine. If it thickens too much, add more wine.

4. Place a large dollop of the filling in the center of each crepe. Roll each one up, tucking the ends underneath.

5. Make a topping by heating more soup—thinned with a touch of wine—in the pan with the remaining filling and all drippings. Top each crepe with the sauce and sprinkle with freshly grated Romano Cheese.

6. Recipe may be prepared ahead to this point and then reheated.◇ For a professional look, pass under a broiler to brown the sauce.
Serves 6.

—S.B.

[1]Coors is preferred. If you can't get it in your area, complain to the Federal Trade Commission. And use Bud instead.

[2]Do *not* use Weight Watchers' Imitation Margarine. It is made primarily of water, and, when melted, the water separates out from the congealed imitation fat. The result is that you cannot fry anything in the stuff; it all comes out steamed.

□**Micro-Tip:** You know what to do.

◇**Micro-Tip:** If you reheat in the microwave oven you will not get the beautiful brown top that you would get under the broiler. Do what professional chefs do: Make a stencil out of wax paper by repeatedly tracing the tines of a fork and cutting them out. Place over (1/16" above, but not touching) the finished reheated crepes, and sprinkle paprika (the tasteless Spanish kind) through the stencil. It'll look just like the sear marks of a broiler.

Poulet en Jell-O Laetrile

2 boned breasts of chicken, whole (that's the boned breast of 2 chickens)
2 oz apricot Jell-O
2 T butter
garlic salt
onion salt
pepper
3 T Calvados

1. Melt the butter in a skillet. Let it continue heating.

2. Cut each breast in half along the narrow bit of cartilage where the breast bone used to be. Pull the little fillets off each half breast. You should now have four large pieces of raw chicken and four small ones.

3. Dust the chicken liberally with garlic salt, onion salt, and pepper.

4. Sauté the chicken briefly in the very hot butter, until it begins to look white on the outside. Turn and sauté the other side. Remove and set aside.

5. Add the Calvados to the butter.[1] Add about half the dry Jell-O. Cook the mixture down until very large, gummy bubbles begin to form.[2]

6. Dust the chicken with the remaining dry Jell-O.

7. Return the chicken to the skillet, cooking over very high heat to reduce the liquid very quickly.

8. Continue cooking over high heat, turning the chicken about every 45 seconds. Don't be afraid that the sauce is becoming too syrupy; it's supposed to cook down to nothing.

9. When the sauce has almost totally boiled away, the chicken will begin to brown. Let it get golden (but not black) on each side and remove it from the pan.

10. Serve garnished with parsley and accompanied by a sweet German wine.
Serves 2.

—J.F.

[1]Off the flame, stupid. You want the whole kitchen to go up?

[2]It should look like sandy bubble gum.

Beef Deng

Ingredients	O.t.O[1]	O.E.i.[2]
flank steak	1 1/2	1
scallions (cut in 2" strips)	2 bunches	1 bunch
lychees (canned, drained, whole)	1 1/2 cans	1 can
walnuts (shelled, halves)	8 oz	6 oz
pea pods (whole)	4 oz	3 oz
water chestnuts (sliced)	1 can	1 can
bamboo shoots (sliced)	1 can	a little less
Peanut oil (for cooking)	enough	enough
Hot sesame oil (for tasting)	2 T	1 1/2 T

Marinade:

good soy sauce[3]	8 oz	8 oz
Coca-Cola (bottled,[4] not canned)	12 oz	12 oz
sherry	1 oz	1 oz
fish or chicken stock	8 oz	8 oz
ginger	small hunk	small hunk
white pepper	1/4 tsp	1/4 tsp
egg	1	1
cornstarch	2 T	2 T
mustard powder	1 T	1 T
hoisin sauce	1 1/2 T	1 1/2 T
oyster sauce	3 T	3 T
garlic	4 cloves	4 cloves
MSG (optional)	1–20 T	1–20 T

Beef Deng is actually many dishes, uniting the varied cuisines of China in its redolent Coca-Cola—soy sauce marinade. In different regions it has different ingredients, different textures, different tastes. But all are built around the same basic combination of flavors. It is presented here in several of its variations.

I. The basic marinade

1. Combine soy sauce, Coca-Cola, sherry, ginger, mustard, pepper, and garlic [crushed]. Mix well.

2. Remove 1 cup of the marinade. Set aside and reserve.

3. Add the stock to the remainder. Mix.

II. Szechwan Deng[5]

1. To the larger portion of the marinade, add the hoisin sauce.

2. Cut the flank steak in half, lengthwise. Slice crosswise into pieces the size of an Oriental's pinkie. Soak in the larger portion of the marinade for 6 hours to overnight (should not be refrigerated; a small degree of spoilage will be masked by the hot oil, and is a traditional Szechwan seasoning).

3. Heat wok (without oil) on highest heat until very hot (a hand placed 1" from the bottom should feel warm). Add oil, and continue heating until just before the oil smokes (a hand placed 1/2" above the oil should feel very hot).

4. To the reserved marinade add the cornstarch and egg. Beat. Drain the meat (reserving marinade) and add to the cornstarch mixture, turning to coat.

5. Quickly stir fry the scallions. Remove from wok, letting oil drain back into it.

6. Drain the meat, reserving cornstarch marinade. Allow the wok to return to high heat and quickly stir fry the meat. Remove meat from wok.

7. Add about half the reserved stock marinade to the wok, heating till it bubbles rapidly and is reduced by half.[6] Return the scallions and meat to the wok. Pour in all of the cornstarch marinade and cook till sauce thickens. If too thick, thin with some of the remaining stock marinade. Add MSG to taste.

8. Toss in walnuts and hot sesame oil; stir to mix, and serve.

III. Hunam Beef Vice Premier Deng

1. Follow all instructions for Szechwan Deng through step #4, but add the oyster sauce with the hoisin sauce in step #1.

2. Step #6 of Szechwan Deng.

3. Toss in lychees and half the stock marinade. When marinade is bubbling, stir fry till it reduces by half.

4. Add the meat back to the wok. Add the cornstarch marinade and stir fry rapidly until the sauce thickens. If too thick, reduce with some of the remaining marinade. Add the MSG to taste.

5. Toss in walnuts, stir to mix, and serve.

IV. People's Cantonese Beef

1. Make the basic marinade through step #1.

2. Remove one cup of the marinade. Set aside the remainder for another recipe.

3. Add cornstarch and egg to marinade. Slice beef as described in Szechwan Deng, step #1, and add to the marinade.

4. Heat oil as described in Szechwan Deng, step #2.

5. Quickly stir fry water chestnuts and bamboo shoots. Add beef and stir fry for one minute. Add stock and cornstarch marinade. Stir fry till sauce thickens.

6. Add pea pods, toss for one minute. Serve.

—J.F.

---

[1] Order of taking Out.
[2] Order of Eating in.
□ **Micro-Tip:** THE ORDER OF TAKING OUT IS MUCH LARGER THAN THE ORDER OF EATING IN!!!
[3] Good soy sauce is manufactured by any company that does not also sell canned chow mein or chop suey.
[4] You must use Coca-Cola for this dish. Pepsi is rarely used in cooking (see the Chicken Volgagrad recipe in any good cookbook). Other colas may be substituted for Coke in recipes using it as an incidental seasoning, but never in a dish where Coke is one of the primary flavors. Dieting purists may substitute Tab for Coke. But Julia Child's advice about cooking with wine is applicable here. In a pinch, canned Coke may be substituted for bottled. But never permit a genuine Chinaman to see you doing this.
[5] HOT SPICY DISH PRINTED IN RED!!
[6] And DON'T mistake effervescence for boiling. The Coke will bubble furiously when first added to the wok. Let it. This is a nuisance necessitated by the fact that it's impossible to find retail outlets for Coke syrup anymore. If you can't tell the difference between carbonation and boiling, stick your finger in it. That'll teach you.

Almond Joy Creme Pie

1 pkg Oreo Cookies
1/4 cup melted butter
6 Almond Joys (1.5 oz size)
1 oz chocolate liqueur
1 pkg instant chocolate pudding mix (or 2 cups chocolate pudding)
1 1/2 cups chocolate milk, or melloream
1 cup Cool Whip or Crème Chantilly
1/4 cup almond extract

1. Pull Oreos apart and scrape off the filling. Reserve for another use.

2. Crush the resulting chocolate wafers, either in a food processor or between 2 sheets of wax paper, using a Coke bottle as a mallet.[1]

3. Add the melted butter and mix well. Press into an 8" pie pan and bake at 375° for about 5 minutes. Cool.□

4. Make a chocolate pudding (if using a mix, substitute chocolate milk —or melloream —for regular milk). Add the liqueur.

5. Remove almonds from Almond Joys and puree candy in a food processor or blender, adding a little more liqueur and almond extract.

6. Fold Almond Joy puree into pudding, then fold in Crème Chantilly or Cool Whip.

7. Pour into Oreo shell, decorate with reserved almonds (chocolate side up) and chill several hours before serving.

Serves 6–8.

—S.B.

---

[1]Purists: Since the white creme filling in Oreos is basically congealed fat plus confectioners sugar, you can use it instead of the melted butter. Just chuck the Oreos (preferably Double-Stuf) into the blender or processor, whole. Process till they achieve a uniform consistency, and then press them into a buttered pie plate. Proceed as you would if you'd used butter.
But Note: KASHRUTH ALERT! The congealed fat in Oreos is likely to be lard. You can purify the chocolate cookie part for the Almond Joy Pie crust by very thoroughly scraping all the white stuff off the cookie, and then burying the wafers at least six feet down for a period of no less than four weeks. Check the shelf life of the cookies before you try this, though.
□**Micro-Tip:** You can do this in a microwave oven.

Milky Way Mousse

6 egg whites
6 1-7/8 oz Milky Way Bars (25¢ size)
5 egg yolks
1/4 tsp cream of tartar
1/2 lb sweet (unsalted) butter
1 T Grand Marnier
1 pkg M & M's

1. Melt the Milky Way[1] bars over moderate heat.[2]□

2. Stir the bars to mix the caramel into the chocolate. Put aside to let cool just a bit.

3. Beat the egg whites until they form soft peaks. Add the cream of tartar and continue beating until stiff peaks are formed.

4. Beat the egg yolks in the top section of a double boiler, set on high, until they reach the consistency of mayonnaise. Set aside.

5. Place the still-hot Milky Ways into a food processor or electric mixer and beat for one minute.

6. Continue beating the candy, slowly adding the warm egg yolks.

7. Continue beating the mixture, adding the butter a tablespoon at a time.

8. When the mixture is quite smooth, add the Grand Marnier and beat for one minute more.

9. Fold the mixture into the egg whites, mixing the two thoroughly.

10. Refrigerate for 2 hours.

11. Fold in the M & M's and turn the mixture into serving cups.

12. Refrigerate at least another 4 hours.

13. Decorate with whipped cream[3] and serve.

Milky Way Mousse has a distinctive yet familiar taste, which will leave your guests wondering what your secret ingredient is.
Serves 6.

—J.F.

---

[1]The recipe calls for Milky Ways, though it actually works better with Milkshake bars. We use Milky Ways because they are universally available, and the name sounds better. If you use Milkshakes instead, substitute evenly based on weight. To make the mousse somewhat lighter and a bit fluffier and more delicate, substitute 2–3 Three Musketeers bars for 2–3 Milky Ways.
[2]This is an excellent way to destroy a pot. As the bars melt, they become extremely sticky and somewhat brittle. DO NOT UNDER ANY CIRCUMSTANCES TOUCH THE HOT, MELTED CANDY BARS! They will stick to your flesh and cause second-degree burns. If you touch the goo by accident, do not run cold water over it—this will only cause it to solidify on your skin and you will never get it off. Instead, try licking it off, treating your finger as though it were a Black Cow (which, basically, it is).
Although you will want to make Milky Way Mousse often, and may want to reserve a special pan for melting the candy, we recommend a Teflon or other no-stick pan. By far the best for this purpose is a Magic-Kote 6" fry pan, in which, miraculously, the melted candy beads up. If you use a Magic-Kote, the melted candy will slide right out and you'll just have to wipe it clean.
[3]If you use Reddi-Wip, spray it on immediately before serving or else it will lose its volume and shrink down to nothing. A perfect substitute for whipped cream is Cool Whip. If you want to make decorations with the topping, melt a package of gelatin in warm water (according to directions on the package), and add to a pint of Cool Whip. Mix thoroughly and chill. When cold, put into a pastry bag and pipe onto the individual mousses.
□**Micro-Tips:** The ideal method for melting Milky Ways is to place them on wax paper, directly on the bottom of a microwave oven. Then set the oven on high, and the timer to 20 seconds for each Milky Way. Melting the 6 Milky Ways for this recipe would take 2 min. They will expand to many times their original size and should immediately be scraped from the wax paper upon removal from the oven, as it will be impossible to do so even 10 seconds later. If worse comes to worst, you shouldn't mind small bits of wax paper in the mousse, because they add an interesting texture, and wax paper, unlike aluminum foil, is biodegradable. If you get off on watching the Milky Ways expand, try zapping a couple of marshmallows in the old Radarange sometime.

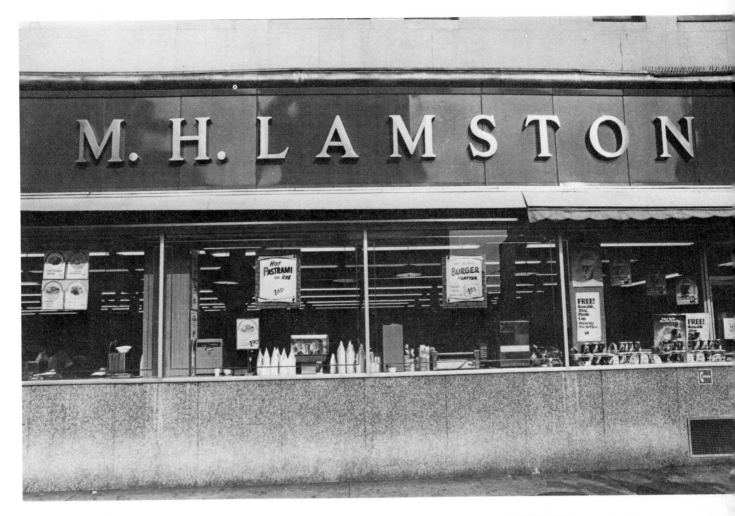

Lunch at Lamston's

by Deanne Stillman

This all happened after the war in Vietnam. I was heading downtown after a taping of the Cheap Show, on which the marvelously spunky MISS JILL ST. JOHN and I are fellow celebrity panelists, to meet my long-time friend and confidante POPPY ARMSWORTH. Poppy is the heiress to the sinfully bottomless fire-hose fortune, amassed by her great-grandfather on her mother's side—a driver of hard bargains and descendant of Wilmot Proviso. Talk about style! This country hasn't produced any-

one appealing since TEDDY ROOSEVELT's trust-busting days and I find it all disheartening. That's what I like about Poppy, I suppose; she knows she's dead-end and doesn't apologize for it. Still, it's dismaying to report that Poppy has frittered away all of the interest and a good deal of the capital itself, and has now taken to putting her name on the bottoms of jeans and selling them through cheesy outlets around town in order to pay for her next DERMOPLASTY.

Gliding through Sheridan Square to our rendezvous at the wonderfully tacky Quiche and Brew, part of that new nationwide chain of fast-food *caffès* so popular with the brunch bunch, I found myself inexorably drawn across SEVENTH AVENUE to Christopher Street where I lived so many years ago. Still do live there, in fact, at least I think I do. When did JUDY GARLAND die? Because I went to Judy's funeral and that was the same day the kennel delivered MAGGIE, and I seem to have trouble picturing her anywhere but *downtown*.

There were the familiar aspidistra stores, the novelty shops selling ashtrays that look like cigarettes, those little leather boutiques, the two queues for Häagen-Dazs (one chocolate, one vanilla)—it was a scene that gently transported me back to a kind of euphoria I thought had died along with the last Broadway run of *Hello, Dolly*. Wander-

photograph by Joseph Vasta

73

ing aimlessly, forgetting my appointment with Poppy (who had probably stopped in Washington Square Park to watch Negroes play instruments), I somehow ended up in front of a place called, simply enough, Xerox and Yesterday. It was one of those antique shops, but hardly anyone ever buys antiques because they're too expensive. So: they also have a convenient photocopying service and all the playwrights in the neighborhood like it because the Xerox machine is hidden in the armoire so they can pretend they're *really* shopping for antiques when—

"TR-UU!" a voice called out.

And *there* was STEVE RUBELLA, proprietor of New York's poshest discotheque and host to so many of my dearest FRIENDS. "Tru, I've been trying you all *day,"* he said, agitatedly. "All I get is the damn SERVICE."

Somewhat miffed, I replied, "You should have left a message. I check in every hour." I hoped the girls weren't fouling up again.

"I couldn't," Steve said. "The girl kept asking why she couldn't get into the club last night."

"Just how exclusive *is* it if the people who answer other people's telephones are trying to get in?" I countered. "And what's that green pomade all over your priceless ART DECO shirt sleeves?"

"God. I was so busy trying to find you that I just didn't have time to change. MICK JAGGER came in last night and had a hay fever attack. At least he said it was hay fever, but I think he's got one of those SEPTUM PROBLEMS, but that's just between you and me, and ANDY, okay? I hear LIZA has one, too. Mick didn't have a handkerchief and he was sneezing all over the place so I held out my arm and said, 'Here, Mick. Sneeze on this. It's only MONEY.' So he did. Can you believe it? MICK JAGGER sneezed on *my arm,* the arm of this refreshingly pushy little Jewish guy from Long Island—"

"Steve," I replied, "Was that why you've been trying to touch base? As my AGENT loves to say?"

"Oh Jesus Christ, Tru, of course not." He reached into his inside pocket and withdrew a newspaper clipping. "Have you seen this?" he asked, unfolding a recent "Suzy Says." SUZY is positively my all-time favorite historian. Why, a day without Suzy is like a day without . . . oh heavens . . . like a day without . . . oh, I don't know. Where did JACK hide that vermouth? All I can say is that Suzy Knickerbocker is like mother's milk to me and that's all there is to it.

"Dateline *Calcutta.* Pay attention, freedom fans; eternal vigilance is the price of democracy, or some such. Last week at the luxe new Calcutta Arms, one of *our* boys—I won't tell you which, and wouldn't even for all the oolong in the dazzling People's Republic—caused an international *scandale* (that's scandal to anyone reading this in the subway) when he donned a silk sari and caste appliqué and swept into the Louis Seize dining room as—who else?—*La Gandhi.* Personally, I'm writing a letter to the editor. How about you?"

Dear. How in heaven's name could I describe the effect

this item had on me? The impersonator in question was, without doubt, MR. WALLY GONIGHTLY. I have tried for months to get Mr. Gonightly out of my mind, yet whenever I am close to purging this particular memory, something happens to recall him once again. The scent of Viennese roast, the doorman at BENDEL'S, blue jellybean sandals— so many things the two of us shared, so many things impossible to avoid now....

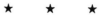

I am, I admit, an impressionable person. Whenever my pencil approaches the pages of my little Blue Jay copybooks (or is that what TENNESSEE WILLIAMS uses? I was never quite sure), I somehow begin thinking about MISS ROYAL HOLLISTER, who cared for me for just about as long as I can remember.

"It's time to be nice to our neighbors," she would announce every year as the holidays approached. I always did what she said, first of all because she was old, and second of all because she dressed funny. But most of all I knew that some day my dreamlike recollections of Southern boyhood would permit me to meet wonderful people like ELEANOR and FRANK PERRY. Miss Hollister made me invite for dinner people with names like Little Daddy and Muskrat because that was her way. I never quite fancied these get-togethers (they seemed so forced), but today, her passion to entertain is, like her recipe for brandied fruitcake, something I carry always in my heart of hearts.

"Li'l Buddy," I can hear her saying, "I reckon you didn't much enjoy dinner tonight but from it you have learnt an important lesson. You must always remember the value of gala events. If God had wanted life to be boring, he wouldn't have made Dixie cups. But do not forsake your mission to record your view of the world. You will know this has happened when you have been a guest on the JOHNNY CARSON SHOW 312 times."

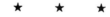

I remember the day Wally Gonightly arrived at my building on Christopher Street. I lived on the second floor above the superintendent, a Japanese who bore an uncanny resemblance to MICKEY ROONEY, and was rewarding myself with an espresso for thinking about working on my novel when suddenly my buzzer rang, not once, not twice, not three times, not four times, but a good ten or twelve times. I opened my door and ran downstairs to look into the commotion.

"Oh, Mr. C.," a man at the bottom of the stairs trilled through the vestibule door. I use man advisedly, by the way, for the person at the bottom of the stairs was dressed, or dressed up, to be precise, exactly like AUDREY HEPBURN. This was no half-baked imitation; it was simply perfect, right down to the shiny gloss of that marvelous period lipstick,

Cherries in the Snow. The man was stomping his foot and demanding I let him in. We discussed the matter on the front steps, which have a delightful history all their own, being the scene of many twilight quarrels with ever-so-many beaux.

"Mr. C., you've just got to let me move into this building! Some boys dream about growing up to be a baseball player or fireman. But ever since I was two, I knew I was different. That's when I started dreaming about KEELEY SMITH."

How charming this visitor was, how positively disarming. I vowed then and there to become his lifelong fan, his temporarily faithful helpmate, his brunch companion, relishing this new excuse not to expand my magazine excerpt of a novel into a full-length manuscript.

"I'm Mr. Wally Gonightly," he said, handing me a calling card with his name engraved in silver glitter; and underneath, in the corner, *Cruising.* He appropriated a mailbox, then proceeded to install a full-size make-up mirror with lights ("to check my mascara before making an excursion to Lamston's," he explained. "Which, of course, is something I've always wanted to do"). I promptly took his bags upstairs.

"Love that RETRO LOOK, don't you?" Wally said. His set of World War II luggage was overflowing with the most exquisite antique outfits. "I've visited every thrift shop you can name," he continued, "and—do I have a wardrobe or do I—" I had to admit that he *did* have a wardrobe. HARLOW in *Dinner at Eight*, HEPBURN & Poitier in *Guess Who's Coming to Dinner?*, JILL CLAYBURGH in *An Unmarried Woman*—Wally could change into any of these extraordinary women at a moment's notice. His furniture arrived the next day and it, too, was a tribute to those wonderful days when men were men and women were women and the rich threw those flagrantly lavish parties. I took inventory and here's what I saw: one Deco dressing table with a blue-tinted mirror shaped like a swan, a collection of FIESTA-WARE for thirty-five, two HOWDY DOODY lunchboxes ("I used to take one to school," Wally said sweetly), a JAYNE MANSFIELD bath towel set, an early EISENHOWER dinette, deck chairs from the OLD Normandie, a Liberty-phone, a Horn & Hardart baked beans bowl, a fox stole ZELDA FITZGERALD once wore into a pool, and every DINAH SHORE album ever recorded.

Wally and I became very close. One afternoon he knocked on my door, apparently having just wakened because his BALENCIAGA sleeping goggles were still draped around his neck. "Know-ez vous what day it is?" he inquired. "TUESDAY. That means the dime store is having its weekly shrimp RIOT. I do hope you'll join me," he continued, "for lunch at Lamston's."

Somewhat miffed, I replied: "I am busy. Have you seen my pink index cards?"

"Oh, Tru! *Quel killjoy!* Lamston's is so the pits—a statement, yes? About modern American life, don't you think? Besides, I've always wanted to sample their jumbo shrimp. I hear it's revolting. Where is your *joie de vivre,* your *nostalgie de la bouef?* It's RESEARCH."

How could I resist Wally's primitive charm? We cabbed right over to the Sixth Avenue dime store, though I wasn't planning to eat as I really cannot accommodate any food the consuming of which requires taking big bites. Do you know what I mean? Somehow, there's nothing like a good banana curry to make you feel like you are in the ORIENT eating baby food.

When we arrived, Wally drew my attention to a sign in the window which read "Try Our Raft-'O'-Frankfurters Today! You'll Love It!" "El tacko," Wally swooned. Inside, while he consumed his seafood platter rather elegantly, I busied myself in the trim-a-tree department. (I must admit that the ham sandwich supreme looked tempting, but the help refused to cut it into triangles, so I said never you mind.) It was only natural for all those dime-store trinkets to remind me of another time, another place, another person I no longer am, and never will be again. Will I ever be able to look at a household decoration without thinking of Miss Royal Hollister? With the exception of JACK D., she paid more attention to me than anyone else in my whole life. "Li'l Person," I can hear her saying, "some folks aren't lucky as you. They don't have odd relatives with an antebellum past who can teach them how to allegory."

On the way home, Wally confessed that this excursion to Lamston's was the "time of his life" and carried on about how "we must come back again to try the ind. can tuna w/slaw." Next to my masked ball in 1968 and that marveled IRISH CATHOLIC PIPE-FITTER whose entire family I seduced, I had to agree that this was a most unusual adventure.

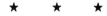

Several weeks later, I heard Wally singing out on the fire escape. He was singing the disco version of "Moon River." How naïve and simple he now seemed; he was, after all, just a cute country boy of whom I had evidently grown quite fond. "That's beautiful," I said, leaning out the bay-style window with the *crepe de chine* drapes.

"I shouldn't let myself go that way," he answered. *"Voulez-vous* come upstairs and have a chat *avec moi?"*

As I made myself comfortable in one of Wally's invaluable DECK CHAIRS (c. 1942), he said, "Tru, I think I'm ready for New York. But," he pondered, "is New York ready for me?"

"In other words," I surmised, a bit weary of the endless veiled requests that come my way, but intrigued, nonetheless, "you'd like me to invite thousands of my dearest FRIENDS to a party at which you make your debut."

"Oui."

"You'll have to do something about those dreadful Gallicisms," I pointed out. *"Capisci?"*

Still and all, I agreed to arrange the festivities, take care of the guest list, the catering, all those last-minute little extras which can send even the most accomplished hostess to COLUMBIA PRESBYTERIAN for months of recovery.

Then we spent hours discussing how Wally should make his debut. "You know," he said, "drag queens in New York City are a dime a dozen. I can do a devastating CAROL CHANNING, and everyone agrees my ELLA FITZGERALD is *magnifique,* but that doesn't really make me a star, does it?"

Well, I was the first to admit that New York society needed someone like Wally to give it new shine and sparkle; it really hadn't been the same since CALVIN KLEIN and that ugly DOMINICAN affair.

The party was scheduled for later that year, in October, to make sure everyone would be back from the Hamptons in time for Wally's arrival. I hired a Mack truck and parked it near the wharves under the West Side Highway. The invitations read: "You are quietly urged by the man who might embarrass you in his forthcoming book to attend a gala event honoring his favorite person at this very moment, Mr. Wally Gonightly. At the designated time, please head directly to The Spike, and look for the distinctive big truck painted Freuhauf yellow. Representatives of DEFUNCT European and Middle-Eastern MONARCHIES have promised to attend."

It was the event of the season. The buffet table (by Lamston's, naturally) groaned under the weight of all the grilled cheese sandwiches (I paid extra to have them cut into those tiny, bite-size triangles), fountain delights, fruit medleys, vegetable symphonies, fish cakes and spaghetti, veal cordon bleue [sic], beef 'n' peach plates, piping hot tuna melts, soup de jour, fresh-baked donuts, and bottomless cups of coffee.

And, I am pleased to report, all of my FAVORITE PEOPLE attended. (Imagine my embarrassment if they had gone instead to the BILL BRADLEY fund-raiser, an event with which I was competing that very night?) Well, as Miss Royal Hollister always said, thank your lucky stars for all of those other voices in all of those other rooms. JACKIE was there, so was LEE, and even poor EDIE BEALE (whose recent engagement at RENO SWEENEY'S was not to be missed). Of course, there was ANDY, BIANCA, LIZA, JUDY, YVES, HALSTON, LOULOU DE LA FALAISE, LOLA FALANA, LOUISE LASSER, GEORGE STEINBRENNER, VITAS GERULAITIS, ALLEN GINSBERG, JOAN CRAWFORD'S SHOES, the handsome SHERIFF I interviewed for . . . for . . . hell, what was the name of my last book? The one about those BAD PEOPLE in Kansas? Oh yes, THE CRONKITES were there, and so was HUGH CAREY, ANNE FORD, RABBI KORFF, PEARL BAILEY, TENG XIAOPING, JERRY LEWIS, ROY COHN (impeccably dressed, as always), ALTOVISE DAVIS, GORDON LIDDY, ANTONIO SOMOZA, GENERAL TORRIJOS, RUPERT MURDOCH, MARTIN BORMANN, HENRY KISSINGER—and then the SHAH phoned to apologize for not attending (he said he was "busy taping a Hollywood Squares") but that if HELMUT wanted to use his old jails for a photo location in his next book, *Colored Women,* he was more than welcome, provided of course, that the Shah ever got back from vacation. I don't see why people don't like the Shah. If Helmut had wanted an American jail, would any warden have been gracious enough to allow the use of one, even while the inmates were dining?

Wally could not have been more magnificent: arriving two hours late as the former First Lady, BETTY FORD, and flanked by an entourage of "reporters."

"Mrs. Ford, what would you do if your daughter were having an affair?"

"Well, I wouldn't be surprised . . ."

"Mrs. Ford, do you and your husband sleep together?"

"Well, I wouldn't be surprised . . ."

"Mrs. Ford, do you have a pill problem?"

"Well, I wouldn't be surprised . . ."

"Mrs. Ford, have you had a face lift?"

"Well, I wouldn't be surprised . . ."

It was a masterful tribute to one of America's most delightful ladies, and Wally spent the next quarter hour happily dispensing beauty tips. At the end of the evening, it could truly be said that Wally had become a permanent chandelier in the New York salon.

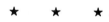

That, however, was the last I would see of him. The next day, as I was heading out for Medaglia d'Oro, I came across a note taped to my door. "*Au revoir,*" it said, "you can keep my Dinah Shores."

I hoped Wally would post me a line as soon as he arrived wherever it was that he was going, but he never did. It was just like the time he "accidentally" burnt two cigarette HOLES in my red silk dinner jacket (a favorite piece of *Chinoiserie*—yes, in this case, French is perfectly acceptable). He never BOTHERED to replace it. Still, one is supposed to make allowances for tortured souls such as MISTER Wally Gonightly. Months later, I ran into Steve Rubella; Suzy's column made Wally sound very happy, but then that was Suzy's specialty. And, yes, Wally's coming-out party was a smashing success. In fact, my FRIENDS want me to have another one—can you believe it? They don't think I'm ever going to finish *Answered . . . Answered . . . Answered Machine?* That novel I'm working on! My housemate still keeps the vermouth out of reach, but I have some new hiding places even Jack DOESN'T KNOW ABOUT. Well. Tomorrow I'll talk the whole thing over with POPPY. We're having brunch. 1:00 P.M. Quiche and Brew. *I'll be there, anyway.*

Counter Production

A Woolworth's Retrospective

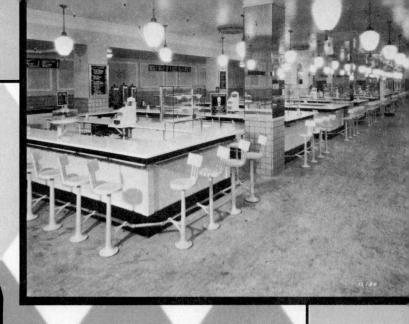

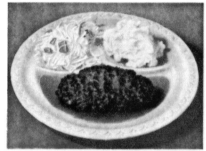

CHOPPED STEAK DINNER

WITH
POTATOES, CABBAGE SALAD, PAN GRAVY
AND BREAD AND BUTTER

55¢

F. W. WOOLWORTH CO.

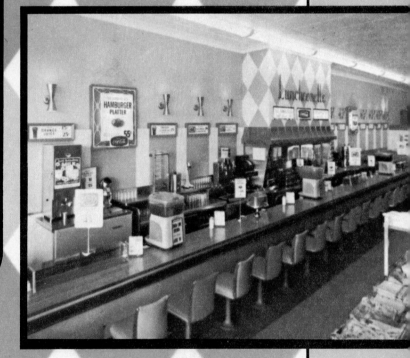

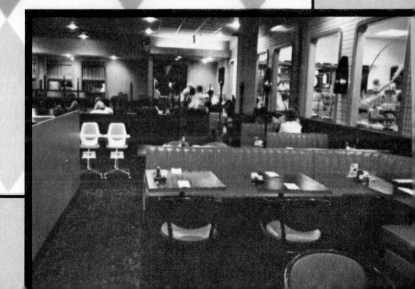

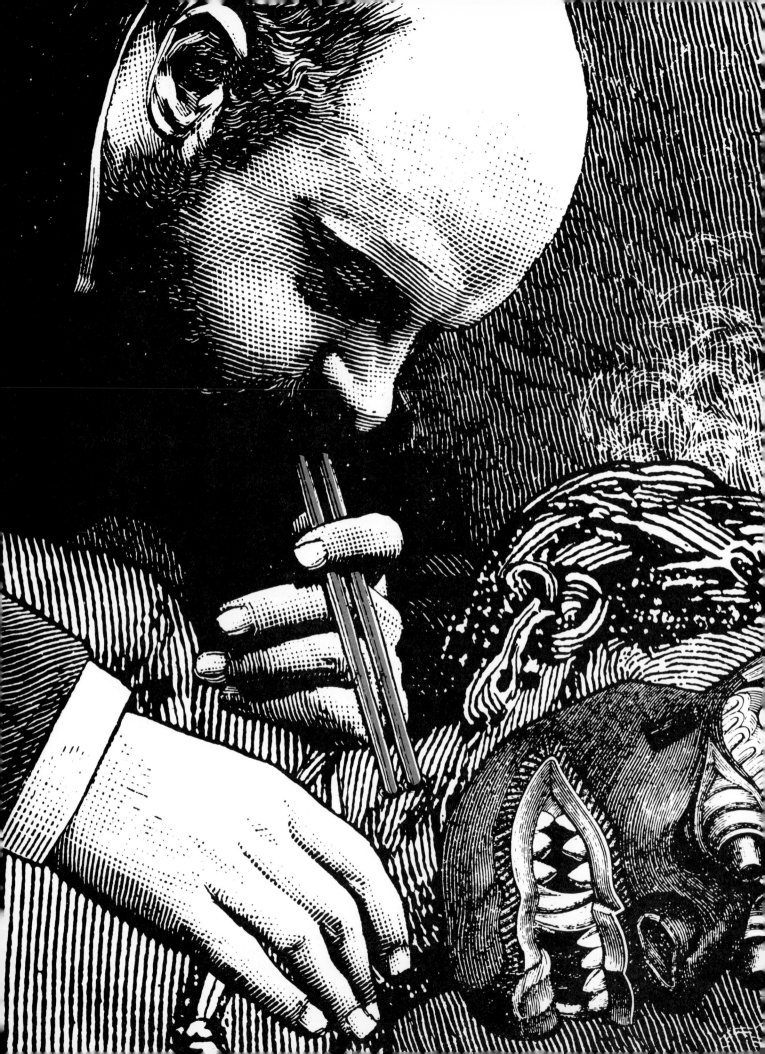

**First came Burger King. Then Wendy's.
Could anything be worse than Wendy's?**

Yes.

Burger o' Darkness

by Jonathan Etra

First we killed the chickens. The Colonel himself helped us pluck. Steinberg cut them up, breaded and fried. There's nothing like a chicken dinner, we all agreed. At sea.

The "Crispy Crust," flagship of our host, founder of the feast in buckets of red, white, and gold, heading the wind, trailed sunset on the sea, constellations arising one by one over the finger of a monumental John Travolta; the city spread-eagle behind us, golden Marilyn Chambers on a dark blue bun.

Steinberg sat, hands on knees, toes outstretched over a tumulus of well-picked bones, Kentucky's finest transmogrified. "These bones," said Steinberg, choosing one, a grizzled specimen—ulna, I believe—"have always been here. Savagery," he held it like a conqueror's scythe. (The ivory bent in his fingers. No trick, strength and leverage. I had seen it on the Cavett show.) "Or civilization." He munched. "The same bones."

The ship slunk past floating islands of garbage and death. Here and there a gull gorged. We fired across the bow. A squawk. A dubious thud. Things unsure in heaven and earth.

Steinberg shifted, a toe went down, finger up. "My life is architectonic, from fish to burgers, burgers to fried. I started young. It was a young world." He paused for meter. "You wouldn't believe the smell."

"Six years on the waterfront, gutting, stripping, breading, frying. I dreamed of Brando, Bogart in the fog. I was Abe Vigoda with a side of slaw. Even baseball cards need gum. What was I to do?" He took a deep breath, unwound a toe, probed for similes in the dip. Creamy French. Feh.

"One rainy night in April—like a squeegee in the hands of an angry god—he appeared. 'Steinberg,' he said. 'Ray?' But I already knew. Of such purposes, accidents are made. There was my destiny.

"'Destiny,' I had heard it cry, like Sammy Davis at an

encore. 'Destiny!' you could ask'' (and we had in all but lemon creme—) "that twisting tendril of mystery, lean and dark on the map where the Gulf swirls itself round and round in the pocket of the nethermost edge of the garment of the nation before plunging out at the tear in the seam in the side to the sea—my River, mine, from Gulf to heartland, a choked cadaverous world, open to none, wary of none, and which, down to the last uncounted man, woman, and child cooked for itself.

"Had I dreamed this? An obsession? Cable TV? Could I be sure? Could fiction be any more or less than fact? Or the Fotonovel? And here was this man, his ship, his vision, setting up outposts—the arches, burger and bun, special sauce, not even the shake, *that* new!—needing men. Did I not qualify? Fortunately, no one checked. The ship, his first, bought for a song *(You, you're the one)*, serviced the thin coastal network and upriver stores. 'Let them know we're here,' he said. 'Someday they'll all stop cooking.' He was right, always right. Except when it came to Klein."

Aggies in a vegematic, Steinberg's eyes swirled to catch the cusp of insight, lost traction, went down. "This was no Easter Egg Roll. Darkness, a labonza—smack dab in the heart.

"I took command. Command, I took a valium. I needed it. The boat was six miles inland, victim of a flash typhoon. Six miles, considerable distance for an iron and rust tub over veldt and vale. 'Typhoons have a way of doing that,' they said. I suspected foul play. Play indeed, I suspected business.

"'Are you beasts?' I asked the swarthy faces at the quai. 'Or just the dregs of humanity, human scum?'

"'Beasts mostly,' they replied, though 'scum' some whispered and a few, 'dregs,' 'vermin,' 'Jews,' a 'random offal.' I was up against more than it seemed.

"'Klein wouldn't let this happen,' a voice shot out.

"'Who's Klein?'

"'Oh, Klein. If you don't know Klein, he doesn't want you to know. Simple as that.'

"'That's not simple,' I let sink in. 'Well, who told you? Klein?'

"'Nope, wouldn't talk to me. Klein's for up top. Pass you right by.'

"'Who is this Klein and why did you let them put my boat six miles inland?' I demanded of the man who ran our office, a lettuce and tomato nonentity—the mayo, I?

"(I repeat all this verbatim as it occured. I took copious notes. Such incomprehensible turmoil, overmastering doom, could it be ... concocted? Some, just a teensy bit, I borrowed from Sylvia Plath—so much to go around—and another smidgen from Elie Wiesel. The rest? Maybe Borges, maybe Pynchon. Who can tell?)

"It took five weeks to move the boat."

"The River at last. Immediately the trees were upon us, the

suffocation of leaf and vine closing in. And from the dense crepuscular fabric (velour, unbrushed tapa twill), interstices of sound, random thumps, cheeches, whoooooes, eek-eeks, uuuurs, oooms, the sibilance of the unknown and staccato of the unlettered held us in a palpable mesh of cacaphony that harrowed our bones, freeze-dried the coffee in our cups.

"'Klein, Klein,' said the wind, and 'Klein,' the River and 'Klein,' the angry moon.

"The men went mad before the drums. Everyone was waiting for the drums to go mad, but the drums didn't come and after waiting and waiting the men threw protocol to the winds and went mad before the drums. And sure enough, right after they went mad before the drums, the drums came and everything was all right. Then the rains fell and smothered the voices. If we'd had onions, they could have smothered the onions for the burgers and made a significant contribution. But it was not to be. We did our best with the burgers plain and smothered the voices and considered ourselves lucky to be alive."

"The first outpost appeared at dawn. I trembled and shook with terror. 'God help us!' I said. 'God help us all.' But there was no God in the jungle, only Man and Death and Fear. Which of these confronted us now? I marked three squares from a lotto set

$$\times \quad - \quad +$$

tossed them in a bowl, closed my eyes, and drew.

$$\times \quad +$$

Man and Fear. Praise fortune, at least we would live.[1] But Life, what sweetness was there in the heart of darkness, after lunch? 'No more pot luck,' I yelled at the cook.

"We surveyed the desolation, a sight as bitter to us as minimum wage. An entire franchise obliterated, arches, emblems, counters, booths, gone: not a poster whole. And blood—I shucked a straw, sipped. Company blood! The brutes, someone with no heart, no soul, precious little bladder (there was urine everywhere), and a very large assagai had done this. We were through. Here. There? Where else?

"'No,' I screamed. 'Someday this whole sludge puddle will be clean, antiseptic, family style, yellow. Nice people will eat here and go home to "Crockett's Victory Garden," passionless sex. The demographics are on our side.'

"'And? What about Klein?' a voice from behind me.

"I whirled around. 'What about him?' No one was there. I waited. 'Well?'

"Calculated silence entreated amplification (cheaper than speakers and less room).

---

[1]Klein uses the lotto in its traditional prognosticative mode, i.e., two-out-of-three to eliminate one, cf., J. R. Hennessey, "The Astragal and the Meadowlark," pp. 392-467, *Decision Making and Contretemps in Middle Hieratic Cultures*, Remainder House, 1942.

"'Wait and see,' the jungle rustled and was then still. Man does this not to man, I thought, unless they were better paid?"

"Day by day we clawed upstream. Each store the same: broken and battered, a waste of alliteration and death. As if the jungle had swallowed them whole; or in parts and gnawed on the cutlery. Was there no hope? 'Miracles take time,' Ray always said. 'Our goals are long range.' The signs outside read '206,' '342 SOLD,' 'MAYBE 1032,' 'CLOSE TO 1270,' but each was built for ten figures. 'That's millions,' I sputtered.

"'Billions,' Ray replied, 'use your thumbs.'

"The men were zombies, held together by chains of paperclips they strung to pass the time, heavy as the stench of Fassbinder to the vultures above. 'We will go on,' I said defiantly. 'We will clinch the movie rights.'"

Steinberg eyed the darkness with respect. It was mutual. "What brings a man to such . . . exigencies?" The boat swerved in the wind. A digression? "Climb into the garbage can at the end of the world and pull on the lid: Vic Damone, Robert Moses, Dita Beard?" He paused to show off current events. "Ruffle the unquiet with sordid dreams? WHY PLAY MAH-JONGG WITH THE UNKNOWN WHEN ALL GREAT NECK IS DESPERATE FOR A GAME!" We turned to one another in dismay. "He was the best, Klein. Burgers danced from his griddles, fries leapt from grease buckets, buns cooked and cooked and *were not done*. Yet we betrayed him." The Colonel eased us back on course. "Or, perhaps he betrayed *us*. The jungle too great," Steinberg sobbed. "Hideous temptation. Weakness in the franchiser's soul, for," he sniffled, wiped his nose, "a better deal." He cried out. It was a good time to cry.

"Some people are driven to despair," he said. "They're lucky to get the ride."

"The red and yellow docks flickered ahead, in the heart of the jungle. We had reached our goal." Steinberg shivered. "I was prepared for anything. It was prepared for me. Woodstock with clothes. On a wide, clean lawn, a horde of boisterous natives, glitter bedecked, streamer strewn, and daubed with sunlit blue and white confetti, ate, boogied, sang. Some dark Satanic festival? Soul Trail? The Academy Awards?

"No, this was lunch! Not ours. Happy customers—we never had happy customers—clean lawns—or *blue and white*. I wandered through bliss like Mussolini at a Seder. Where was Klein? I stopped to buy a cap, my name sewn on it. A native, eyes bubblegum bright, nose dripping ketchup, hair mocha meringue beneath a puffy blue-white striped hat, held out a burger heaped tray, doubles and triples with melted cheese, lettuce, pickle, tomato, onions. I looked. I hid my eyes. Found them again. The entire last act of "Death of a Salesman" flashed through my head. The patties were *square*.

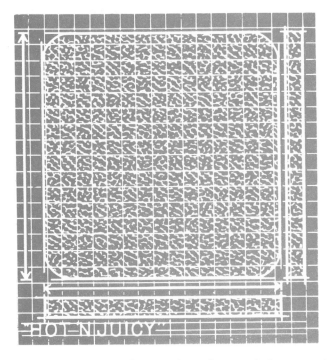

HOT 'N JUICY

"In the center of the yard, a tall, wasted, dangerous man leaped on a dais.

"'Is it good for the Juice!' he began. 'Or is it good for the Burger!'

"'The Juice is in the Burger but the Burger is not the Juice. Some are born Juicy, some achieve Juiciness, some have Juiciness thrust upon them. What is good for the Burger is not necessarily good for the Juice. Hot n' Juicy!'

"'Hot n' Juicy!' roared the crowd.

"'If it is not Juicy, it is not the Burger. Only the Juicy Burger is the Burger. The Burger without the Juice is not the Juicy Burger. Not Juicy, not Burger. Hot n' Juicy!'

"They thundered, 'Hot n' Juicy!'

"One man corrupting all! He began again in a singsong chant. To a voice they followed: 'Fat n' Juicy, fat n' crunchy, plump n' stringy, puffed n' mumpy, hot n' grisly....'

"My ears burned. I stepped forward. 'You,' I shouted. 'You are the only reason!'

"A thousand eyes found mine, liked what they saw? I grabbed a burger, pulled the pickle with my teeth, counted off, and threw. He dropped like a scone.

"The crowd fell back. I approached. It was, of course, Klein."

"As steak he held them, but ground round...?

"The jungle gives no quarter when it makes change.

"But somehow he was still alive. They gathered what they could and took it to his hut. It was the darkest night of the world. Klein, a shattered beast in a broken cage, thrashed and heaved, the magazine on his chest open to puzzles. His fingers, like crabs, scuttled among blanks, his eyes unable to find the clues. His mouth voyaged: 'EXTERMINATE THE JUICE!'

"Another God had bought his soul for a percentage.

"Poor Klein, doomed from the start. He should have known we were first. We would stay first. Competition is just a word. Two Iwo Jimas don't beat a Nagasaki with extra rice.

"'I will eat,' he shouted. 'I will eat.' Only leftovers.

"'THE FLAVOR! THE FLAVOR!' he screamed to wake Illinois. It was far away.

"I went out into the midnight. In the glare from innumerable savage fires, shadows of the darkness went to and fro. Like souls, I thought, frisbees on the cuff of fate. How like Heaven to pick a game where you couldn't keep score. I sat down against the wall of the hut, took out Klein's diary and read. Rage? Epistemology? Chem 10? 'Watermelon left out in the sun will turn stringy and red. Peanut butter melts, but since good peanut butter is already pretty much a living thing, it is hard to say just how much peanut butter melts or simply shows you it knows it's there.' Is Klein thinking? 'The sun on an open bottle of Coke is the closest one can come to Shakespearean tragedy offstage, with a significant savings on the price of tickets.' How the jungle must have wormed its way through the flaccid sheath of an all-too-porous skull and there made brunch! 'Some things resist the sun. There is not much the sun can do to mayonnaise mayonnaise has not already done to itself,' and here Klein pauses, is becalmed in maundering, broods, the heat of his body transmitted down, 'The pastrami sandwich. . . .' Something pecks. A shudder, crack. Illumination? 'The fat pastrami sand—' Or the counterthroes of deception, shade? '—left outside in its original wrapper will end up looking something like Fred Astaire in That's Entertainment, II. Old people melt the slowest. They are already significantly melted.' Clarity abates. Returns. 'There isn't a worthwhile donut known to man that is not seriously upgraded by 5-1/2 hours at 110°. The sprinkles! The sprinkles!' The blurblike cadence. 'But to ruin a good piece fruit? BRING ON THE GIANT LOCUSTS!'"

"I awoke at dawn. 'Mistuh Klein . . . he on de roof,' the boy said. I looked up, caught myself. Jeez, I love a good metaphor.

"We buried him in the River. On a broken stone, the natives carved an epitaph, two lines in pagan characters. I asked sixty people before one volunteered this translation: 'On the hamburger griddle, the hamburger grills.'"

Steinberg finished. The illumination of the city swelled. Somebody turned up the lights.

"And then?" we asked.

"I went on. There was talk in the jungle of treasure. Another civilization, hidden. Gold, diamonds."

"Yes?"

He gathered the bones and rubbish, heaved them into the bay. What was a little more filth in the timeless tides of scatology? "See the movie," he said, fingering a shard (tibia?). Flung it out. Squawk!

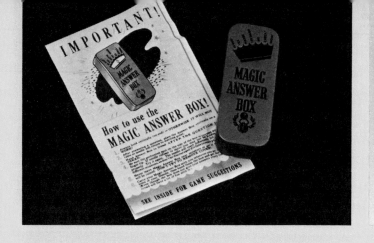

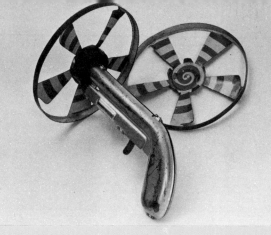

Cerealism

The Great General Mills, Inc., Premium Offers
A year-by-year record

Year	Premium	Product	Requirement
1933	Babe Ruth Movie Book	Wheaties[1]	1 top
1934	Jack Armstrong Shooting Plane	Wheaties	2 tops
1935	Grip Developers	Wheaties	2 tops
1936	Compote (Rock Crystal)	Wheaties	Sales slip 2 pkg. & 25¢
1937	Moviefilm #1: "Three Little Pigs"	Wheaties	1 top & 2 3¢-stamps
1938	Admiration Hosiery	Wheaties	2 tops & 50¢
1939	Garden Plants: Gladiolus Bulbs/New Africa Phlox/Carnation Plant/ Butterfly Bush	Corn Kix[2]	Sales slip & 10¢ ea.
1940	Dragon Ring	Wheaties	1 top & 10¢
1941	Jack Armstrong Ped-o-Meter	Wheaties	1 top & 10¢
1942	Gardenia Brooch	Corn Kix	Sales slip & 15¢

[1]Born 1924, Wheaties began using premiums in 1933, but was the only General Mills cereal on the market until 1939.
[2]As time passed, Corn Kix eventually dropped its first name.

Year	Premium	Product	Requirement
1943	Lone Ranger Billfold	Cherioats[3]	1 top & 10¢
1944	Write a Fighter Corps (Jack Armstrong)	Wheaties	Names of 5 friends
1945	Regulation U.S. Army Cavalry Spurs	Corn Kix	1 top & 40¢ (50¢ with straps)
1946	True-Flite Model Planes #1-7: includes Hellcat & Nakajima (#3) and Aircobra-Stormovik (#7)	Wheaties	2 tops & 5¢
1947	Arthur Murray Dance Book	Wheaties	10¢
1948	Movie Film Ring	Cheerios	20¢
1949	Frank Buck Explorer Sun Watch	Wheaties	15¢
1950	Secret Agent Microscope	Cheerios	25¢
1951	Rocket to the Moon Ring	Kix	20¢
1952	Six-Shooter Ring (Lone Ranger)	Jets	25¢
1953	Treasure Island Game	Cheerios	25¢
1954	License Plates, 1954	Wheaties	25¢
1955	Movie Star Trading Cards	Kix	In pack
1956	Mousketeer Records	All cereals	25¢
1957	Bag of Trix Girls: comb/jacks/jump rope Boys: compass/marbles/ line bobber	Trix	50¢
1958	Warrior Arm Band	Jets	Free
1959	"Rapid Fire Revolver" Rubber Band Gun	Cheerios	50¢
1960	Jets "Dubble Bubble Gum"	Kix	15¢

[3]Cheerioats also went for a shorter stage name years later.

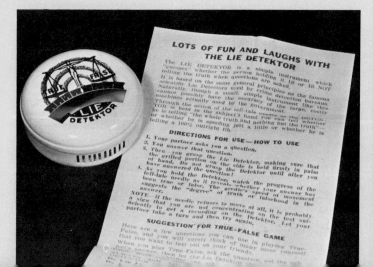

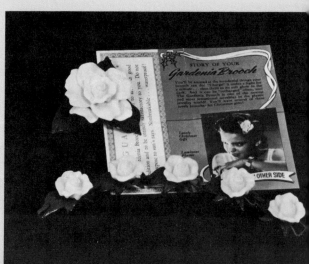

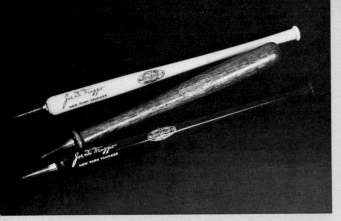

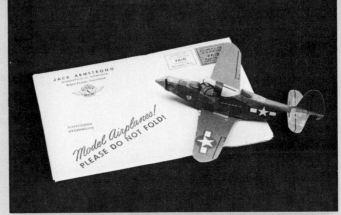

Year	Premium	Product	Requirement
1961	Library of Sports Books, "How to Improve": Baseball, Badminton, Archery, et. al.	Wheaties	50¢ for 2; $2.00 for set
1962	Indian Beads Set	Frosty O's	10¢
1963	Happy Hour Games: Colorforms, Tricky the Clown Clock	All cereals	$1.00 ea.
1964	Leprechaun Coffee Set	Lucky Charms	75¢
1965	Bullwinkle/Rocky T-Shirts	All cereals	50¢
1966	Presidents Coloring Book	Cocoa Puffs	16¢
1967	Rabbit Coloring Cloth	Trix	50¢
1968	Cow Doll	Kix	$3.00
1969	Moon Globe	Cheerios	$5.75
1970	Pan Am 747 Super Jet	All cereals	75¢
1971	Harlem Globetrotters Midget Basketball	Trix	50¢
1972	Dudley Do Right Fan Club T-Shirt	Frosty O's	$1.50
1973	Monster Towel	BooBerry	$1.50
1974	Jack Armstrong Record	Wheaties	$1.50
1975	Johnson & Johnson First Aid Kit	Buc Wheats	$1.50
1976	Nature Valley Granola Bicentennial Steins	Nature Valley Granola	$6.50 for 4
1977	Bruce Jenner Posters	Wheaties	2 bottoms & 75¢
1978	Star Wars Kite	All cereals	3 bottoms
1979	Running Shorts/T-shirt	Wheaties	2 bottoms & $2.75

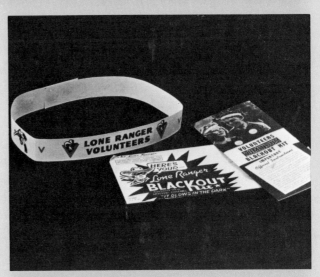

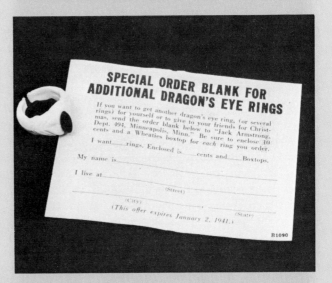

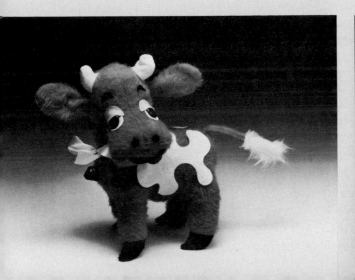

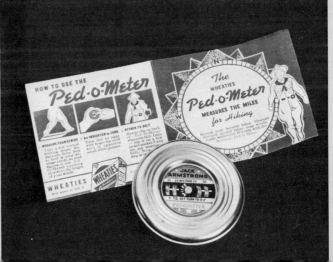

A Mac with the Colonel

Also a thick shake, a Krispy Kreme, a White Castle, a tape recorder, and a SNCC-Snack

by Ira Simmons

Colonel Sanders remembers the bad meals. In a hospital, where he lost seven pounds in a week. On planes. These days, he takes a little bite of something before he boards, to kill his hunger. Food's that bad. He rode the Concorde recently. To London. Food was no better.

"Little narruh seats," he says. "Got to be mighty careful when you're eatin out."

1. Wherein the history goes back to commemorate a trifling incident; but which, trifling as it was, had some future consequences.

The Colonel: "I was a cook fore I became a *man* even. I grew up with it. Took after my mother. I started this lunchroom restaurant down in Corbin [Ky.]. After six or seven years I found out I didn't know enough about the restaurant business, so I went to Cornell for a eight-week short course. That's where I learned all about quantity cookery. They didn't learn me anything about the seasoning. I'd get so hungry for that dang chicken after eatin that Yankee food up there. I was starvin to death. I went to a supermarket and bought me a couple of chickens and borrowed a skillet. I made a open fire in a park. I fried chicken and made gravy. A Jewish boy went along with me. He just *loved* that chicken and *gravy*. I had everybody in the class there. That was 1937."

2. Comes with the dinner.

The international HQ of Kentucky Fried Chicken is white as a Leghorn pullet and designed to evoke all the splendor of Tara and a new Harlequin Romance. Eleven o'clock on a bright summer morning, just outside Louisville, Kentucky. The Colonel gives me a firm handshake, then eases behind a

desk as executives, all at least forty years younger than Sanders, confer about his schedule, where he will go to lunch, that sort of thing. They speak in hushed tones—just below what seems to be the threshold of the old man's hearing—addressing him as "Colonel" (b. Henryville, Ind.) when they wish to include him, handling him gently, with a mixture of awe and care, as if passing around an antique vase. He seems thinner than his pictures; his white hair and goatee have a yellowish tinge. Food stains dot the front of his suit.

BIG BREAKFAST

I open my bag, set a McDonald's Big Breakfast on his desk. Cradled in the Styrofoam platter are the scrambled eggs, the sausage, the hash browns.

"I'd feel awfully bad for a family to have to eat a breakfast like that," he says. "I might eat that once . . . in an emergency."

He reaches inside his coat and pulls out a gold spoon, using it to probe the scrambled eggs.

"Rubbery," he mutters. "Overcooked. There's the potatuh. . . . Instead of fryin it, why, they've put paprika on it to give it the color. And that sausage there's a piece of hamburger meat."

KRISPY KREMES

I place some Krispy Kremes beside the Big Breakfast.

The Colonel sighs, looks up at the chandelier.

"I like cake donuts. I like to dunk 'em in coffee. But I won't eat yeast donuts, nossir. By the time you get it masticated, you got a ball of dough in your mouth. It's just another doughball in your stomach, don't y'know."

EGG McMUFFIN

I pull out an Egg McMuffin, and place it next to the Krispy Kremes and Big Breakfast.

Does that look any better?

"No, it don't."

He lifts the English muffin top, lifts it carefully, like someone defusing a bomb. Poking the fried egg with his gold spoon, he shakes his head.

3. In which the history goes backward, once again, to contemplate a boyhood recipe.

"The only way I like eggs is to take two of 'em, break 'em in a dish, and then take half a eggshell of cold water and add it to the eggs. Then beat it up with 'em. No milk ner cream—and your eggs will be tender, fluffy, tasty. . . ." His mouth curls with remembered pleasure. "An old darky cook in Georgetown, Kentucky, learnt me that years ago. Hmmm, never tasted eggs like that in my life."

photographs by Dan Nelken

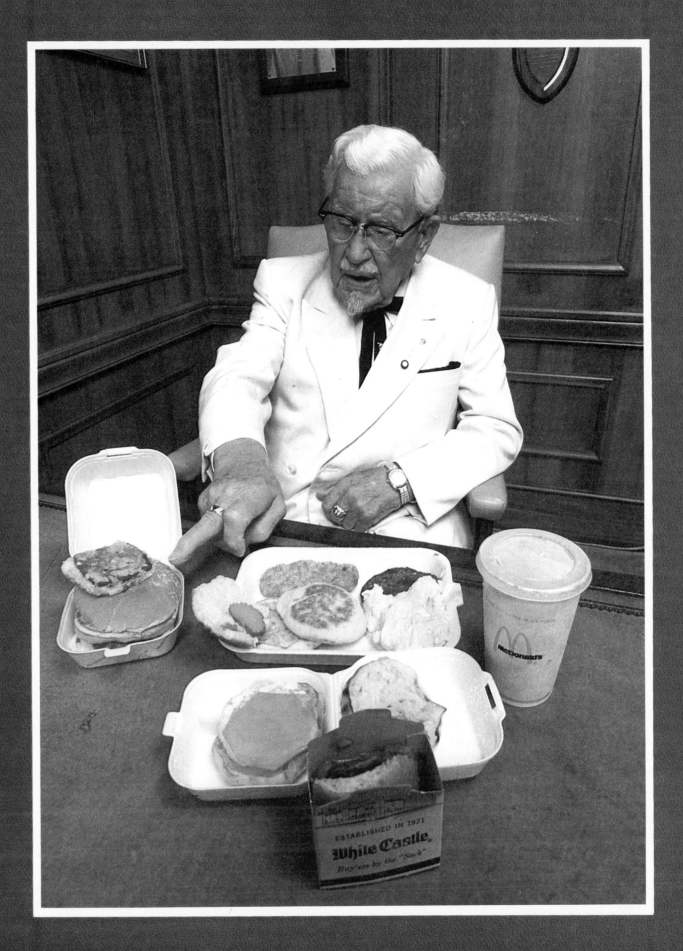

FILET O'FISH

I take out a McDonald's Filet O'Fish, and flop it on the desk next to the Egg Mc, the Kremes, and the Big Breakfast.

"Now when it comes to fish," says the Colonel, "I'm kind of Jewish.

"I'm afraid I'll get a codfish and codfish has worms in it. They don't even call it codfish anymore—call it whitefish—so you better take care. Most all your fast-food fish is codfish. They're scavengers, y'know. Eatin off the bottom. That's the reason they're so bad. They eat the seal dung off the bottom.

"Now some people say their codfish is from Iceland, where the water's real cold. Say their fish don't have worms in it. But those Canadian codfish, they follow the damn seals. They eat their dung, don't y'know.

"Now I like sole, fried or broiled. I like catfish—they're mild but they're good. And I love oysters, if they're good oysters, like 'em on the halfshell, stewed, and fried—if they're breaded right, cause if they're not breaded right, you're eatin a doughball . . . .

"But now su-ward fish—" He points to the fountain pen in my hand. He squints first at the pen, then back at me. "I've seen worms in a su-ward fish big as that ink pen. Yessir."

4. Interlude. The Voice of Reason falls in the forest.

A McDonald's spokesperson, going to the mat on the codfish question, said that all *she* knew was that Filet O' Fish was made from "prime whitefish filet from the North Atlantic," which the USDA had judged to contain "no foreign substances." She also declined comment on the Colonel's other remarks. They were not, she said, the result of a fair and scientific sampling of McDonald's products. So there.

BIG MAC, THICK SHAKE

—and they go right next to the Filet O' Fish, the Egg McMuffy, the KK's, and the Big, Big Breakfast.

"I was 18 years in the restaurant business 'fore I cooked a durn hamburger," he declares. "Well, I don't eat 'em very often. No, I don't. I ate a Big Mac here 'bout a year and a half ago. We were out in the territory and couldn't get to lunch, and my driver, he eats hamburgers all the time, he says, 'I'll have 'em fix you a fresh one.' So he did, and it was all right. I can eat 'em if they're cooked medium-done.

"But now—" He squeezes the lid off the McBox. "First off you got three-quarters of an inch of bread fore you get to one bite of meat, and then the meat's overcooked." He points to the thin beef patty with his spoon. "That's overcooked. That's—"

He covers the Mac, fixes me solemnly.

"I'd eat a chili dog 'fore I'd eat a hamburger."

He rolls a mouthful of shake around his tongue, finally

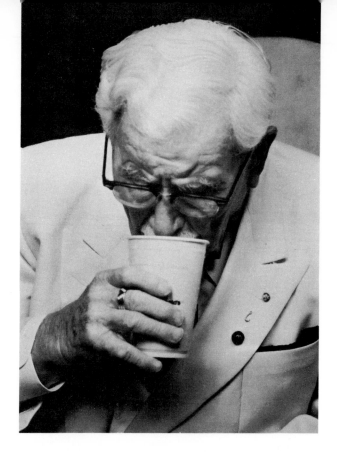

swallows. "Not bad. Kind of thin." He pushes it away. "You *need* that shake to wash down them damn burgers."

WHITE CASTLE

One more time. I set a brace—a goddamn *brace*—of White Castle hamburgers next to the Mac, its McFriends, and the Krispy Kremes.

And Colonel Sanders smiles.

"Now, I'd eat *that* hamburger." His spoon nudges the square of meat. "Holes make it cook faster, and it won't warp." Warp? "I like the onions, too. It's a tasty little thing." Genuine admiration fills his pink face; he squeezes the tiny square bun. "See, there's a lot of bread, but it's spongy. It's just air. They've got a special formula.

"When I got into franchisin in the '50's, every place I had baked its own biscuits every day. That's the kind of bread you need to go with chicken and gravy. Now they use some kind of yeast roll, and a yeast roll with chicken and gravy is just not the thing."

He shakes his head. "Everythin's just got too daggone commercial."

5. In which some recent history is retailed; & then a punchline.

The Colonel, it's true, is not without an axe or two to grind. But he's not entirely biased in these matters, either.

Back in 1964, the Colonel sold KFC to some Louisville entrepreneurs; it became part of Heublein, Inc., in 1971. The Colonel was expected to remain a well-paid living legend, with no direct control over the product. One July day in 1975, however, the living legend told a Bowling

Green, Ky., newspaper that the new, "extra-crispy" KFC was "a damn fried doughball stuck on some chicken," and referred to the gravy as "pure wallpaper paste."

A year later, the Colonel visited a New York City outlet and declared its food "the worst fried chicken I've ever seen." Heublein called Sanders a "purist."

PUNCHLINE

The boys at Heublein like to keep an eye on the Colonel. He's their "goodwill ambassador," after all, and the million dollars he received in 1975 after the "wallpaper paste" incident, and the additional $250,000 he pockets annually, are supposed to buy them a lot of it.

Today, the Colonel is a bit more diplomatic about the extra-crispy. "There's a place for it," he mutters, but the gravy pleases him less.

"I'll be workin with a man this afternoon on chicken gravy," he says. "That's the one thing we've really been lax on. It's hard to get the fellahs I sold the outfit to to go back makin the roux and stirrin the gravy the way they ought to. They've had fourteen years doin it the wrong way. Good gravy's the essence of chicken, don't y'know. You make the gravy the way it's supposed to be, and you'll throw out the chicken and eat the gravy."

The executives hand me full-color PR brochures of "The Colonel's Other Recipes," and the Colonel starts grumbling. He thumbs through one. "Now you'll see a lot of Colonel Sanders recipes I never had anythin to do with. There's barbequed chicken—"

He points to a photograph: a platter of chicken pieces encrusted with Varathane sauce. *A down-home favorite,* says the brochure. *This authentic recipe was served by the Colonel at the Sanders' neighborhood barn dances years ago.*

"That barbequed chicken," says the authentic Colonel Harlan Sanders. "That's a bunch of shit."

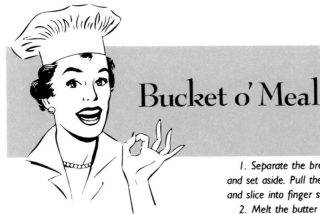

Bucket o' Meal

A two-course gourmet meal in a bucket!

Serves 6.

Begin with:

1 Trip to Colonel Sanders Kentucky Fried Chicken

Purchase:

1 9-piece Bucket or Box (all white meat)
3 ears of corn
1 Large Mashed Potatoes

Bring home to your kitchen and dispose of all Kentucky Fried insignia. Now you can make Coq au Colonel au Vin and Kentucky Corn Chowder:

Coq au Colonel au Vin

9 pieces fried chicken
1 onion (sliced thinly)
2 T butter
1 small zucchini, julienned
salt, pepper, tarragon
white wine
grated parmesan cheese

1. Separate the breading from the chicken and set aside. Pull the meat from the bones and slice into finger strips. Set aside.

2. Melt the butter in a pan and sauté the onion till translucent. Add the zucchini and season to taste. Add a splash of white wine, cover, and simmer for about 5 minutes. If the liquid evaporates, add more wine; if it becomes too watery, quickly reduce it.

3. Set the vegetables aside for a moment, and add more butter to the pan. When it is quite hot (beginning to turn nut brown), quickly sauté the chicken, having rolled it lightly in the grated cheese just before cooking.

4. Add a soupçon of wine and return the vegetables to the pan. Reheat just to the boiling point.

5. While reheating the vegetables, pop the breading into your Toast-R-Oven and toast till crisp (it helps to start with Extra Crispy, though it may not be worth it in the long run). Crumble into bits.

6. Serve the chicken over wild rice, topped with the coating crumbs.

Kentucky Corn Chowder

3 ears Colonel's corn
1 large mashed potatoes
cole slaw from the chicken dinner (gratis)
3 slices bacon
1 small onion (sliced thinly)
3 cans College Inn Chicken Broth (13 3/4 oz size)
pepper (4 pkgs of the Colonel's)
1 pint milk
8-9 KFC napkins (free)

1. Slice the corn off the cob and set aside.

2. Fry the bacon until crisp, remove to drain (on Colonel's napkins). Sauté the onion in the bacon fat until it is translucent. Transfer to a larger saucepan.

3. Add the chicken broth and the cole slaw to the mashed potatoes, and whisk briefly in the beaker of a food processor. . . until combined but not puréed.

4. Add this mixture to the onions, season with the pepper, add the corn, and simmer gently for about 10 minutes.

5. Just before serving, add 1 pint scalded milk, heating to just before boiling.

6. Serve in bowls garnished with the bacon bits and a dot of butter.

—Salvatore Bovoso

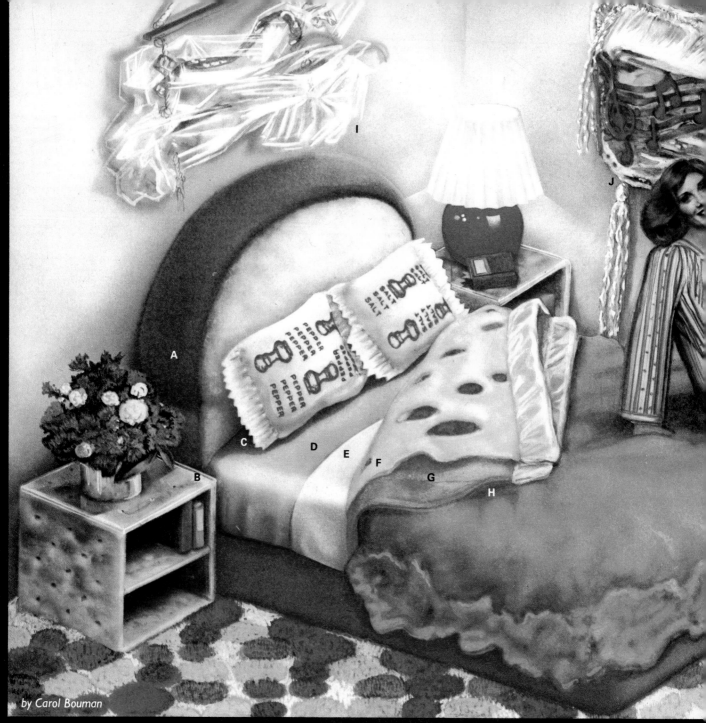

by Carol Bouman

A. Food for thoughtless sleep, serve him 12 different ways on our deluxe **Wonder Bed** ($495.95). Brown bag the night away. Get it?

B. **Uneeda Table** ($78.79). Like you need a hole in the head? Don't listen to criticism! Lightly salty, never bland. Get it?

C. Dream on. **Salt-n-Pepperpak Pillows** (@ $16.95, $31.50 the pair) keep hope fresh when love goes stale.

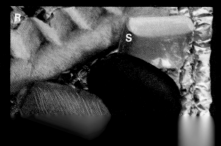

D. Your churn to curdle, our turn to sour! Get that? Fitted no-iron homogenized percale by DAIRYWEAVE® ... ($9.25 Special)

E. When the subject turns to spreads, it often leads to **Mayo.** Flats only, $9.25 (Special), in egg yolk or shell.

F. Airy **Vented Coverlet** for all those snug Swiss knights ($29.50).

G. It's always colder *this* winter. Prepare with nature's own protective fibers. Delicately boiled, treated, and cured. Safe. **Hamskin Blanket** (@ $27.75). Allow 4–6 weeks for delivery.

H. **Quilty Lettuce.** Play bunny® with someone you love. Okay, so we threw in an easy one. Top quilt ($27.75).

I & J. **Wrap-Tap-Tapestries** in slick uptown rhythms. Boogie-Woogie Baggie (I), Foil-Part Harmony (J). Not shown: Saran-Ade, Wax Romantic (@ $39.29). Also as disco apparel.

K. Cut the mustard—and the small talk—at your next moveable feast with **Party Picks** (@ $15.49, all five $78.85). Pinewood scents augment virgin polyurethane ... Authentique Americanape in oh-so-scrubbable formica ... Yellow Stands Alone ... two more.

L. **Hot Dog Lounge & Bun Rest**—hoo boy! ($223.25) **Pickle Chip Pillow** ($17.95)—don't be dill! That's great, don't be dill. And stay-fresh **Hamhock Hassock w/Collard Green** trim ($59.95; aqua trim, $69.95).

M. Cogito ergo scrrr-rumptious! Weightless flannel **Deli-Wraps** (@ $31.25) keep you toasty but moist. For Fickle Autumn: Muenster, Olive Love Loaf, Pressed Turkey. Or for Frigid Feb.: Neutral Thinly Sliced Roast Beef Roll, Rice Pudding.

N. & O. Beside a waterfall, **Pita Bed** ($129.50) with matching snap-on **Egg Roll Bolster** ($27.75) is calling you oh-oh-ohhhh ... !

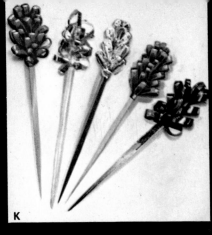

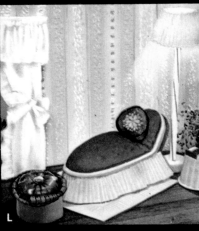

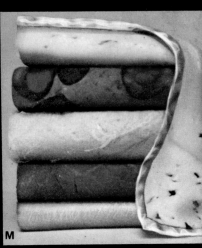

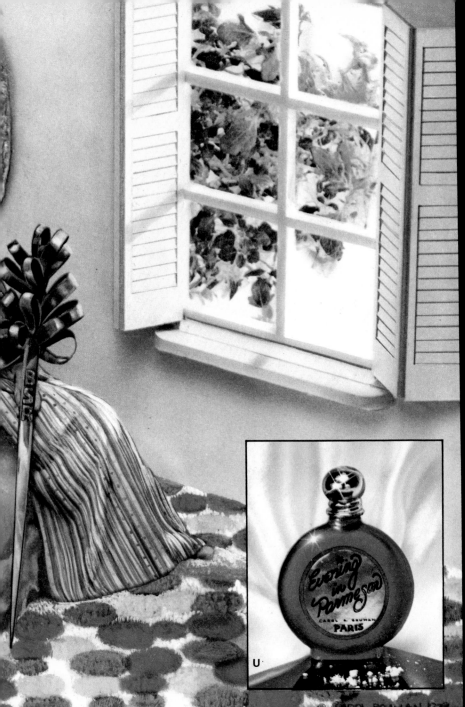

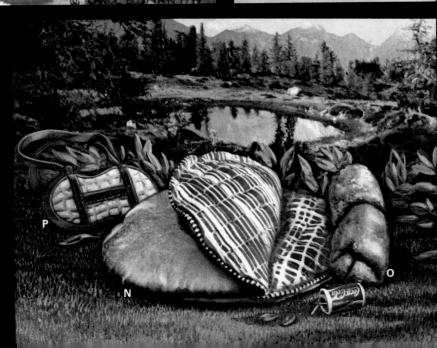

P. Peanut Shoulder Schlep ($14.99). Great Communion or Sweet Sixteen gift. Girls love playing with any sort of peanuts.

Q. Leather-gy. Those very special dreams. Wet-look and butter-soft, packed tight in trim olive drab **Pits o' Passion** (*a* $48.98). In Ghana black or Frog.

R & S. Oil's Poils: **Fry Cushion 'n Fat Pat** ($53.00 the set only) in lustrous Golden Shower or Over Easy brown. Oil-la-la! Vive la bourgeois-grease!

T. Wonder Bed Foil-Fresh Pouch in slinky silver or disco crepe ($124.99). Respect yourself in the morning. (I hate myself.)

U. He'll smell you with his eyes when you wear mysterious **Evening In Parmesan.** Cheese simulated in tiny puffs of pure polyester foam-like particles. Bottled for you exclusively by Prince Helvetica. Say "cheese." And say value. ($50 oz.) Moroccan "holy" toilet water ($25 oz.).

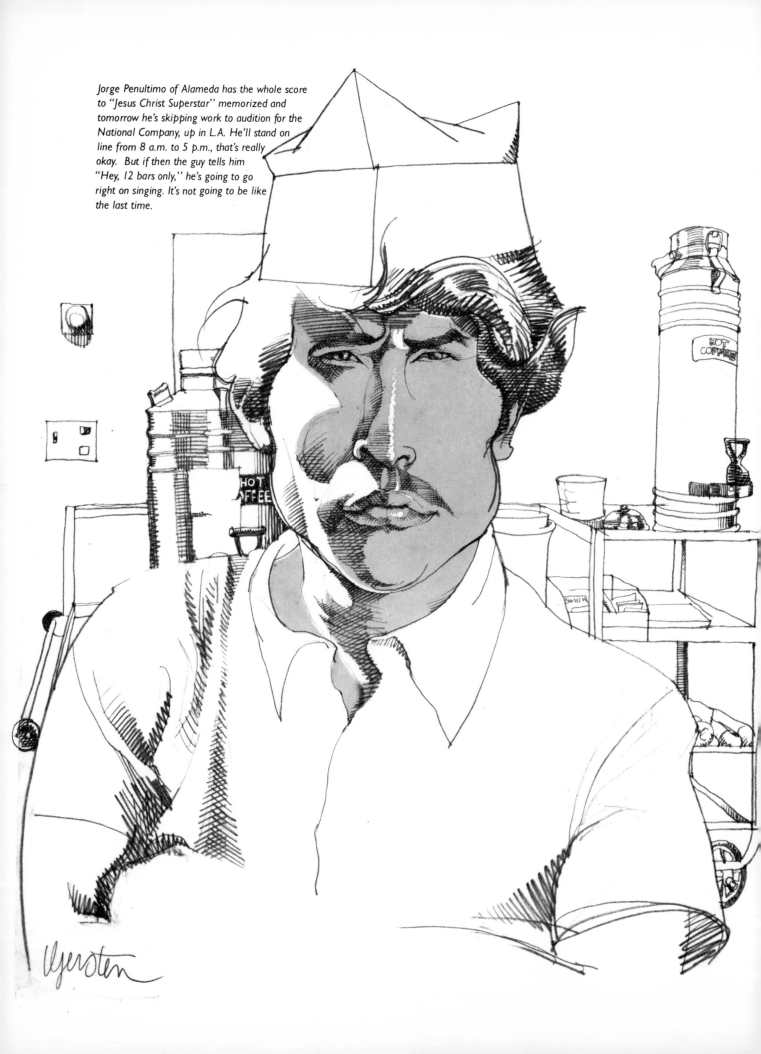

Jorge Penultimo of Alameda has the whole score to "Jesus Christ Superstar" memorized and tomorrow he's skipping work to audition for the National Company, up in L.A. He'll stand on line from 8 a.m. to 5 p.m., that's really okay. But if then the guy tells him "Hey, 12 bars only," he's going to go right on singing. It's not going to be like the last time.

TV QUERY TREE

By Ed "Golden" Retriever

Q.—Did Sean "James Bond" Connery walk past a "Nathan's" in the encore performance of "Doctor No"?

A.—James Beard, the famous chef, is often seen munching a "dog" in "Nathan's." Sean Connery walked past a "Nathan's" in "Goldfinger." James Bond is a fictional person.

Q.—What were the exact words to the old "Kentucky Fried" jingle that went: something "HAPPY YOU" something "FOOD" blumpity blumpity, nah-hah-num? And where can I buy the music?

A.—Tum-ta-toom-ta "THE BABY MULE LIKES HIS—" *Dum*-something "WARM AND"—I'm stumped, friend.

Q.—There's a cafeteria I enjoy patronizing. It's not too fancy but they treat us cabbies like kings and the food is first-rate. One night while viewing the closed-circuit tv I could've sworn I saw Johnny Carson come in with his tray. What was he eating, and how can I order it?

A.—Stars cannot always separate one meal from another. However, Johnny says, if his memory serves him, it was "some ordinary fish thing." Hope that helps you out next Friday.

Q.—My father has disappeared. We found mother's body in the washing machine. The agency lady is coming over. Why did those men take our rugs away?

A.—This column cannot answer questions that do not pertain to tv.

Q.—Why aren't people ever shown biting their fingernails? Do the sponsors make them take it out?

A.—Rhoda told Brenda she was so nervous, she was biting her whole *hand*. McGarrett said "This case is a nail-biter." Merv said "Don't palm that off on me" (ad-lib). *Bum-bum*-something. "CRUNCH, HAPPY YOU—" . . . damn.

Q.—I've written a great "Dairy Queen" commercial. Now what?

A.—Be prepared. Admen often have limited visions. They tell you "Humor is out" or "Why is this funny?" *They* say. Sometimes you were the top humorist on your college paper and they still tell you this. I suggest you learn to expect a little less from life.

Q.—To settle an argument, is Ronald McDonald a clown or an angel?

A.—Ronald is a *boy*, hence he must be a clown. If this opens up a theological debate, I'm going to be very annoyed.

Q.—Where can I write for a picture of that great Xmas dinner they had on "The Walton's" last night? And were there any leftovers?

A.—CBS replies that no photos of that dinner will be available to the public. There were no leftovers, either. TV people work hard to get where they are, many after years of struggle. They shouldn't have to share their food with anyone.

Q.—With five bucks on the line, was that Farrah in a cameo at the "Dunkin Donuts" counter? My sister says so, but she's a cunt.

A.—No kidding. You win.

Q.—On a "Kojak" two-parter, a car chase completely totalled an "International House of Pancakes." My wife and I are about to take a long drive out West. Has the IHOP been repaired?

A.—Long ago. A spokesman for the pancake corporation says: Stay away from cable tv reruns and don't waste their *time*. Ditto QUERY-TREE's. It's 13 channels and 100 pancakes, right, IHOP? Not vice-versa!

Q.—Did the actress who plays "Edith Bunker" get mutilated in a bottling accident at the "Doctor Pepper" plant?

A.—The mongers are at it again. I keep vowing not to mention these ghoulish rumors but this one is so patently twisted it demands my denial. YES, Dr. P. cans WERE withdrawn in four southwestern states. But those were just GLASS SLIVERS inside! Christ, you people make me sick!

Q.—For a long time I used to go to bed early. Sometimes, when I had put out my candle, my eyes would close so quickly that I had not even time to say "I'm going to sleep."

A.—IF YOU ATE A LITTLE LESS, YOU WOULDN'T BE SO DAMN SLEEPY.

Due to the increasing volume of mail, this column regrets it can no longer make personal replies. You may, however, continue to mail us stamps for that purpose. Please do not lick the gum off the stamps. They don't count.

Angry Candy

by Sean Kelly

If only Keats, that poet laureate of groceries, had not been taken from us so soon! Had he but lived, say, another 150 years, how he could have added to his list of sweeties to be served on St. Agnes' Eve:

. . . Oreos round, and mello Mallomars,
With fudgicals, mouth-melting M&Ms,
Elfwitches magic, tempting Twinkies, too . . .

But, by an Irony of Fate, the very bards fit to praise the wonders of this Century O' Progress were dead by the time it dawned.

Last of the old-line Poets (with a capital P), only W. B. Yeats survived, with the aid of certain glandular transplants, into the age of junk food. And he wrote only one ballad on the subject, published posthumously in his *Words For Muzak, Probably:*

I went to the confectioner's
To buy a paper, nothing more,
And saw a bloodshot eyeball
In the sawdust on the floor.

Hippety hop to the candy shop!

Today's men aren't like yesterday's,
Today's men spit and spat.
Unlike O'Leary, Burke or me,
They'd miss a thing like that.

Hippety hop to the candy shop!

Among the jelly baby jars,
The gumdrops and the mints,
The third eye of a seer, or of
Some cyclops Celtic prince.

Hippety hop to the candy shop!

I picked it up, and saw within
That visionary ball,
Reflected and reflecting
An old humbug after all.

Hippety hop to the candy shop!

The young Ezra Pound and ancient Yeats wore matching brown shirts there, for a while, but soon slouched toward separate bedlams. Unless one counts the several Chinese take-out menus Pound published verbatim in the later *Cantos*, one finds few poems celebrating junk food in his work, but here's one:

And returned to America:
* never asylum more political,*
But not for the wine of the country.
Hardly αμβροσια the barbarous vintages
(Hollywood grafted unto Vine)
* "Gallo" or "Almaden" to E.L.P.*
* (he'd drunk Il Duce's health*
* in Bardolino)*
si fueris Romae:
Nor for the godam "health foods"
viz, escarole ripped off for ill-got salads
vide Chavez . . .
re all organic victuals was Ez
emphatically CONTRA NATURAM.
Au contraire,
* The sage demanded*
* Goodly fare:*
Bagels his deli bread now
* si fueris (perfidious) albi . . .*
& noshed for crow knishes,
fressed latkes, humble pie,
* "side order peppers, mebee*
* a glass seltzer"*
Slide home and safe
from Circe's porcine trayf,
* 'Til by Yeshiva Eng. Lit. grads*
* Discovered dead &*
Strictly kosher . . .

Like his friend James Joyce (frustrated sloganeer for Guinness Stout), T. S. Eliot tried his hand at advertising copy; in the case of the rather less Dionysian Mr. Eliot, however, the products flacked were soft drinks:

I

Because I did not deposit,
I cannot hope to return.
Dead soldiers, empty, wait
To be disposed of thoughtfully.
* The Yogi said:*
* Jug jug. Yoohoo! Yoohoo!*
Dr Pepper, so misunderstood, has a bad cold,
Nevertheless is — how shall I say — original
In the whole, wide, world . . .

II

A tin pan alley jingle
Pollutes the pianola
Catholic in his tastes,
He orders RC Cola.

print by Frances Jetter

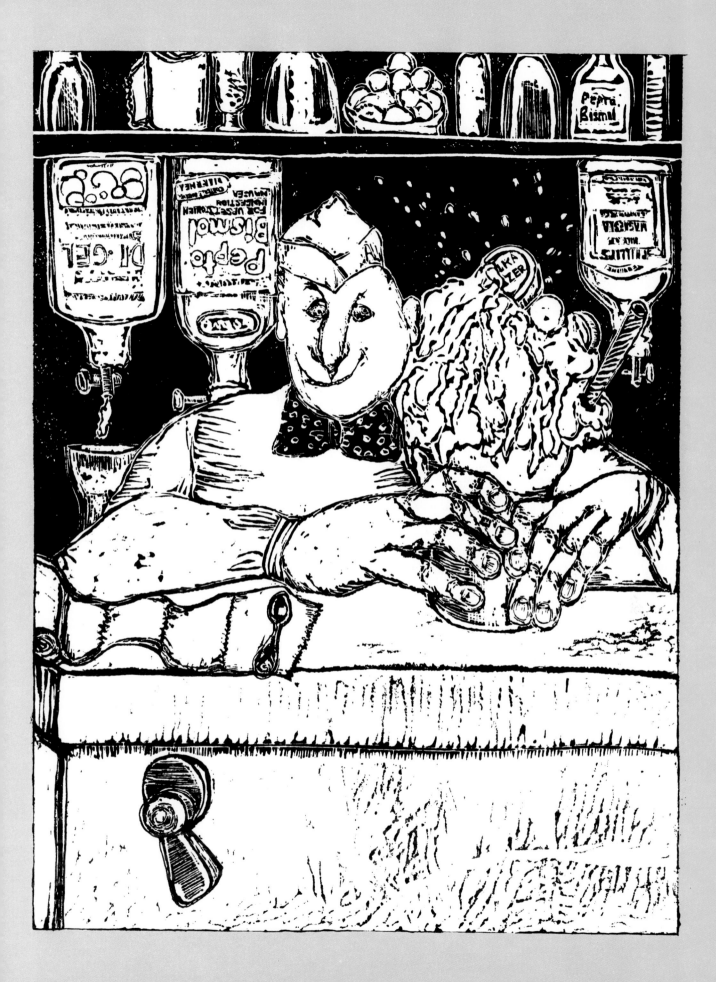

III

Between the dry old man
And his dry mouth falls,
    The pause that refreshes.
And I will show you
Ice cold mountain dew,
And teach the world to sing
In perfect harmony.

IV

Oranges crushed, and bitter lemons,
And the ginger dry . . .
Can Mr Pibb from clutching roots
Make beer?
A Pepsi generation come alive?

Of the suppressed "Hershey, Pennsylvania" episode of Hart Crane's epic *The Bridge*, only a fragment remains, a first draft of a single stanza discovered on the back of an extremely bitchy letter to Ivor Winters. Of the infamous "Queens Tunnel" sequence, there is to be found, mercifully, not a trace . . .

Caked stakes the sugar sky fudge, ice, with smoke—
An almost edible calligraphy,
Above Thee, Hershey, toothsomest of towns!
O, almond joy! Bitter or semi-sweet
Each street a high or milky way to Mars!
O Henry! Reggie! We three musketeers
Here snicker and take quick brown chocolate kisses
From chocolate soldiers in each chocolate bar!

Doctor Bill Williams often demonstrated that disdain for the rules of good nutrition so characteristic of American physicians. . . .

On a white
plate
the peanut
butter sandwich
with one
bite
gone:
what did you
want—
jam on it

. . . whereas Wallace Stevens, in the insurance game, put a premium on long and healthy lives for all his customers. . . .

Eighty-six that baked alaska, Jack,
A whey to go and hold the curd, Haha!
Bring us a round around of bitter milk,
Fetch fat-free yummies pour les filles et moi.
Let anorexic heiresses delight,
Consuming inconspicuous calories.
The only king is the king of frozen yogurt.

e e cummings went on record early that freedom was not a breakfast food. He later elaborated the theme in one of those weird verse forms he insisted on calling sonnets:

that juice is colored very like a orange;
the cereals (at least) named after wheat;
the syrup on them pancakes tastes like maple;
them fried things by the eggside smell like meat;
but that aint milk yer pourin in yer coffee;
nor is that powder sugar tho its sweet;
so put a lot a toothpaste on yer toothbrush
an start yer day off with a bite to eat

Sylvia Plath (the late Ms.; maybe you saw the movie?) was nothing if not a devoted mother. ("Nothin' says lovin', etc.," as she used to sing.) To warn her soon-to-be-orphaned children against cavities, she bequeathed them this cautionary verse:

I am that skinny kid
All ribs and knees,
Who's always eating—
Never gains a pound.

I am the sugar vampire,
Like my poems thin,
And burning
With false energy.

Spoiled rotten
By the Nazi candy man—
Give her some cola, cookies, anything
To shut her up.

My sweet teeth feed.
And one by one,
I'll starve myselves
To death.

But the times they are a-changin', as was first observed by the folk-rock bard (whose own composition, "Baby Ruth Munchie Surrealistic Blues Revisited" was a significant contribution to this field). As our century fades out to the crackle of granola and fizzle of Perrier, the poets have tempered their traditional fulsome praise of unhealthy edibles and potables. Consider Gregory Corso's recent and cautionary "Tootsie Roll Sutra," which concludes:

All that trash rubbish you're always shoveling in, boy!
I'm telling you, America, you're getting fat, watch it!

So, in mankind's quest for that chimera, some thing that tastes good and is good for you, poets will continue to show the way. In the brief 17 syllables of a *haiku*, Gary Snyder leads our Graeco-Roman culture down the path of Zen:

In a sushi bar
Eating deep-fat fried eels. O,
Tempura! O, morays!

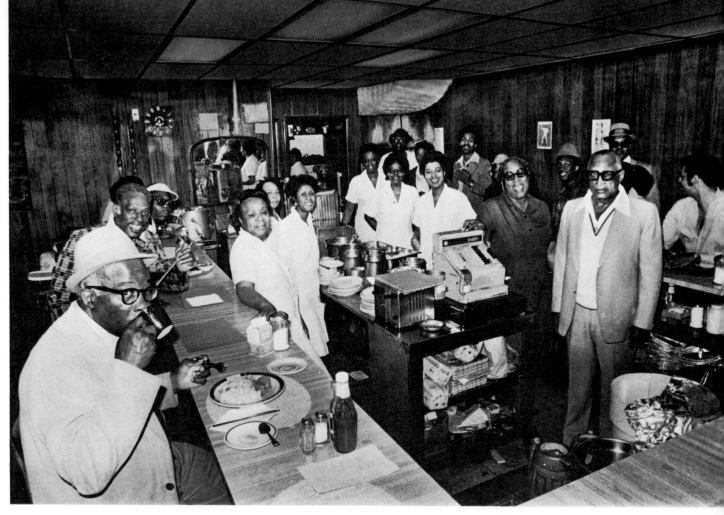

Les Matthews with sources and regulars at Adele's on Seventh Ave. near 118th St. in Harlem. That's Les on the left, with the coffee.

Mr. 1-2-5 Street Eats Out

by Les Matthews (Mr. 1-2-5 St.)

Harlem's Red Rooster Cafe on Seventh Ave., a favorite drinking spot of the late Congressman Adam Clayton Powell, Jr., sponsored a Nostalgia Evening at the Renny Ballroom. A number of former performers, a chorus line of boys and girls doing the Charleston, and Jerry Wayne, the sexy body-wiggler from the Bronx, were featured.

A recent testimonial for one-time tumbling artist Baby Joyce, now living in a Far Rockaway nursing home, brought back memories of Harlem's theatrical heyday, when she performed with her husband, Bobby Goins, at the Lafayette Theater on Seventh Ave. at 133rd St. And, bound up with these memories, thoughts of the pri-

vate clubs once located throughout Central Harlem, and of their 'tater pies, fried chicken, chitlins, and spiked tea with fruit coloring to evade the police, as Prohibition was still the order of the day. The popular spots stood right next door to each other on W. 132nd, 133rd, and 134th between Seventh and Lenox Aves.

Small's Paradise, which was known as Sugar Cane when the late Ed Small operated it on Fifth Ave. at 135th St., will undergo extensive alterations. Small's, later owned by Wilt Chamberlain, was at one time the swankiest supper club in Harlem. Stage and screen stars would drop in to watch the show and eat the delicacies prepared by a Chinese chef. Ed Small was a small man with a soft voice who could get things done by conferring with the right politicians.

Among the clubs were Jimmy Daniel's, Connie's, the Baron's (where the Roy Campanella liquor store now stands), and Stella's. Regular guests were Clara Bow, Harry Richman, Tallulah Bankhead, Clark Gable, Mayor Jimmy Walker, George Raft, James Cagney, and Ziegfeld. Pop's and Jerry, on W. 133rd St., was the club where Billie Holiday made her debut when she arrived here from Baltimore as a 15-year-old girl. She sang from table to table with that sexy, moaning voice of hers.

Ellsworth (Bumpy) Johnson, one of Harlem's best-known badmen, died while eating in the internationally known Well's Chicken and Waffles night spot on Seventh Ave. at 133rd St. Joe Wells, the proprietor of the club, which opened its doors in 1938, said Bumpy was eating and all of a sudden he keeled over and died. Bumpy, who was an associate of

photograph by Cheung Ching Ming

Dutch Schultz's in the numbers racket, was also a Shakespearean student, and could recite some of the great writer's plays from memory. He said he studied Shakespeare while serving a decade in Alcatraz.

The Cotton Club was on Lenox Ave. and 143rd Street. That was where Charlie Banks, the song and dance man, performed with Lena Horne, Cab Calloway, and Edna Mae Holly, who became Sugar Ray Robinson's first bride. Under the Cotton Club was Jeff's Club, featuring Southern cuisine, where the performers mingled with the customers. There was also Mike's at 143rd St. and Seventh Ave., Dominick's on Lenox Ave. and 126th St., and an after-hours club complete with kitchen in the basement of the Apollo Theater at W. 125th St.

William Rogers, 38, wanted to be a comic M.C. He could provoke laughter among his friends and he convinced Honi Coles and Bobby Schiffman at the Apollo Theater that he was what they were looking for. They gave him a chance. He scored a hit with the crowd, but his jokes were vulgar. Though the audiences frowned, they loved it. During a slow week just before the new year, Rogers went to work as a bartender at the East Village Hollywood Social Club, 181 Second Ave. A gunman walked into the club and announced that he was sticking up the joint. Rogers, a fearless man, did not believe it. He refused to comply and was shot to death. Det. Eugene Paturzo of Homicide Zone I is seeking the killer.

The boys and girls who performed for a living would meet at the Hotcha Cafe, a small and cozy club on Seventh Ave. at 134th St.

In the Bedford-Stuyvesant section of Brooklyn, they are talking about how gunmen walk into after-hours joints, rob and kill the patrons, and get away with it. Recently, three men walked into the Chess Club at 2168 Fulton St. and ordered everyone to lie on the floor. One woman who quickly dropped to the floor reportedly said, "I'm glad we didn't have to strip because the stitches

are still in my stomach from my recent operation." The gunmen shot Clarence Winnham, 30, of 930 Herkimer St., who died from the wounds, and Simon Johnson, 21, of 3000 Surf St. They also wounded shapely Melonie Blount, 20, of 72-A Sommers St., and David Tracey, 27, of 1322 St. Marks Place.

White and black musicians, singers, and writers used to meet nightly at Minton's Playhouse at West 118th St., in the Cecil Hotel, to sip, eat, and listen to the sounds. The non-participating musicians would sit at the tables, where they would be joined by waitresses with a "Your order, please" look in their eyes.

Bill Robinson, the gun-toting tap dancer, enjoyed playing pool but he did not like losing. He would play in the poolroom near the Lincoln Theater where he performed on 135th St., which was Harlem's big street. Black Harlemites did not frequent 125th St., they would confine their buying to 135th Street and attend the movies and theaters around the upper Harlem area. The movies around 125th St., like the Alhambra, Regent on 116th, Loew's on 125th St. and Seventh Ave., would only allow blacks to sit in the balconies.

Lloyd Pendleton, 30, a cook in a midtown restaurant, could not control Mrs. Cecilia Brown, 37, mother of five, and they argued constantly. He reportedly left his wife and child to shack up with Mrs. Brown in her apartment at 576 E. 165th St., Bronx. The couple argued constantly after the new year made its appearance, and the arguments stopped when Mrs. Brown's head was hammered in and she was also knifed. Det. Pat Harnett, who is assigned to Homicide Zone 7 in the Bronx, took Pendleton into custody, and he has been indicted.

Charlie Bank's parents went to the Alhambra to watch him perform and they had to enter by the 116th St., Jim Crow entrance. The same theater had a number of apartments, with elevators, but did not allow blacks.

Queens police are looking into the

hit murder of Herbert (Shep) Jennings, 59, in Mr. Ugly's Bar, 190-20 Linden Blvd., to see if it's connected to narcotics. Jennings was known to the police as a gambler, but rumors have it that he was into drugs. Police said a masked man walked into the crowded bar and executed the smiling Jennings.

There were a number of restaurants on 125th St. Some were known throughout New York, like Frank's, which specialized in thick, juicy steaks, Child's, and the Waldorf, but they did not allow blacks. But the blacks welcomed the whites to eat in their restaurants.

Ronald Young, 18, drove Gerald Polite and Joseph Matos to the pizza shop at Tremont and Sampson Aves. in the Bronx and was trailed by two cops, who gave them summonses when they returned home and entered the Throgs Neck housing parking lot. Polite said the cops were not polite. He said they pulled their guns on the three young men and told them they were under arrest. Mrs. Inez Polite observed the police and ran down from her second floor apartment to find out the trouble. She was told the young men were arrested for littering. The police said they threw a shoe out the window of the car. The youths said they wore sneakers. The youths also said police officer 2566 threatened to take them to the police station and Jap them.

Restaurants in the Harlem area were the place to mingle with stars like Eartha Kitt, Cab Calloway, Bricktop Conge, Ethel Waters, and Louis Jordan. The clubs and restaurants did not refuse, but some of them did not welcome, the black trade because they wanted to have their places ready for the big spenders.

Luther (Red) Randolph, former proprietor of Carl's Corner and the Shalimar Supper Clubs in Harlem, will shortly open his latest club, The Quinessence, on West 46th St. The club will feature French and American cuisine, and it will be a membership club. He will also have top entertainment.

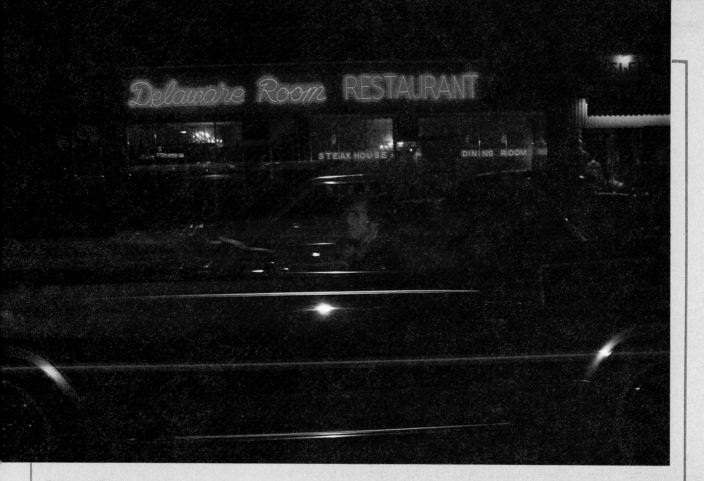

Delaware

by Joseph Vasta

Every day, stripside America skims a little bit more off the top of roadside America. Helen's been running Helen's Lunch for four years now. She ran the snack bar in the Ames shopping center first. "I don't want to run nobody down, naturally," she says, meaning Hardee's, Wendy's, "but one man came in and wanted to know if he could have a hamburger in a minute. I told him yes, if he wanted it raw. Because I don't fix nothing but my vegetables ahead of time." Her specialties are "Tubs of Fried Chicken, Pressure Fried," and "real potatoes," not instant.

"Get a lot of comments on that," she says.

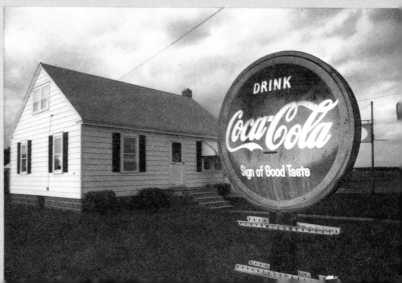

Helen's Lunch, Rt. 113, Millsboro

Billy's Carryout, Rt. 1, Bethany Beach

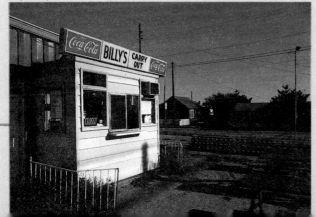

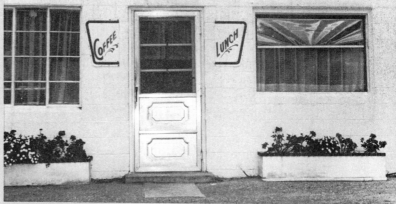

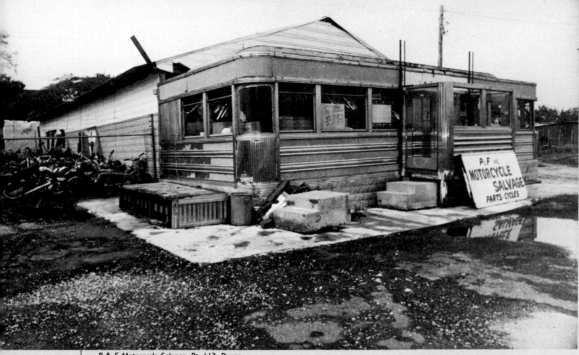

P & F Motorcycle Salvage, Rt. 113, Dover

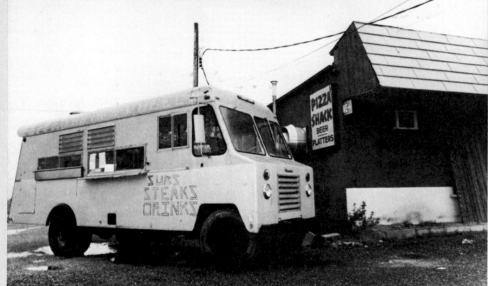

Pizza Shack, Rt. 113, Milford

SCRUMPTIOUS FOOD

Red Barn, Rt. 13,
south of Smyrna

CHILI STEAK FISH STEWS SOUPS RED BARN STEAK SUBS FISH CLAMS GUMBO

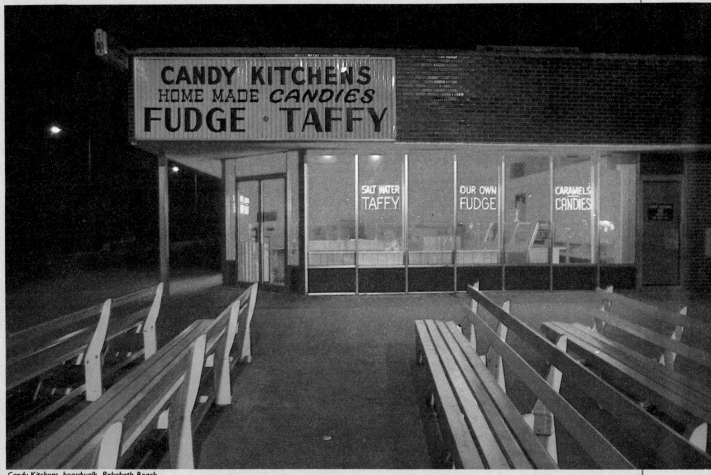

Candy Kitchens, boardwalk, Rehobeth Beach

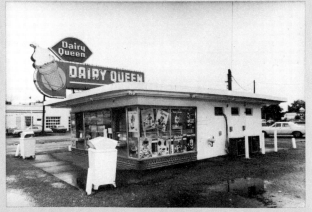

Twin Kiss Drive-In, Rt. 13, south of Harrington

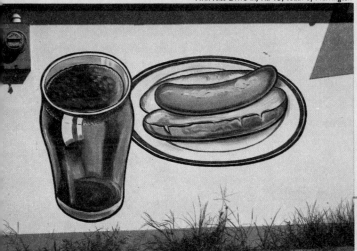

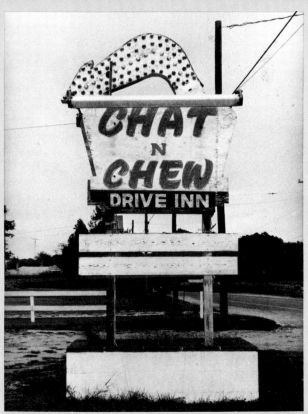

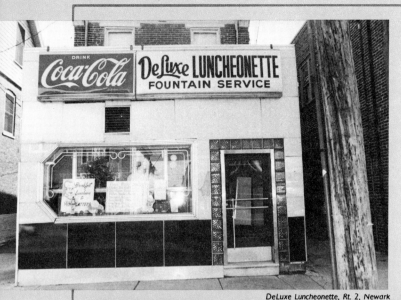

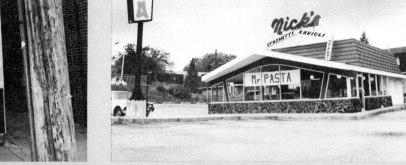

DeLuxe Luncheonette, Rt. 2, Newark

Nick's (Mr. Pasta), Business Rt. 13, Holly Oak

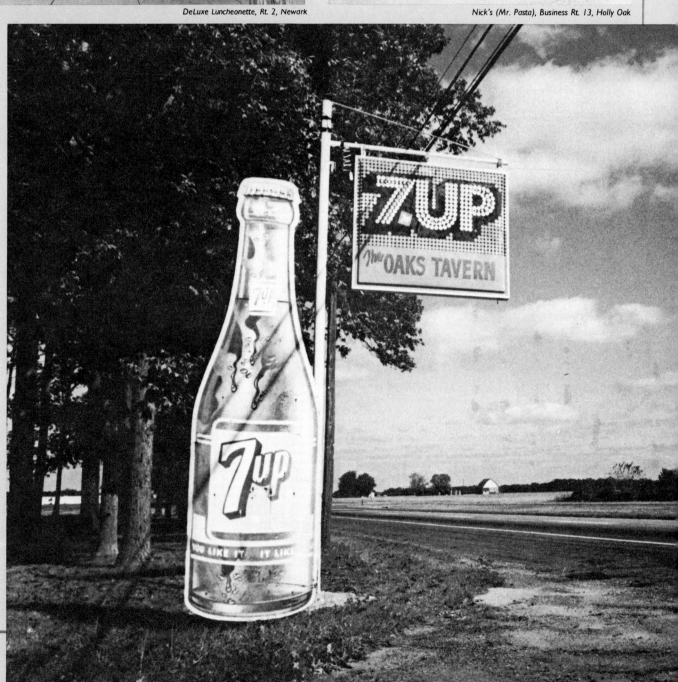

Carbo-Loading

by Max Apple

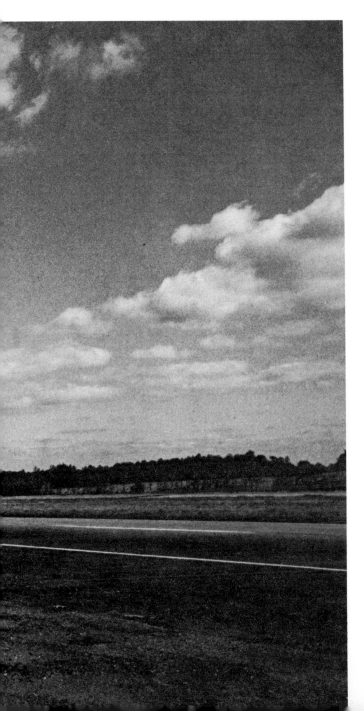

My first significant carbohydrates came from beer. Mom was a miler, but to nurture embryonic me she didn't even walk stairs. She spent eight hours a day in bed. While nursing she developed a taste for beer. Vaguely, I recall foam at the nipple. Dad sat beside us and sipped from long-necked bottles.

"He'll be a hurdler," they thought, judging by my stride. As they cuddled me they stretched my tendons from the ankle to the knee. Dad wanted a sprinter, Mom hoped for distance. When I was 30, she got her way.

By then I had been a beer man for a decade. When I finally started to run I felt like a washing machine. The beer swirled within amid the colorful jungle of entrails. I had no stamina for a final sprint, no burst of glucose for the hills, I was always on rinse and hold.

My doctor said that because of my drinking I had developed little pockets of beer, not just the well known belly, but beer bulge at the wrists, behind the ears, between the vertebrae. As I ran these bits of beer quivered like dangling earrings.

Dr. Isle is a runner too. He figures that if it increases his working life by just four years it will make him $1,000,000 richer. So he cut the million from life insurance and added it to malpractice. He runs 15 miles a day. Lots of times he's too mellow to diagnose. Tumors and arrhythmias float by as unnoticed as dull movies, but he perks up for a stretched Achilles tendon or a swollen knee joint.

After he drains my pouches with a long needle, Isle looks me in the eye. "Cut the beer," he says, "if you ever want to run a three-hour marathon."

Sweet Nurse Phillips bends to lace my Nikes. I hobble into the waiting room and crush my last six-pack in an ashtray.

"Good for you," Nurse Phillips says. There are bright tears in her eyes. The patients cheer.

For the next two weeks I take Gatorade intravenously and run on a treadmill beside the bed. Then, during my first outdoor ten miles, my hair turns the color of autumn, my legs cramp, and my ankles crackle like chestnuts.

"Carbohydrate depletion," Dr. Isle says. He gets me into a reclining position on the examining table. Nurse Phillips spoons dry Cheerios through my wind-chapped lips.

"10,000 cc's," he orders.

Her tender feeding revives me. The Cheerios that fall to my legs she spears on the point of a long fingernail. She does an impromptu cardiogram by putting her ear at nine different spots on my chest. Her tight curls tickle. When she embraces me I respond.

"It's normal," she says.

Isle prescribes a box of unsweetened cereal for dessert every day. "Load up on carbohydrates," he says, "protein will never get you more than ten miles. Amino acids are selfish. They want to stay the way they are. That's why I don't believe in life on other planets. Protein is insular and xenophobic. It's all left-handed. It's expensive and hard to maintain. I hate it as much as sugar, but what can you do? It's all there is.

"After twenty miles the body eats itself."

Nurse Phillips hands me a plastic packet with professional samples of bee pollen, desiccated liver, and Body Punch. I ask her to go out with me on Saturday night.

"The Boston Marathon is in two months," she says, "I'll be doing stretching exercises every minute until then."

"I'll see you in Boston," I say, "at the finish line." We make a date for the 27th mile.

"I hope you'll really be there," she says. "I hope you've got what it takes."

"I'll be there," I say. I pat the top of her nurse's cap.

What it takes, I learn, is more than what you have. I learn this from all the experts. The books confirm what Isle says. He has not deluded me. Carbo-loading will only get you 20 miles. For the last six you eat your heart out. In my training, even with Gatorade and bee pollen and $70 heel inserts, I can't make it past 20 miles.

I think of Nurse Phillips in Boston moist and anxious at the finish, seeking me. Still I can't get past 20. I think of Jesus on the Cross, martyrs on the rack, witches at the stake, but my own misery is not diminished by the suffering of others.

In desperation I bone up on personal cannibalism. The Prime Minister of India drinks his own urine, various ladies have sampled their breast milk, and all of us suck blood from our snake bites and swallow great quantities of phlegm and saliva. But none of this historicism helps.

Finally, at the advice of an experienced marathoner, I check into a running clinic. There I am immediately weighed naked under water and am relieved to learn that only 9% of my person is fat. This is better than average so I have no excuse there. Furthermore my resting pulse is 40 and I can hit alpha waves at the mere mention of the word peace in any language.

I am a difficult case. The Director assigns me to a running therapist. "Pick your speed," the therapist says, "stay comfortable, don't try to impress me. You will for a while in middle distance try to model yourself after me. There may even be a passing boyish crush, a temporary identity crisis. Don't worry. By fifteen miles or so it will be over. You will learn to identify a stride and a gasping pattern that is totally unique to you."

The therapist has a gray beard as I expected, and wears conservative dark gray shorts. He takes notes on a dictaphone no larger than a digital stopwatch.

My parents and childhood take the first five miles. We hit puberty at about 13. I talk on the exhale. Every three miles we take a two-minute break from analysis. During the rest I jog in silence. He encourages me to have pastoral fantasies during these intervals. "Pretend you are a gazelle," he says, "a gazelle along the verdant banks of the ancient Tiber; or a sleek antelope galloping toward some lush African watering place."

He is right. I do admire his long authoritative stride. I am enthralled by the way he hears me out, knowing exactly when to press the dictaphone. To him my lack of endurance is just a job. When I am finished he'll shower and take on someone else. What strength he has, what dedication. He reads the admiration of my silence.

"Look," he says, "body language aside, I don't think this should be a block for you. Let's just go on. By sixteen or seventeen miles it should be over. Believe me, it's just sort of oedipal."

I get nostalgic then about my early training, my blue Adidas Dragons, the high school track, my first seven-minute mile.

"Speaking of time," he says, "you're doing an 8:14 pace and we're at the nineteenth mile."

I know that he will stop at 20. "The last six you're on your own. Even in therapy," he says, "I can't take you all the way. But I think you're ready."

At 20 miles an orderly in a golf cart is awaiting him. The orderly pours a bucket of water on my head, gives me a cup of Gatorade, and takes my therapist back to the clinic. "Good luck," they shout.

I am in the deep woods now and it is almost dusk. Certain primal fears try to grip me but my heart is too busy for fear. Twenty-one passes. This is all new territory. It's like suddenly growing four or five inches and having to relearn old habits like the length of a step. In my pride at having passed 21 miles I stumble on a tiny tree root. I am unable to stand. When I'm not at the clinic as expected the therapist himself comes out for me in the golf cart. He loads me onto the seat. "Nothing seems broken," he says, squeezing my right tibia and ankle. "There are obstacles in everyone's path. You'll have to be more wary in the future, but I think you'll make it."

And that, my friends, is as close as I came to 26 miles 385 yards until the day in Boston. Yes, I ran slow tens and twelves. I did sprints and fartleks. I ran hills and trained my breath on the steps of the football stadium. People who knew me in the beer days, even in the three- to five-mile stage, were in awe of my leanness. At the track I lapped those who used to be my peers.

In Boston it's true I was alone and far from home. I had a bad night in a lumpy motel room. I was stiff and eager and maybe slightly overtrained. But I had eaten for the race. It was Monday. From the previous Sunday through Wednesday I had nothing but protein, meat at all three meals. At McDonald's I threw away the bun and held the double beef patty and melted cheese in my bare hands. Instead of Coke I carried my own powdered beef broth which I mixed with boiling water. Then from Thursday through Sunday I loaded carbos. With Dr. Isle's permission, of course, I had a six-pack on Sunday night. "Lots of carbos," he said, "and it will clean you out before the race." I ate miles of spaghetti and bought bread by the pound.

On Monday morning, 26 miles from downtown, I was ready. The stars of the distance world were all there pretending it was just another day in rural Massachusetts. Frank Shorter ate a Ding Dong and a banana, Bill Rogers munched on gingerbread. Way up front, in the under-three-hour grouping, I thought I spotted Dr. Isle, but I couldn't reach him in the throng. The one I really looked for, Nurse Phillips, was somewhere in the herd of four-hour women stretching their backs against trees, adjusting straps, fine-tuning themselves.

"Well," I thought, "I'll give it all I've got." Those were my words to myself at the start. I said them over and over for the first four miles. I studied faces as they passed, then I switched to subjects. I did philosophy from miles five to eleven, trying to form one discriminating sentence about Socrates, Kant, Spinoza, Kierkegaard, whomever. When I came to the authors of *How to Be Your Own Best Friend*, I knew my mind was wandering and let go of systematizing. I listened to the rhythm of my breath, which was unsteady as early as 12 miles into the race.

By 15 miles lots of women were passing me and I understood that I might not make it. Without despair I continued step by step.

If not for the nurse's cap I might not have recognized Miss Phillips as she pulled alongside. Her stride was lively. The insides of her thighs puckered. "Take one of these," she said, slipping me a brown tablet. "Dolomite."

I hesitated.

"It's just magnesium and calcium, it will help with the cramps." Though I could barely talk, esprit de corps was in my eyes. She ran alongside me, my inspiration and my pacer until I ran out of myself. She says it was after 24 miles. My feet just stopped taking orders.

In the sudden stillness I thought someone had put me into the sidecar of a motorcycle. I heard the static of a CB radio. Eight or ten horsepower seemed to be propelling me. It was Nurse Phillips. In charity she had entered my nervous system.

"Women have more stamina," she said, "I knew it before liberation."

I could feel that layer of feminine softness give of itself cell by cell. Her generosity moved my heart.

"Save something for later," I moaned, "for childbirth and famine." She held my hand.

"I can't make it," I gasped.

"There's more to life than the marathon," she said. "There's the 25 kilometers, the hillclimbs, the 5-kilometer sprint, the half-marathon."

"I'm too old," I said.

"There's the submasters and the masters. There's Golden Age jogging and finally trots in the sunset."

"Without you I couldn't make it," I said. "The therapist told me the last six miles had to be alone."

"There will still be loneliness," she said, "swollen joints and arthritis, varicose veins, arguments over money."

The finish line was in sight—the Prudential Building, the great tower of insurance.

"For you," I said with my last breath, "I did it for you." At the finish line I collapsed in her arms. People all around were doing the same. It looked like World War I in underpants.

She doused me in Gatorade and slipped bee pollen under my tongue. "At any pace," she said, "there is infirmity and disease. Carbo-loading will never be enough."

We bronzed our shoes and toasted one another in Body Punch.

"When our electrolytes balance," she said, "maybe we'll live happily ever after."

We showered and went into training.

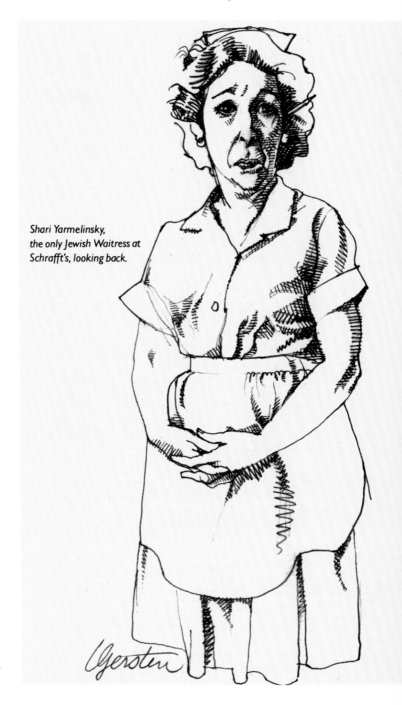

Shari Yarmelinsky, the only Jewish Waitress at Schrafft's, looking back.

Food Fight

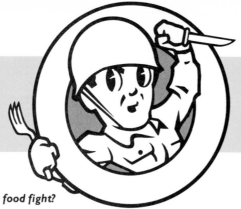

Q: What was your most memorable food fight?

PETE HAMILL, tough guy: "Where I came from, food was a triumph. Nobody fought with it—they ATE it."

R. COURI HAY, gossip columnist, National Enquirer: "This goes back . . . almost ten years, about 1969. This was still the 'reckless '60's'—and there I was in Monte Carlo with 'Princey' Baroda, who is the Prince of Baroda, and Princey Baroda and I went off in the Maharani de Baroda's cream Rolls-Royce down to a restaurant in Monte Carlo called 'The Pirate.' I think it's 'Le Pirate,' I'm pretty sure. It may just be 'The Pirate.' I'm pretty positive it's 'Le Pirate,' but 'Pirate.' But Arndt Krupp, who is, of course, the Krupp heir from the German—the movie **The Damned** is about him, incidentally—so he was giving a little party, and there was this mad group of us. And all of a sudden, the entire contents of the table were flung at everybody. I mean, just everything just went. They had these trees—it's outdoors—this big tree with roping in it, like on ships? And suddenly people were climbing up in there, including myself, I was throwing down big pieces of soufflé from a dish at the people underneath. Originally I had a magnum of Dom Perignon that I would shake and then spurt down, and this was like $100 a bottle, you know, and people were hurling things back at me, the whole restaurant was suddenly being heaved at each other, to the point where chairs were all smashed, some of

them thrown into the barbeque pit and all burned. . . . They have a feature in the restaurant where various animals are brought through by trainers, well, sometimes we managed to break the animals loose from the trainer. So you have all these sheep and different animals, lamb and sheep and things running madly around the restaurant, you've got burning chairs and all the table accessories, five or six people in the trees. I was all dressed up—this was the time of the Gypsy period, I was there in a Giorgio di Sant' Angelo Gypsy outfit—it was worth a lot of money. [Laughs.] Arndt was in Yves St. Laurent and Princey Baroda was in one of these Maharani Indian looks, the rubies and jewels. And I took the bottom of my shirt and just filled it with all this fooood, and climbed up and was throwing it—it was a chocolate soufflé with heavy vanilla white cream at the top. And I heaved the soufflé full force at the Prince, who had made a comment that I thought was catty, something about my outfit. [Laughs.] The Maharani was famous for her jewels, and the Prince used to borrow them. We were all, you know, 17, 18, 19 . . . and the soufflé just ruined this incredible silk caftan. We always called him Princey. And there was Princey dripping emeralds and dripping soufflé. It was just vaguely mad. And further extended by the fact that Arndt had to pay somewhere in the vicinity of, I think, $7,000 for the resulting damages. Why it started? Too much champagne . . . and a kind of boredom that comes on you in Monte Carlo at a certain point. It's a boredom that means—every night, you go out, something exciting's gotta happen. We were very much into making things happen in the '60's."

JF: What had brought you to Monte Carlo?

Couri: "Oh, I always spent August in Monte Carlo, for years. It was June in Capri, and July and August in Greece and . . . but my more recent food fight was in this restaurant in China, the Empress Imperial Restaurant, so here we were in this restaurant with all this history, marvelous history. We were in this special room, in China you find they have private dining rooms a lot, so we were in this private room about to partake in a banquet that was some twenty-seven courses, that would take seven hours—this was our last meal in China, we were going to really do it up there in the Imperial Restaurant, we were really ready for the whole number. And of course we were drinking all their famous little drinks that they drink, these little tumblers full of, I think it's called tai or maui, or something like that. Mao Tai is what it's called. So we were throwing back the Mao Tais and we're dining on smoked fish surrounded by cucumbers done like flowers and cold duck and the Dowager Empress's bean curd cakes, and 100-year-old eggs, and Dragon's Mustache, which is a marveous dish with abalone and chicken and asparagus all in it, all white, then rhinoceros surrounded with lotus eggs, and sea beaver with peanuts, served Szechwan style, and fish, sort of silver carp caught right out in the lake outside, covered with little onion pearls and all these marvelous things, and the Mao Tais were flowing and Tsandra had done herself up, she's always rather extravagant, she'd really outdone herself this time and she had on one of her $3,000 chiffon numbers with the little pleated jacket, and her blue and green hair and the little pink streak going, and the jewels, and we were really dressed to kill. And I was in one of my new black silk padded Chinese jackets and one of my new silk Chinese shirts and one of my new silk Chinese scarves—we were both done up to death, making our last grand banquet. And all of a sudden, I get this 100-year-old egg in my face. So I picked up a glass of Mao Tai and threw it at her. The next thing, the Dowager Empress's delicate bean cakes started flying across the room as I raced around the table and hid behind one of the couches and picked up the sesame buns, and holding the minced pork—which you make into little sandwiches, like putting the minced pork in the sesame buns, it's a whole thing with the sesame buns—and BANG, BANG, BANG, and we started running around the table, and the buns were flying, and the rhinoceros horns started flying, and the lotus eggs all around that started flying and, you know, the whole room looked like it died. Well, in the middle of this, was the knocking at the door. They always knock. I ran to the door and pushed a couch in front of it: 'No! No! No!,' meanwhile the Peking Duck things that are wrapped, these are flying, the little shrimp that are still in the things, they are flying, pieces of cauliflower were going. And there was Tsandra's $3,000 chiffon dress dripping lichee nuts, raisins, and warm oranges and pineapples, it looked like a painter's smock done in food. And they're banging on the door and we're going, 'Oh, no, no, no! Everything is o.k., come back in an hour! We're enjoying everything!' And there was the Empress's beautiful Imperial yellow dishes done with crimson lotus leaf designs—then I threw a plate and that ended it. And I looked up and said, 'My God, what are we doing? Here we are in Red

China: I'm the first American tourist ever into China, after the normalization of relations. Here you are, a British subject. What is the Queen going to say? What is the President going to say?' I looked around the room and said, 'My God, Tsandra. This could be a diplomatic incident.' "

ROBIN MOORE, author, The Green Berets: "When I was in Rhodesia and ran the American Embassy there —I made myself the ambassador there, y'know, there was no official title— every Saturday we had what was known as 'The Saturday Afternoon Bun Fight,' which was for all the Americans who were fighting in the Rhodesian army. Anytime they could get in the Embassy, they'd come in. It started out with beer, booze, and hamburgers, and they took to throwing the hamburgers and buns at each other. We threw for two years, usually for half an hour. We had a swimming pool, too, and we'd throw it into the pool. It was quite a mess. I miss those fights. I miss being in Rhodesia, as a matter of fact."

LAWRENCE PARKE, agent of Mae Clarke: "Over the years, the grapefruit has become the one thing that has held her desirable, let's say, in things, and she feels the grapefruit is really Jimmy Cagney rather than Mae Clarke. And she has felt exploited sometimes, just doesn't like to be opportunistic, I suppose, in terms of exploiting the grapefruit

that was simply part of a scene with Jimmy Cagney and when they can't get Jimmy Cagney, sometimes they want Mae Clarke because of the grapefruit. She did 102 films, but people always say, Public Enemy. Now, this is her situation: she would perhaps grant an interview if there were money involved, but in so many of these things, there is no money involved at all, and she simply says no. And the minute the grapefruit came up, she'd just say, 'I want nothing to do with it. . . .' "

HAROLD HAYES, editor: "There used to be watermelon fights in Boy Scout camp down South. After supper, the camp would provide ten or twelve watermelons, and we'd cut them up and just start clobbering each other with them. It usually lasted half an hour or longer. You'd just sort of bash each other with watermelon rinds. I think this was fairly traditional down South about forty years ago."

QUENTIN CRISP, raconteur: "My parents were invincibly middle class. That is to say they hated one another but never raised their voices. They never hurled adjectives—let alone food. Now I live on a preparation called Complan. This is a whitish powder which, mixed with water, obviates the need for any other sustenance. It also does away with all cooking, all washing up, and almost all shopping. I recommend it."

Wheaties

by Marc Onigman

Cub trainer Andy Lotshaw used to rub Guy Bush's arm with Coca-Cola.

In 1938, Lou Gehrig, Joe DiMaggio, Joe Medwick, and Charlie Gehringer all endorsed Wheaties.

The American Association was the first league to sell beer in its parks, in 1883.

Of course, baseball food differs from country to country. Red wine and pizza are available at Italian games. The Japanese can get sushi and diced eel sandwiches. In Hawaii, Pacific Coast League fans eat noodles with pork broth, pork and onions, steamed yeast dough stuffed with pork, and salted plum and cherry pits. Hey, get your pits. Hey, pits.

A late '40's New York Times cartoon, warning what would happen if "[Mexican] Beisbol Should Cross the Border," showed a vendor selling hot tamales in the stands.

Babe Ruth often placed a lettuce leaf under his cap to keep his head cool on hot days. The Babe was also known to chug a half dozen franks and sodas as the team changed trains on the road. At the peak of his gluttony, he missed much of the 1925 season with what the sports pages dubbed "The Bellyache Heard Round The World." But it was most likely syphilis.

Mickey Mantle's Hall of Fame induction speech quoted the slogan of his (failed) Mickey Mantle Fried Chicken chain: "To get a better piece of chicken, you'd have to be a rooster." Mantle made that up himself. Mantle and Roger Maris used to be called the "M&M Boys."

Walter Johnson boasted that all he ate on the day of a game was a quart of ice cream.

Lou Gehrig also once endorsed Huskies, another breakfast cereal. "To what," asked the radio announcer, "do you owe your amazing strength and condition?" "Wheaties," replied Lou.

When Bill Veeck owned the Milwaukee franchise during the war, he served free milk and cereal at all the team's morning games.

As part of its summer, 1923, campaign to substitute paper containers for bottles, the American Bottlers of Carbonated Beverages cited frequent newspaper accounts of "beaning" the umpire with soft drink bottles.

Germany Schaefer liked distracting the opposition by eating popcorn from his position in the first base coaching box.

In the early days of baseball, the poorer teams were called muffins.

Smiling Mickey Welch credited his pitching effectiveness to the consumption of beer, saying "Pure elixir of malt and hops, beats all the drugs and all the drops."

Atlanta built its stadium for the Braves in just 51 weeks, a tidy rush job, which probably explained why there were still a few bugs to be ironed out when the place opened in 1966. The stadium food came in for its share of abuse. After the season, building engineers discovered that one of the restroom pipes was leaking down onto the hamburger grills.

Eddie Collins stuck his chewing gum on the underside of his cap when he batted.

Charlie Faust, a New York Giant mascot and good luck charm who hung around with the team in 1910 and 1911, ate pie for all three meals and before retiring each night.

Roberto Estalella reportedly ate ham

and eggs three times a day for a month because none of his Washington Senator teammates realized that this was the only dish he could pronounce.

Ballplayers were slept two-to-a-bed in the early days, to cut expenses. Pitcher Rube Waddell once had a clause inserted in his bedmate's contract forbidding the man from eating soda crackers in bed. Of the same Waddell, a manager once said: "I could have stood his drinking, maybe. But I couldn't forgive the fact that he wouldn't get serious."

At the turn of the century, cherry pie, cheese, planked onions, and tripe were ordinary ballpark fare.

President Herbert Hoover was allegedly displeased by "We Want Beer" placards at Shibe Park, during his visit there in '29.

Nabisco's Shredded Wheat—not Wheaties—was the original "Breakfast of Champions," before 1900.

Ty Cobb honed his bats with steer bones.

"Baseball steak" commonly refers to a poor cut of meat.

Meat has also been used by catchers as a sponge between the mitt and the hand.

Mordecai Peter Centennial "Three Finger" Brown lost the other two fingers while chopping meat as a youngster.

For the last time, the Baby Ruth candy bar was not named after Babe Ruth, but after President Grover Cleveland's daughter, Ruth—the first baby born in the White House, which meant something, once. In fact, when Babe and some noble dreamers tried marketing "Babe Ruth's Home Run Candy," the Curtis Candy people appealed to the U.S. Patent Office and had Babe enjoined from using his own name. Nice.

Now Reggie Cleveland's nickname when he came up with the Cards was "Double Cheeseburger." And when they traded him to the Red Sox, it changed to "Snacks."

In 1914, the Brooklyn Federal League

painting by Ronald Dixon

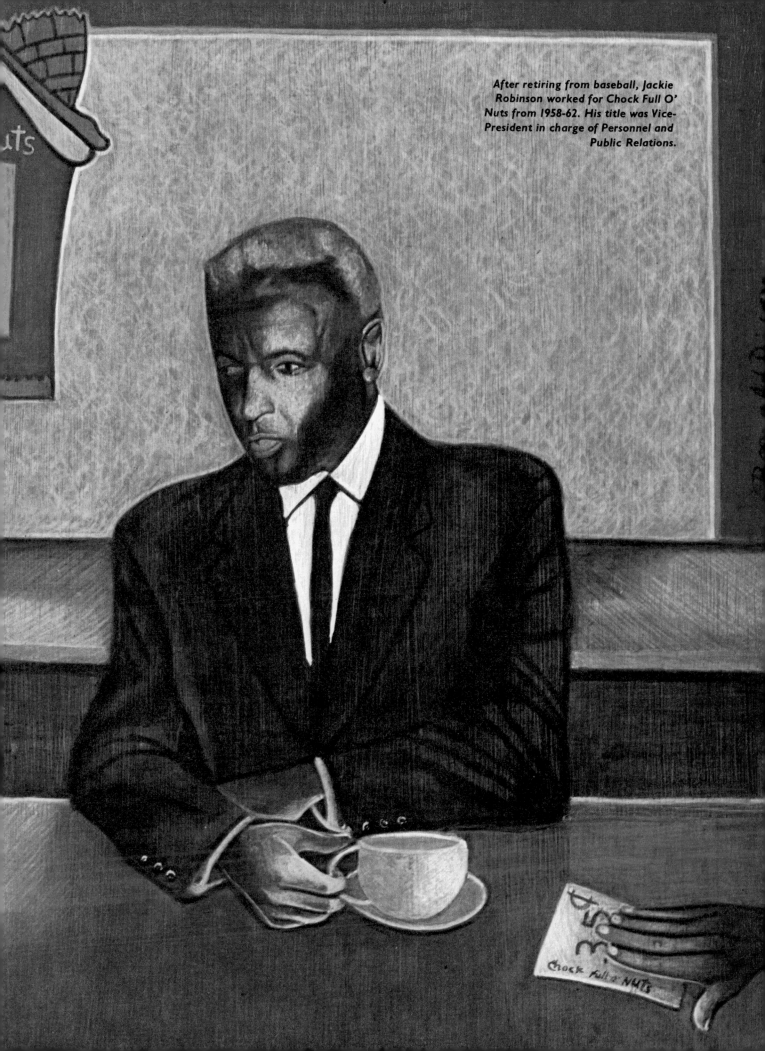

After retiring from baseball, Jackie Robinson worked for Chock Full O' Nuts from 1958-62. His title was Vice-President in charge of Personnel and Public Relations.

entry was nicknamed the "Tip-Tops." Because the owner also ran a bakery.

A device called a "German Distributor" was popular in the 1880's. It was a keg of beer located strategically in foul territory near the third base bag. Any player who got that far was allowed to reward himself with a cold dipperful.

Harry Coveleski carried a piece of bologna in his back pocket and secretly ate it while on the playing field. It was a difficult habit to break, despite the fact that other players mocked him constantly. He ultimately left baseball, rather than give it up.

Harry's brother, Stanley, allegedly used alum on his spitball. Other pitchers have used licorice, slippery elm, and cough drop juice on theirs.

Cincinnati used to serve free German lunches on Opening Day.

Some of the Reds—about four, five years ago—advocated chewing the "gumball," which is one part eating tobacco and two parts bubblegum. Merv Rettenmund once offered columnist Red Smith his favorite recipe: "Take two large sticks of sugarless gum and one stick flavored. Chew them into a moist, adhesive wad. Sit on the bench, take out the gum and spread it on the knee to make a big square. Place three fingers of tobacco on the middle of the square, fold the gum around it, and stuff the glob into your cheek."

Some great bubblegum card faux pas: The 1969 Aurelio Rodriguez (#653) is really the batboy. Dave Bennett's 1964 Rookie Card (#447) reads: "This 19-year-old curveballer is just 18 years old." And the 1966 Dick Ellsworth (#561) depicts his teammate, Kenny Hubbs. Unfortunately Hubbs had been dead for two years. Topps Chewing Gum, which has been turning out baseball cards since 1951, just shrugs that last one off. See, they'd been preparing this special memorial card and . . . .

Chocolate-coated marshmallows with peanuts were popular in 1911 at many baseball parks.

The trainer for the Detroit Tigers favored a rubbing compound which came to be known as "Go Fast." The mixture consisted of Vaseline and Tabasco sauce. This was many years ago.

Nap Lajoie, Rube Waddell, and Walter Johnson endorsed Coca-Cola in the early 1900's. Waddell: "More than once a bottle of your Coca-Cola has pulled me through a tight game." Lajoie: "It is the most refreshing beverage an athlete can drink, and after a hard game I make my way to a Soda Fountain and get a glass." The company ad: "Refreshing and invigorating when one is in training and has none of the 'let down' qualities of alcoholic beverages. A few bottles on the bench will quiet the nerves when the game is close."

Baseball Steaks, etc.

BOOZE: Clarence Beers, Pop Corkhill, Brandy Davis, Tinsley Ginn, Sherry Magee, Charley Ripple, Gene "Half-Pint" Rye, Larry Sherry, Johnny Walker, Highball Wilson, Bobby Wine

APPETIZERS: Oyster Burns, Soup Campbell, Crunchy Coonin, Pea Soup Dumont, Chile Gomez, Juice Latham, Grapefruit Yeargin

HORS D'OEUVRES: Smoke Herring, Peanuts Lowrey, Pretzels Pezzullo, Cracker Schalk, Cheese Schweitzer

SALAD: Walker Cress, Tomatoes Kafora, Vinegar Bend Mizell, Oil Smith

MEAT: Ham Allen, Liver Ancker, Eddie Bacon, Stew Bolen, Meat Brosnan, Herman Franks, T-Bone Giordano, Ralph Glaze, Pork Chop Hoffman, Lyman Lamb, Raw Meat Bill Rodgers, Coot Veal

FISH: John Bass, Jess the Crab Burkett, Jim Crabb, Catfish Hunter, Thornton Kipper, Cod Myers, Shad Roe, Chico Salmon, Bobby Sturgeon, Dizzy Trout

POULTRY: Partridge Adams, Goose Goslin, Goose Gossage, Duck Shifflett, Chicken Stanley, Turkey Tyson

STARCHES: Spud Chandler, Pat French, Pete Fries, Hot Potato Hamlin, Del Rice, Noodles Zupo

VEGETABLES: Cuke Barrows, Bill Bean, Hap Collard, Harry Colliflower, Hubbard Perdue, Lerton Pinto, Squash Wilson, Yam Yaryan

DAIRY: Fats Berger, Tom Butters, Frank Buttery, Eggie Lennox, Greasy Neale

CONDIMENTS: Pickles Dillhoffer, Jelly Jelincich, Howard Maple, Mayo Smith

SPICES: Garland Buckeye, Jim Curry, Pepper Martin, Salty Parker

BEVERAGES: Sugar Cain, Jack Coffey, George Creamer, Moxie Hengle, Punch Judy, Coco Laboy, Bob Lemon, Buttermilk Tommy O'Dowd, Bosco Snover, Sassafras Winter.

BREAD: Oats DeMaestri, Bill Cissell, Bun Troy, Zack Wheat

FRUIT: Bananas Benes, Strawberry Bill Bernhard, Ken Berry, Peaches Davis, Apples Lapihuska, Prunes Moolic, Frank Pears, Peaches Werhas

DESSERT: Goobers Batcher, Honey Barnes, Doughnut Bill Carrick, Candy Cummings, Brownie Foreman, Puddin' Head Jones, Cookie Lavagetto, Peach Pie O'Connor, Sen-Sen Sensenderfer

EXOTICA & GAME: Goat Anderson, Sweetbreads Bailey, Moose Bowler, Frank the Crow Crosetti, Bucky Dent, Harry Eells, Grasshopper Lillie, Rabbit Maranville, Moose Skowron, Whale Walters, Possum Whitted

MISCELLANEOUS: Heinz Becker, Harry the Cat Breecheen, George Burpo, Icebox Chamberlain, Chuck Churn, Doc Cook, Joe Crisp, Jake Freeze, Nemo Gaines, Joe Garagiola, Dinty Gearin, Johnny Grubb, Lick Malloy, Billy Muffett, Pussy Tebeau.

Official Major League Stadium Food Statistics

	Price of Coke (C) /Pepsi (P) (Large)*	Price of Hot Dog*	Local Specialty	Vending Force	Vendor Gender Average (Girls: Boys)	Vendors per Patron
Atlanta Braves	C 60¢	65¢	Chick-fil-A, $1.40	150	.111	250
Baltimore Orioles	C 60¢	65¢	Crab cakes, 90¢	200	.111	250
Boston Red Sox	C 50¢	65¢	Pizza, 60¢	100	.000	335
California Angels	C 50¢	75¢	Helmet sundae, 90¢	90	.052	477
Cincinnati Reds	C/P 45¢	60¢	Mettwurst, 80¢	100	.666	523
Chicago Cubs	C 75¢	60¢	Smoky Link, 60¢	150	.052	300
Chicago White Sox	C 95¢	70¢	Tacos, 85¢	180	.111	250
Cleveland Indians	C 55¢	75¢	Roast beef, $1.35	200	.111	385
Detroit Tigers	P 70¢	75¢	Hot Dog, 75¢	150	.000	353
Houston Astros	C 75¢	75¢	Nachos, $1.00	200	.176	225
Kansas City Royals	C 50¢	60¢	Polish sausage, $1.10	200	.250	204
Los Angeles Dodgers	C/P 75¢	70¢	Peanuts, 25¢	80	.000	696
Milwaukee Brewers	C 60¢	60¢	Bratwurst, 60¢	300	.111	183
Minnesota Twins	C 45¢	75¢	Bratwurst, $1.00	200	.000	245
Montreal Expos	C 50¢	85¢	Pizza, 85¢	200	.000	300
New York Mets	C/P 75¢	65¢	Knish, 60¢	200	.538	250
New York Yankees	P 95¢	75¢	Pizza, 70¢	500	1.000	110
Oakland A's	C 65¢	60¢	Colossal Dog, $1.25	200	.053	200
Philadelphia Phillies	C 75¢	65¢	Pizza, 60¢	325	.053	188
Pittsburgh Pirates	C 65¢	65¢	Roast beef on roll, $1.40	150	.538	333
San Diego Padres	C/P 45¢	75¢	Chili, 75¢	165	.666	312
St. Louis Cardinals	C 75¢	65¢	Steak 'Umm, $1.50	180	.250	278
San Francisco Giants	C 75¢	75¢	Almaden wine, 75¢	250	.111	220
Seattle Mariners	C/P 75¢	70¢	— — —	125	.053	472
Texas Rangers	C 55¢	75¢	Nachos, $1.25	250	.250	168
Toronto Blue Jays	C 55¢	75¢	Sausage on bun, $1.50	125	.053	368

*Prices as of March 1, 1979.

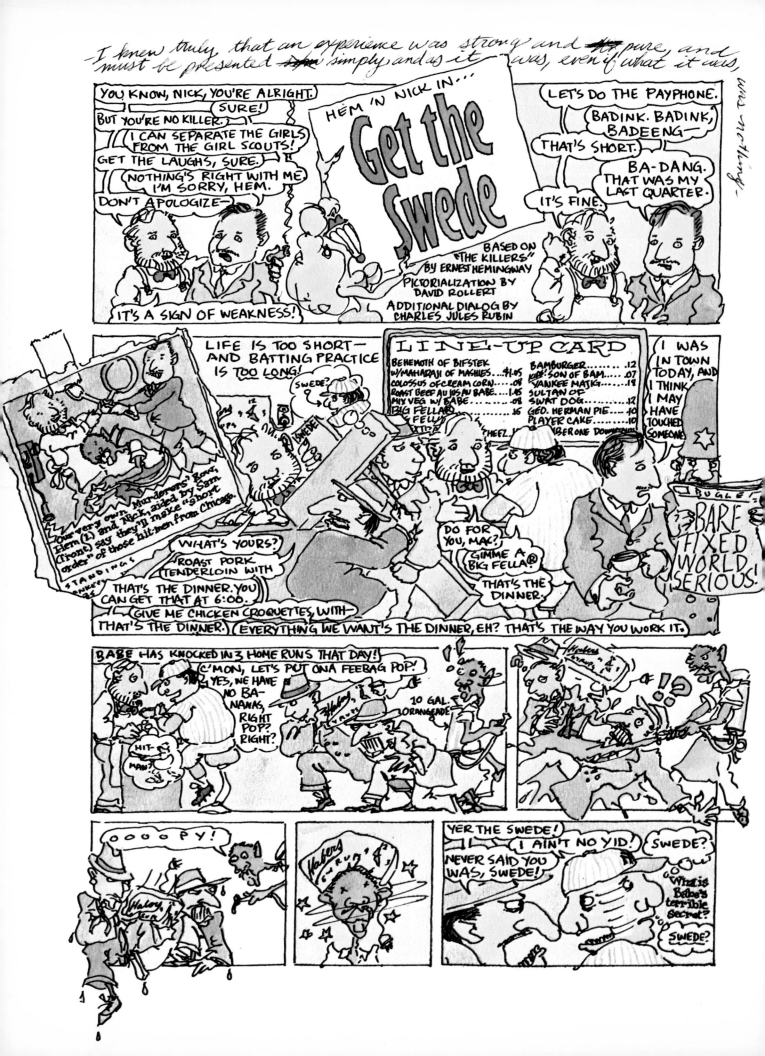

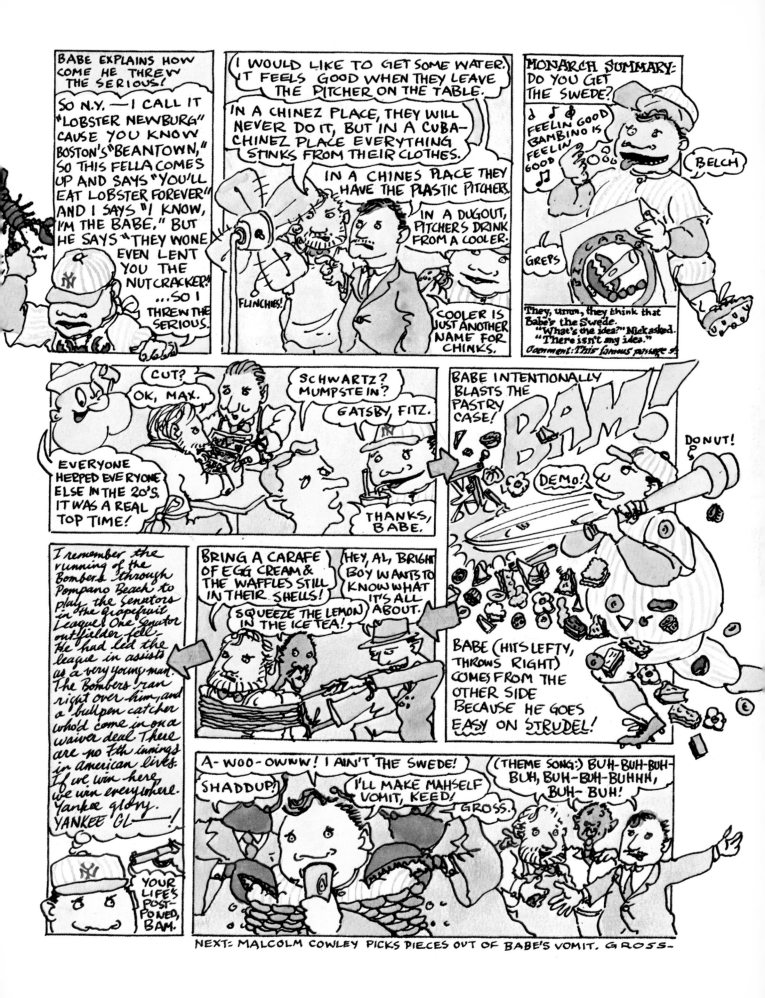

NEXT: MALCOLM COWLEY PICKS PIECES OUT OF BABE'S VOMIT. GROSS—

The Special at the Please-U Café in Prairie City, Iowa

by Douglas Bauer

During the months, from early spring to late fall, when "the men were in the fields," my mother prepared each day a noon meal of such proportion that one had every reason to assume she was cooking for a number considerably larger than four. But in truth there were only four of us and the appetites that mattered belonged to my father and grandfather, who were out there, faintly visible from the kitchen window, steering their tractors through monotonous raking patterns on the Iowa horizon. When I was growing up, too young to join them, I sat on the long front porch and watched them move, slow as a minute hand, across the edge of the earth, while Mother, glancing frequently at the kitchen clock, brought the day's cooking to a high finish. Almost exactly at 12:00 the tractors, distant insects, could be seen turning toward the house. Dad and Grandpa were heading in—for "dinner"; not for "lunch."

I didn't know about "lunch" until I went to college and asked a girl, as we left our 11:00 class, if she'd like to have dinner. "All right," she said. "About seven?"

"Hell, no," I told her. "Just you and me."

Lunch is something light, unobtrusive; chilled air on lettuce. Food you can eat without your stomach even noticing. Try lasting an afternoon, on a tractor pulling the season's particular implement, after "lunch."

So we sat around the kitchen table and ate a hot, huge meal—egg noodles and stew beef, mashed potatoes, escalloped corn. Then, while my grandfather sucked the sap from his toothpick, coffee was served, and pie or cake or fresh pudding. Our average dinner weighed about 50 pounds, which, since the only part of the work day I participated in was the eating, was about half my weight at the age of ten.

What all this has to do with the Daily Special at Snub's Please-U Cafe in Prairie City (other than proximity: Snub's, on the square in town, is four miles from my father's farm) is the custom and the temperature and, until you look closely, the appearance of the food. For 31 years Snub has offered the 1200 citizens of Prairie City a noon-hour menu that includes — besides the hamburgers, fries, fast-frozen pizza, the usuals — a hot "dinner." Snub's customers are farmers, or children and grandchildren of farmers who've moved into town but whose hunger remembers those days in the fields. It's a habit that wants, at noon, hot, thick food. The Special; each day's fare written on the blackboard on the Please-U's east wall. Creamed beef on biscuits. Tenderloin with gravy. Ham and Beans.

Ninety-five cents.

"Special!" shouts Snub above his own kitchen noises as he plops a plate on the serving sill of the open window through which he looks, from his stove and his pots, to the noon-filling restaurant. From the other side of the window, the customers' side, Snub is framed in aesthetic imbalance, a bust in profile in the lower right corner. Frequently, when things need to be stirred, or flipped, or quickly rescued, he goes out of the frame altogether, ducks to his stove, then pops up again into view. The closer to noon, the larger the crowd, the more frequently he bobs in and out.

The restaurant is long, narrow; an alley of Formica history. It runs, 5' x 80', or so it seems, until lights can't help, appears not so much to end as simply fade, like the landscape at sundown, to a darkness at the back of the building. There, if you know the architecture, you can fumble for a handle to the back door. Beyond the door, Prairie City again. The dimensions of the Please-U are original and secured against change—flanked on either side by thriving local businesses: on the left, the pharmacy; on the right, DeWit's Grocery, owned by Snub's brother Don, who employs himself as his own skilled butcher, and who will reach the Please-U for lunch at 12:07, emerging from the backdoor dimness, having left his meat-cutting room at the rear of the grocery moments before.

"Special!" And again: "Special!"

Snub's waitress props two Specials on each arm, holds them in a position of poised flight, and heads down one side of the horseshoe-shaped counter. A few stools are empty, no more, and the back room tables are filling quickly.

"Special," announces the waitress and a plate comes off her arm. "Special here?" Another, two stools away, and two more around the bend. She sheds her plates like seasons.

Let us study the dish, itself; dissect its genius. The topography appears authentic: mounds, and gravy lakes, and steam-exhaling *slabs* of things. The plate looks filled, crowded even. And it unarguably is. But what's finally worth admiring is not the size of the portions but the cunning of the arrangement; the ratios.

Start with a pure white plate, diner-thick. Pour instant potatoes into a pot. Water them. Scoop them, mashed-appearing, onto the plate. Quarter-fill it. Uncan a vegetable from a stout, wholesale drum. Heat it, ladle it, half the potato portion. Wedge the meat—a small piece of pork, ham, cube-cheap beef—into the composition. In there next to the potatoes where empty plate still shows. All right, now take the gravy ladle, dip it low into the pot and bring it up full. Lower it into, not just onto, the potato hill, creating as you do a movement of geological certainty—a reservoir for the gravy and simultaneously a plate-filling food slide that runs to the edible rim. On an accompanying smaller plate, stack four pieces of white bread, pats of butter. Into a dish set a jello square in one of two flavors—Red or Dark Red, depending upon Snub's attention to the chemistry. There you have it, a Special, all its consistencies mixing and eddying as it travels along on Snub's waitress' arm.

Snub's illusion fools no one, and doesn't really try to. His motive, as a merchant and a son of the place, is to keep the price low and, at the same time, present a Special vaguely reminiscent of the ancestral dinner. Which he does. His Special weighs as much as any meal my mother ever cooked. So no one really minds if the Meat Loaf, 95¢, is mostly "loaf." Or almost no one. No one who lives here and understands the terms of the offering.

About 11:00, or 11:15, Snub comes out of his kitchen carrying the day's first Special. It is his. He is his first customer. He sets the plate on the counter, fills his coffee mug, swings around the end of the horseshoe, and climbs up on a stool. "Damn french fryer," he mutters, removing his "grease goggles" and wiping his eyes. Snub is of average height, thick-chested, with sandy-colored wings of hair that rise above his temples. He devours his Special at starvation-speed. He is not really hungry, just in a hurry. To Snub, food is fuel. Fuel and his merchandise, nothing more. He holds his fork in a childlike grip—thumb along the shaft, like the bottom hand of a golf grip—and shovels the Special home. "God," he growls, cornering the last speck of meat loaf with a piece of bread, "I'm glad that's over. Now I can get on with the finer things in life." He lights one, and draws from the cellar of his lungs.

Once, a storekeeper who had been having some trouble with the meat loaf offered Snub his wife's recipe.

He replied, "Do I look like Betty Crocker?"

Snub refuses all recipes as a matter of policy—has never read a cookbook—this is his way of keeping a curb on business. "I've got a bigger noon crowd than I can handle," he explains. "What would happen if the food got better?"

Which is not to say he doesn't care about the food, is not solicitous of his customers. He even plans his menu with the season's vegetables in mind. So to speak. For Jean Troisgros, that means inspecting provincial produce stands every morning; for Snub, it means substituting canned peas for canned corn when the autumn grain harvest is at its peak. "The poor devils," he says of the farmers who head over to the Please-U after delivering wagonloads of corn to the town's grain silos. "They see so much corn this time of year. Last place they want to see more of it is on their plate."

Several years ago Snub remodeled the Please-U. He gave it a new facade and, inside, covered its surfaces—counter, floors, table tops, a new layer of tile and plastic, like generational rings of a tree. When the bills came, he met them with cash. "That's the way," he says. "Anybody buys things on credit doesn't own them, he owns *at* them." His philosophy extends to the bottom of his meal checks, where he asks a customer for the amount, plus tax, and refuses anything else. "I'm in the restaurant business, but I don't believe in tips. Tips are an excuse to starve your help."

He says, "Oh, maybe if we go down to the Gold Buffet in Knoxville [a place whose special appeal is a long buffet table crammed with twelve flavors of beef, gelatin salads in all the pastels, and an open invitation to return for extra helpings], I'll leave a dollar. They almost shame ya into it down there after you've gone back for your third plate of meat."

The front door of the Please-U swings open and a group of local men, dressed in dark suits, enters.

Snub asks them, "Who died?"

"Elton Montgomery," says the first man.

The 11:00 funeral has let out. Eleven and two are the popular times and, in a rural midwestern area whose early citizens have not traveled far, the times are often elected.

The dark-suited men take two back-room tables, order Specials. Seeing them, Snub knows that the young undertaker (he only recently bought into the funeral home) will be along shortly, having tended to the janitorial details. The undertaker calls Snub's tenderloins "cardboard specials." "He says you can't tell if it's pork or cardboard inside, with all the breading around it. He's right. You can't. He's a real character," says Snub, "when you know him."

A man wearing a suit is a rarity in the Please-U at any time, but especially if his face is unfamiliar. Prairie City has never been a magnet for tourist curiosity, and its commerce is fairly self-contained. But since the interstate highway cut, east and west, through the middle of Iowa, Prairie City has seen, now and then, a traveler who's left the road at the Colfax exit, seven miles north, made a wrong turn, and wound up in the flat, bleak center of the village. The Please-U, at that point, seems a logical place to ask directions.

Not long ago, a man came through the door, looking spectacularly lost. Entering Prairie City, he had no doubt noted the empty vistas, spreading from ranch-style homes on the fringes of town; had sensed the weight of sky and open spaces lying like a tent canvas on the town; the low, treeless sweep; the spare geometry. He'd taken it all in and, from the expression on his face as he entered the Please-U, feared that English was not the spoken language.

It was about 11:30. The place was nearly empty. The traveler was tall, thin, conservatively dressed in a dark blue suit. His gray hair was combed straight back from a sharp V at his forehead. It was reasonable to suspect he might have been from another state. He might even have been a Democrat.

He approached Snub, who was sorting silverware at the base of the horseshoe.

"How ya doin'?" Snub asked. The traveler explained, and Snub advanced simple directions involving a few left turns. Then the stranger decided he was hungry.

"Well, great," he said, clasping his hands. "As long as I'm here, I may as well get some lunch." (Did you hear that? Lunch.) "What's good?"

"Oh," Snub growled, holding a bouquet of spoons. "What's good is that I've been burnin hamburgers for thirty-one years and nobody's died eatin the stuff yet." He smiled radiantly.

The stranger eased himself onto a stool.

Snub said, "Actually, we got the regular sandwiches, fries. And," nodding to the blackboard, "we got a Special."

The traveler followed Snub's eyes, turned on his stool and saw, in chalk:

Special

ham and beans

95¢

"Ham and beans," he said softly and tried as casually as possible to see if any of the customers had ordered Specials. No one had. Roger, the delivery boy at DeWit's Grocery, was methodically devouring a double order of french fries, a ketchup-covered bluff. Two farmers, on the other side of the Please-U, were perched forward on their stools, sipping coffee and staring, wholly mesmerized, at the traveler, as if he were a television show. Snub had turned away to wipe the counter, grumping, "I'm so busy, I don't know which ashtray to empty first." The traveler straightened his tie. He asked, "What sort of, um, *beans* are they?"

"*Beans,*" Snub said. "You know. Soup beans. Like lima beans, only smaller. Pale, kinda pink-colored beans? Ham-and-beans beans."

"Right," said the stranger. "Fine. I'll have the Special."

"One Special," said Snub. "Coffee?"

"Please."

"Cream?"

"Yes. Cream."

"One Special. One coffee, one moo cow." Snub hurried back to the kitchen.

The traveler rocked around on his stool, trying to

seem at home. The farmers leaned forward radically, as if they'd later be required to describe him in detail. Feeling their eyes, he turned to meet the full blade of their stare.

"How you fellows doing?" he asked.

"Oh, fair and warmer," went the reply.

Lord. English was *not* the spoken tongue.

He squinted at the big clock hanging above Snub's cooking window. The businesses of Prairie City had rented advertising space around its face. It was 20 minutes till Dee's Beauty Salon. The traveler swiveled warily toward the door, like an inmate contemplating a dash past a sleeping guard, but as he did, the door flew open, and that's when John Shuey came bustling in.

Shuey has lived in Prairie City all his adult life and is something of a legend in Jasper County. He sells livestock, and his work takes him to all the small towns that dot the table-smooth landscape, making him, in comparison with most people here, who travel from their farms to their towns and back again, positively cosmopolitan. If you do not know Shuey, you know about him, have heard stories of some practical joke, real or apocryphal, the distinction blurs; or of his merciless memory. People say that if Shuey has caught you in a bit of foolishness, or has heard of some, he will sooner or later enact it for you at the exactly inappropriate moment. Everyone in Jasper County likes Shuey; they have to.

He's in his 50's but looks younger. Black, neatly combed hair tops what was once, clearly, an athlete's frame.

Shuey walked to the counter and nodded to the farmers.

"Hey, John," they said together, bravely smiling.

Shuey nodded again and sat down beside the traveler. He briefly took him in. Here, he knew, was a man who'd made a wrong turn.

The traveler smiled at Shuey and said, as if in explanation, "Having a little lunch."

Shuey smiled approvingly. "Having a little lunch, myself."

"The Special," said the traveler.

"Oh," said Shuey. "What's today? Barbequed watermelon?"

"No. Ham and beans," he said. "You know, *soup* beans."

"Right," Shuey said. "Watermelon's Tuesday. I forgot. You know, I better wash up." He left his stool and made his way around the counter, passing the farmers. "Garrett," he said to one, "You better get home. I drove by your place. Your fences are down and your wife's got out." He disappeared toward the back of the Please-U, into the dark.

Snub came out of the kitchen, bearing the traveler's Special. "Here you go," he said, and set it before him. He gave him utensils, refilled his coffee cup, withdrew a napkin from the dispenser and placed it beside the plate. Without a word, he headed back to tend his grill.

The traveler examined the Special from several angles,

drawing by Gerry Gersten

as if for a little flag marked START HERE. He eased a fork into the jello—Dark Red, that day—and took a small bite. Then he turned his attention to the ham and beans and shifted them around a bit. The ham had to be unearthed, it was just a few translucent strands wound through the beans. As usual. And beneath the beans, swelling them to a small hummock on the plate, were mashed potatoes. The traveler, daunted, got by on spinster-bites, chewing carefully for clues.

A few minutes later, Shuey returned. He stopped at the kitchen, accepted a Special from Snub and, after a long instant, carried it back to his seat.

"How is it?" he asked.

"Oh, fine," the traveler said. "I've been wishing for some soup beans."

"Good," Shuey said, and took a big bite. "Myself, I like the ham. Umm, that ham's good, isn't it?"

The traveler glanced at Shuey's plate. He saw, nearly hiding the beans, huge cubes of ham—pink, dominant, as if a block wall of ham had collapsed on the plate. He glanced back at his own Special, at the five strands that lay across his beans like tiny shadows.

Looking everywhere but at his neighbor's dish, Shuey added, "Ham and beans is one of Snub's best Specials. Lucky you stopped today."

The traveler ate silently. He took a bite, looked to Shuey's plate, took another. Shuey matched him stroke for stroke, staring straight ahead at a vision of angels, and acknowledging no more than the certainty of weather to other customers now entering and packing the cafe. At precisely irritating intervals, however, he would mumble, almost inaudibly, "Mmm." And when he did, the traveler's face would flush to a deeper red, so that, by meal's end, it had all the hue of a new flavor of jello.

The traveler ate every bean, every bit of the Special, and when the waitress delivered his check, he asked if he might see Snub.

Shuey smiled up at him as he waited, and said, "You ate fast. Musta been hungry. I don't know if I can finish all mine."

Snub came hustling out. He was puzzled and slightly peeved to be summoned from his stove at the day's most crowded moment. The traveler faced him, rod-stiff. He told Snub, "I just want you to know that your blatant condescension towards anyone other than local has not been lost on me. I may have been lost, but I assure you, sir, I am not stupid. Here is my check. Ninety-five cents, plus tax." And from his pocket he produced a handful of change. "And here, for your labor, is a tip. One nickel." With that, he strode dramatically from the Please-U.

Snub watched the traveler get into his car, then scanned the insult he held in his palm. He turned to Shuey, who by now had polished off the evidence and was managing a sudden interest in the ads on Snub's clock.

Finally, Snub just said, "What the hell was that about? A *tip*? That guy was more lost than I thought. Where'd he think he was? The Gold Buffet in Knoxville?"

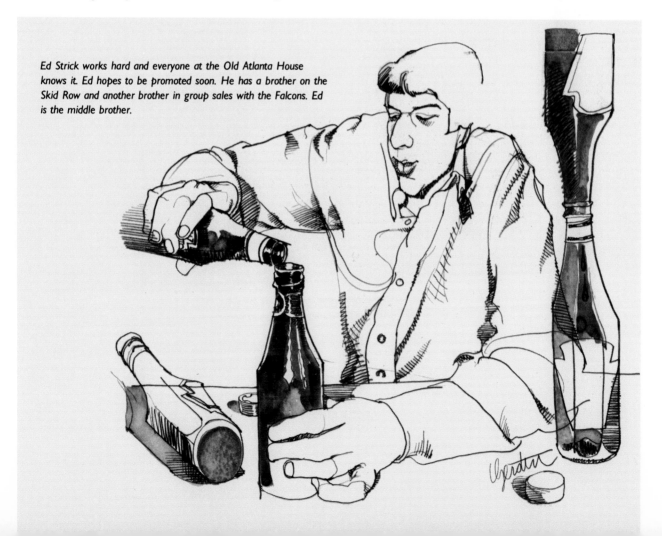

Ed Strick works hard and everyone at the Old Atlanta House knows it. Ed hopes to be promoted soon. He has a brother on the Skid Row and another brother in group sales with the Falcons. Ed is the middle brother.

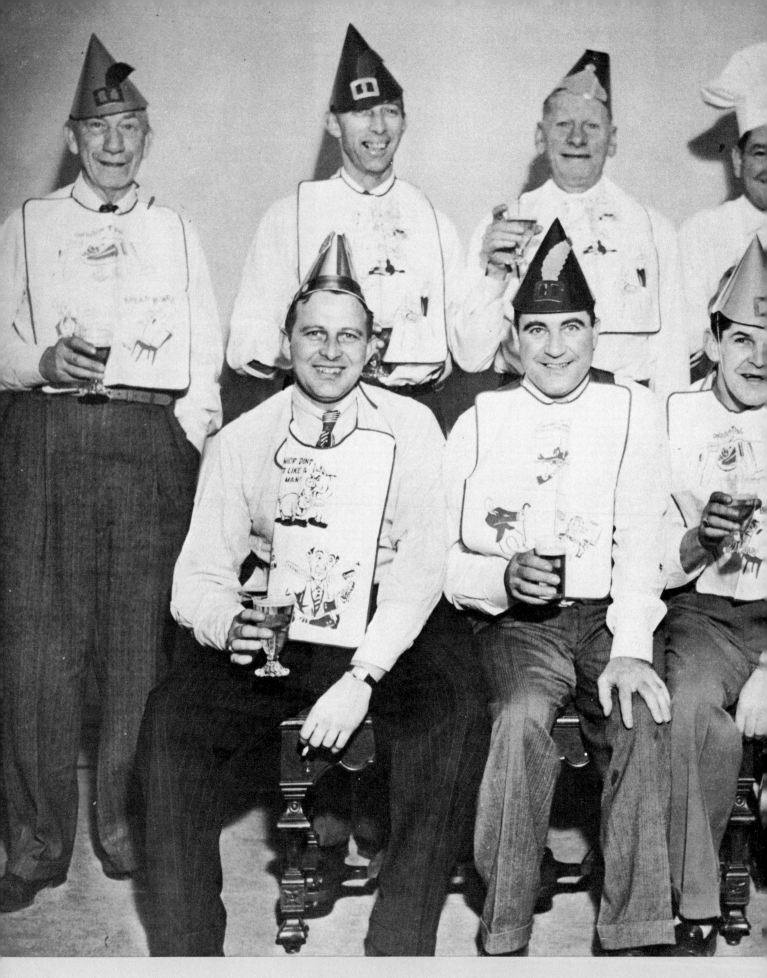

Animal Alcoholism

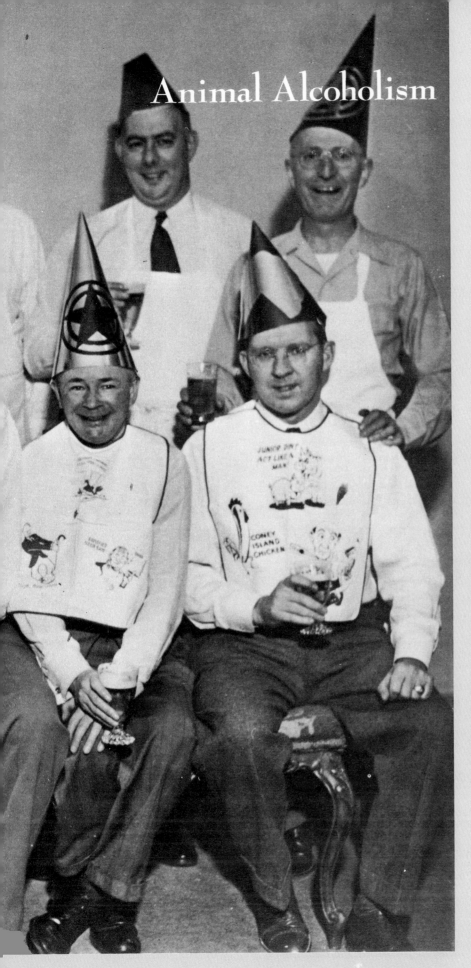

"With all me faults there's still wan thing I niver done," said Mr. Dunley, leaning across his bar.

"And what's that?" asked Mr. Fennessy, as he stepped into the Jughead Road establishment for the first time in over half a century.

"I niver sa-arved a dhrink to annythin' 'twas on all fures on th' way in, so help me hivins," said Mr. Dunley.

"Have ye been samplin' ye'er wares agin, Dunley?" replied Fennessy.

"Come now, Finnissy, haven't ye anny idea why 'tis we're seein' mure an' mure of the Good Lord's babby creathures squished an' decapotatoed alongside th' highways? What with th' speed limith gawn down all th' time?"

"Can't say that I have," confessed Mr. Fennessy.

"Cause the animals be dhrunk! And do ye know who we've got to thank f'r this sorry state of things?"

"I haven't a clew," said Mr. Fennessy.

"It's the industhry boodlers. Ye kin be sure they're ma-akin' a gr-rand livin' off little livers! Whin I heerd tell iv th' new push-open beer ca-ans, I cud niver in th' wurruld iv imagined 'twas f'r some pinty-snouted or horney animal t'poke his shnoot in there an' toss wan down. 'N those roadside establishments plunked down in th' middle of some gawdf'rsakin stretch o' th' counthryside—ye think it's people they're sa-arvin'? Why, whin th' slaughterin' iv huntin' sayson rayturns, th' game will be in th' same condishun of robust bad health as th' la-ads in th' blinds. Meself, I cuddent see me doin' nawthin' to help a phaysant be self-bastin'. Bedad, 'tis an onwholesome an' injoorious situashun f'r th' whole animal kingsom, an' a thricky wan f'r th' bist iv human ba-artinders."

"What is there to be done?" cried Mr. Fennessy.

"Me, I giv the man from the Animal Alcohol Abyoos Comity me word I'd be sa-arvin' no customer in a bear suit 'cept he kin take it off. But unless all me associates in th' profession do likewise, th' raysult cud be a lost winter f'r th' la-ads."

—Gary Lippman

The Multinational Corporation Cookbook

United Fruit Salad

600,000 tons bananas
500,000 tons pineapples
300,000 tons sugar
275,000 tons mangoes
100,000 gallons guava paste
1 Honduran Presidente
2 million dollars

Pick bananas, mangoes, pineapples fresh from harvest at lowest possible cost. Add sugar and guava paste. Mix together in large freighters. Clean 2 million dollars thoroughly, using Swiss bank, before adding to Honduran Presidente underneath table. You may add a touch of CIA to reduce flavor of nationalization to taste.

Serves corporate board of 10.

ITT Chilean Coup Stew

1 head Marxisti Red cabbage
39 innocuous fronts
1 oppressed populace

1 large bundle frozen assets
1 fresh supply liquid untraceable assets
409 seasoned cloaks-and-daggers
1 pickled American Congress

Funnel liquid assets into innocuous fronts, then stir up populace. Using an official disclaimer, add cloaks-and-daggers while squeezing appropriations from pickled American Congress. Let it come to a boil. Now it should be easy to shred Red cabbage into tiny bits. Defrost assets and extract juice.

Serves congressional committee of 8.

Exxon Kebab

17 lean Saudi sheiks
4 million barrels crude oil
12 bankloads mixed petrodollars
500 million consumers (pressed)

Carefully skewer the consumers and baste in crude oil. At the same time, give yourself plenty of allowance for oil depletion. Season sheiks with petrodollars, cover with military

aid (add jets if necessary), and let stand in large tankers just offshore until price rises to top. Serve with lots of tax and add kickbacks to taste.

Serves nation of 250 million.

Seoul Fried Porkbarrel

1 pocketful of envelopes
1 quorum congressmen
handfuls of refried foreign aid (in tens and twenties)
1 pig's eye

Stuff envelopes with refried tens and twenties. Add to congressmen and stir until votes can be skimmed off top. Let it get hot, but don't burn your Tong. Place on bed of hooker and serve in a pig's eye. Good for a picnic in the Park. One helpful Tip: wait for porkbarrel to cool off before serving to gullible press. Add immunity if necessary.

Serves a foreign interest of one.

Chase Manhattan De-Lite

1 portfolio South African investments
40,000 gold nuggets
40,000 gallons whipped Negro blood

Stuff investments with gold nuggets and garnish with fancy swirls of whipped topping. Raise the prime rate if not high enough. Goes nicely alongside Oysters Rockefeller.

Serves interlocking directorate of 4.

Pepsi Kremlin Punch

30 million bottles Pepsi (nonreturnable)
40 million bottles vodka (Stolichnaya)
800 million bushels wheat

Mix together in large samovar until wheat disappears. Add a touch of strained détente and SALT to taste. Serve in diplomatic pouches.

Serves summit conference of 18.

—Rex Weiner

collage by Gary Friedman

drawing by Rick Meyerowitz

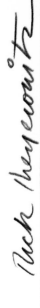

ANOTHER GREAT MOMENT IN CORPORATE RESPONSIBILITY

Tom Carvel is always doing things for people. He can't help himself. His Carvel ice cream stores in the New York-New England area are always sponsoring one giveaway or another. In the early '70's, once yearly, it was ponies, according to a source close to the corporation. Unfortunately, National Velvet loses some of its sock around the wide open spaces of Bridgeport, or Teaneck, or Worcester, and many of the ponies went unclaimed, or were returned by parents frustrated by the upkeep, or their own stupid inability to turn an elevator shaft into a corral. So what to do with all these ponies piling up, was the problem confronting the Carvel Corp. Meanwhile, T.C.—to his friends—had begun constructing a whole community in Pine Plains, N.Y., up in Duchess County, called Sports City. It started off with a wild animal menagerie and an amusement park, and was eventually supposed to include a retirement village and a golf club. When the bulldozers came in to lay the sewer system, however, they unearthed a cache of bones. T.C. had just gotten tired of all those unwanted ponies standing around, the source continues, so he had them slaughtered and fed to the wild animals.

Given a chance to respond to this allegation, Glenn Keegan, house counsel for the Carvel Corporation, denied the story, reminded JUNK FOOD that he had warned it against the inclusion of the Carvel name in any book calling itself JUNK FOOD, and said, "We deny that the ponies were even on the property," adding, "The property is posted against things like hunting," and finishing up, "Really, this whole pony and wild animal business doesn't bear commenting on."

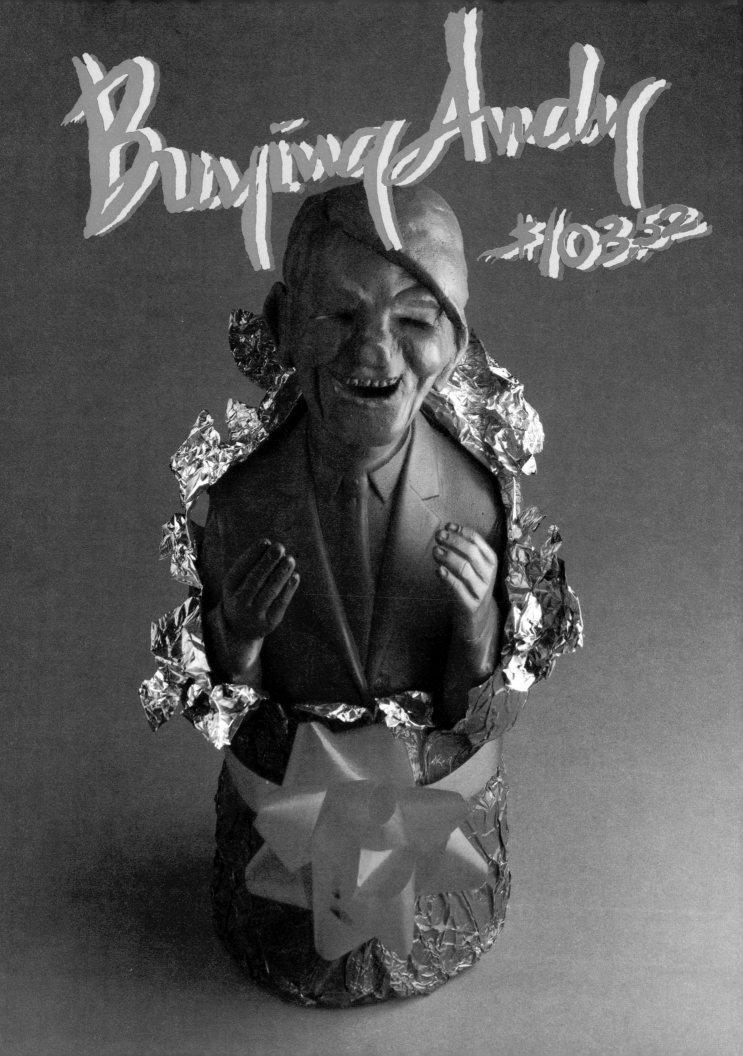

by Jonathan Etra

Andy eats. Andy eats in little bites.

I surmise that Andy cuts in little chunks, paints in little dabs.

Some are born to junk food . . . some must subscribe; Andy gets house seats. "The most beautiful thing," he says, "in Tokyo is McDonald's. The most beautiful thing in Stockholm is McDonald's . . . in Florence is . . . ." Oy, basta! His own franchise— Andy-mats—impends: a chain of frozen-food sit-down supermarkets, inexpensive, efficient (pneumatic tubes deliver everything), entertaining (a TV at every chair). Million-dollar funding eludes, but Andy is not discouraged. There is always candy. As a child, Andy receives a Hershey bar for every page colored in his coloring book. Two pieces of bread, candy in the middle, that's a sandwich.

We wish to lunch with Andy. Who are we? the secretary asks. Replies are insufficient.

It is Andy's birthday. We send five pounds, solid milk chocolate. He calls us.

We appear at the Warhol Factory, 860 Broadway, a shopping bag of penny candy along for support. Volunteers separate out the chocolate for Andy, who prefers Chunkies: Andy, a bottomless face, riveleted, gouged, indented like verse.

Other gifts are suggested and we comply. Now they know us. We are buyers, they are bought.

Lunch is set. We are sent to McDonald's. A cheeseburger and medium Coke forgot, we are sent back. At table, finally, in the Factory's mahogany dining room, Andy, Paul (Morrissey, dir. Trash, Flesh, AW's Frankenstein), Rob (Geddes), Bridget (Polk), Ronnie (Cutrone), we. The food comforts Andy—it is all wrapped. Andy will not eat unless he has viewed all wrappers, packaging, art.

"Not even a slice of pizza," says Bridget, "until he sees the box."

	TAB
5 lbs. chocolate	$25.00
tax	2.00
1 shopping bag assorted candy	21.60
1 Fraser-Morris smoked turkey (frozen)	34.95
delivery	1.50
McDonald's lunch for 6	8.56
medium Coke and cheeseburger	1.09
umbrella (forgotten)	3.00
Spiderman kite	5.40
string	.42
Andy's Price (as of 10/78)	$103.52

Lunch is opened.

ROB: They're going to have to do something about the Filet o' Fishes.
PAUL: You know, they're not good. You ever read what they do to make this fish?
RONNIE: They grind up the whole fish.
ROB: Isn't it called. . . .
PAUL: It's not, it's dolphin. . . .
ROB: Dolphin! Dolphin's too expensive. It's called sea trout. It's called sea perch and sea perch is the name for all the fish that they grind up. It's like pressed meat or something. Head cheese.
PAUL: They bleach it. It's all bleached.
ROB: I'm sure it's all crappy dark meat from a whole mess of fishes and they just bleach it. Ketchup, please.

BRIDGET: Who got the candy?
ANDY: Uh, Benjamin.
ROB: Do you hear that, Andy? How they make that fish?
ANDY: No, how do they make it?
ROB: They take any old fish they can find, any old salt water fish they can find. And usually it's just crappy dark meat or something. And they bleach it and they press it. . . .
ANDY: No, that's not true.
ROB: Yes, it's like head cheese.
ANDY: No, it isn't! They don't do it this way, it's called, ah. . . .
PAUL: No, this is not fresh.
ANDY: No, it isn't? Are you sure? Are you right?
ETRA: I'm not sure, Rob is sure. I'm vaguely sure.
PAUL: No, I read about it. This is. . . . If you look at it you can see it's not fresh, but it's bleached.
ANDY: No, it's not bleached.
PAUL: Yes, it's bleached white.
ROB: I wonder what kind of fish it is?

Everyone wonders.

1

ROB: Are there any good barbeque houses in New York?
PAUL: That's poison, barbeque. It's cancer.
ROB: Listen, what Bridget's eating is cancer, the sauce on the Big Mac.

2

College

PAUL: You know what's the sickest thing? In England, whenever you get chicken. . . . I mean I thought I was dreaming, but it tastes and smells like fish. I happened to mention it to somebody who said, look, all the chicken is fed with ground up fish manure. So the chicken tastes exactly like fish and smells like fish. Which is really sick. Also in England, they recycle all their sewerage and drink it.
ANDY: Oh, they do that there?
PAUL: Yeh, they've been doing that for years.
RONNIE: And drink it?
PAUL: Yeh, and drink it!
ROB: And here too.
ETRA: I heard yesterday that Larry Flynt drinks his urine. I thought that should be shared.
ROB: He's in a wheel chair!
PAUL: That's done by the Prime Minister of India.
ANDY: That's right, we know a lot of people who drink it.
PAUL: Isn't there a bar in New York where they do that?
ROB: Yeh, one just closed down.

Beverage banter.

BRIDGET: Does that fall into the category of junk food?
ETRA: It is—recycling waste material!
ROB: You must have gone to Columbia?
ETRA: I should have, simply for the access to some vague life.

3

ETRA: We need a watermelon. Is there any place that will send up a watermelon?

ROB: Yes there is.
ANDY: We've decided you're not a good host. This is your lunch.
ETRA: I am deeply apologetic.
ANDY: You'll have to do it again another day.
ETRA: We will have to have a repeat.
ANDY: I know.
ROB: But turn off the phones and lock the doors and have a big feast, a big one.
BRIDGET: I mean even if you had bought me 60 McDonald's hamburgers—
PAUL: You know it was a big decision whether to become a chicken joint at McDonald's.
ROB: What?
PAUL: Because the cancer scare.
ROB: About what?
PAUL: The fried hamburgers. McDonald's might go chicken.
BRIDGET: McDonald's might go chicken? Have you heard that?
PAUL: They talked about it, I saw it in the paper.
ROB: Have you ever had that Kentucky Fried Chicken?
ANDY: They have that artificial banana thing, and then they'll go out and give a quarter to leukemia victims.
PAUL: Isn't that funny. Isn't that ironic.
RONNIE: Not to mention the microwave ovens. That's another thing.
PAUL: They're leaking.
ROB: Leaking? What do you mean leaking?
PAUL: They leak and give you cancer.
ANDY: They do?
RONNIE: Everything gives you cancer. Except they've just found a cure.
BRIDGET: What? This new interferon?
RONNIE: Yeh.
BRIDGET: Have you heard about this new thing?
ANDY: No, what's that?

4

BRIDGET: Well, there's something in human cells that when you get, say, a virus or something, these cells produce this stuff called interferon, which fights off the virus. But the trouble is, it doesn't produce enough of it. They think it might work with cancer. It has to be human interferon.
RONNIE: Of course, anything you can possibly get you can fight off, naturally. But the problem is overpopulation.
ROB: Sounds like a rip-off.
PAUL: The problem isn't overpopulation. It's overpopulation by the wrong people.
ROB: Right.
RONNIE: Shall we decide who are those people?
PAUL: Everyone should pull their own weight, as Archie Bunker said.
RONNIE: The welfare state.
PAUL: Yes.

5

ROB: I told you about seeing Frank Perdue, last week, dancing? He's the best dancer you've ever seen.
ANDY: Really?
PAUL: Who is?
ROB: Frank Perdue.
ANDY: But he killed somebody with his car last year?
PAUL: The old man is a good dancer?
ROB: Frank Perdue! He's a fabulous dancer.

model by Jim Wilson, photograph by Carl Waltzer

PAUL: Where did you see him dancing?

RONNIE: Where could he possibly be dancing?

ROB: Uptown.

PAUL: What do you mean uptown? At an uptown discotheque?

ROB: Yeh.

BRIDGET: Where is he, at 54?

ROB: Uh-um.

RONNIE: When I went to see the play *Dracula,* he was there.

PAUL: People recognize him?

ROB: Out on the block.

PAUL: Guess that's part of his job . . . to go out and be seen?

RONNIE: (bleeds in) . . . Dom De Luise plays the lead!

ROB: Somebody saw him on 72nd Street, on the block.

PAUL: (turns) I always see Dom De Luise.

RONNIE: And I like him.

ANDY: I think he's very funny.

PAUL: He's in all the old movies. Other than that, he's always on the talk shows. And all he talks about is having sex with his wife on the talk shows.

ROB: Who?

BRIDGET: I don't know who he is?

PAUL: Dom-ee De Luis-ee. Dom De Luis-ee.

BRIDGET: He looks like Koch?

PAUL: No, he's round.

ROB: Frank Perdue's handsome.

BRIDGET: What?

PAUL: Oh, Koch? Yes, Perdue looks like Koch.

BRIDGET: He does look like Koch.

ROB: Yeh, but he's more handsome.

PAUL: He is not.

ROB: He is so.

BRIDGET: Oh, say, you've gotta be. . . . you're nuts today.

RONNIE: Did you watch Johnny Carson?

ROB: I am not.

BRIDGET: You've said the nuttiest things I've ever heard you say, today.

RONNIE: They're doing this summer repeat, the best of Johnny Carson. It looked really excellent, so good.

ANDY: Yeh, well, why don't you tell us about your summer. . . ?

RONNIE: I always hated Sammy Davis, Jr., until I saw him on Johnny Carson.

PAUL: I always hated him till I met him once. He's so sweet. You get to watch him in person, he's the most untalented human being on the face of the earth.

RONNIE: No, but he really sang well, the other night. Oh, really, like, you know, I watched it last night. He's fabulous.

PAUL: Did you see what John Simon. . . . He's in a show where he plays a "Little Chap," this character in some *Stop the World,* called "Little Chap." John Simon said they should call him "Little Chimp." They took it out of the review. Then the following week he said, my editors made me take out "Little Chimp" and put in "Little Chump."

RONNIE: But he was so fabulous on Johnny Carson last night.

ANDY: Who? Dom De Luise?

RONNIE: No. Sammy Davis.

ANDY: O.

PAUL: Singing and dancing. . . .

RONNIE: I always hated him. I always hated him. . . .

PAUL: Singing and dancing, he's good?

RONNIE: He was . . . no!

PAUL: Talking, he's good?

RONNIE: No, he sang. He was good.

PAUL: He can't dance.

RONNIE: He sang for about five or six minutes last night and it was incredible. He's *so* good. I always hated him. I always despised him. But he really sang well. He did all these jazz, you know, up-tempo-down type of blah-blah-blah, and he really sounded great. And then he started talking, and for the first time on TV he brought his wife out.

PAUL: What color is his wife?

RONNIE: Black. Now.

6

PAUL: Schrafft's is totally gone? Does Schrafft's exist in ice cream or something?

ANDY: A little bit, yeh.

PAUL: Remember Schrafft's logo?

BRIDGET: I love Schrafft's. The old Schrafft's.

PAUL: Schrafft's had a logo. You must remember their logo, that little line under Schrafft's? It used to say, "Where tradition lingers." That was Schrafft's logo.

ROB: Do they still have those fancy restaurants uptown, Schrafft's?

ETRA: There's one Schrafft's left.

PAUL: There is?

ETRA: There's two, there're two. There's one a block south of the Public Library on Fifth Avenue. And there's one opposite the General Motors Building on Madison.

PAUL: Opposite General Motors!

7

ANDY: (fingering gift box of Russell Stover) That's the best candy made now.

BRIDGET: There's one at 58th and Madison.

ROB: It's better than Godiva?

ANDY: Yeh.

ROB: Russell Stover?

ANDY: Yeh, it's really good.

ROB: I don't get to eat this mass-produced candy.

PAUL: And what about poor Horn & Hardart's, totally gone.

ETRA: There's one.

PAUL: There is?

BRIDGET: 42nd.

ETRA: Yeah, 42nd. They put a side in the Smithsonian.

PAUL: They don't have the little. . . .

ETRA: They have little windows, yeah.

Barbara Allen stops by to say hello.

ROB: Columbus, Ohio, is supposedly the mecca for fast food. It's where a lot of them rear and die. It's supposed to be *the* American city.

BRIDGET: Is Roy Rogers good?

ROB: Oh yeh! They're really good. You've never been to Roy Rogers?

RONNIE: They make their sandwiches roast beef and hamburger, too. That's the worst thing I ever heard. They make their hamburger patty with slabs of roast beef on it.

ROB: You ever been to Arby's? Those are really good.

BRIDGET: I haven't been to anyplace but McDonald's and Arthur Treacher's.

ROB: They have great barbeque sauce. That's the worst, Arthur Treacher's.

PAUL: Isn't it funny how Arthur Treacher's, they use the name and he's been dead for so many years. I mean, who are they impressing?

ETRA: He'll be back.

PAUL: No, but I mean, why bother to promote the name if a man is . . . nobody remembers.

RONNIE: Everybody remembers him.

PAUL: Think so?

RONNIE: Yeh.

ANDY: Well, he was on the Merv. . . .

PAUL: Merv, Merv Griffin.

ANDY: Yeh, I met him.

RONNIE: He was Merv Griffin's sidekick and Merv Griffin—

PAUL: I guess he was. He was, he was . . . good. I ran into Betsy the other day, she's doing the costumes for Ruth Gordon. She said Ruth Gordon is so old, she's 83, and she doesn't have anybody helping her around, and she keeps getting locked in rooms, the poor thing.

RONNIE: Oh, really? She keeps getting what?

PAUL: She locks herself in rooms and people can't find her. She can't turn the knob cause she's got arthritis.

RONNIE: She's totally gone, totally gone.

PAUL: She's great.

RONNIE: She's my favorite actress.

PAUL: Do you know that she came to New York in 1915, by 1917 she was a star. It's a long time. And then she went and had her legs broken and sawed up to correct her bow-leggedness.

8

RONNIE: I didn't know that.

PAUL: When she was very young she had her legs broken and tried to have them sawed into straight and it never worked. She still is bow-legged today.

ROB: That's why she locks herself in rooms.

PAUL: Is [this book] just about junk food?

ETRA: Well, it's about the junk food ethos. I mean, I consider this to be junk food central. But. . . .

PAUL: Junk food what?

ETRA: Central.

PAUL: Central what?

ETRA: Andy.

PAUL: Andy doesn't eat junk food.

ETRA: Andy is junk food.

BRIDGET: Uh-uh.

ANDY: I don't eat it.

PAUL: No, he doesn't.

ETRA: I thought he eats only at McDonald's.

RONNIE: He doesn't eat anything except a McDonald's hamburger.

BRIDGET: O God, he looks at every label like a maniac.

9

ANDY: O yeh, you know they haven't had different labels on, they don't have a label on this? I mean how come they don't have the name on this and on that?

10

PAUL: And what's in every can.

ANDY: And what's in every can and stuff. I mean how do you know it's true?

PAUL: You know they never said what's in Häagen Dazs? You ever notice that?

BRIDGET: Do you know, everything is junk. You know, what's the thing that makes vanilla Häagen Dazs, chocolate Häagen Dazs, boysenberry, have all the same flavor? That's the chemical. They all taste alike.

PAUL: Häagen Dazs lists no ingredients. I think you only list ingredients if you want to sell in the state of Pennsylvania? Is that right?

Reflection.

PAUL: Well, why do, then, little people put their poisons on their labels?
ROB: Because, it's, you know, probably, you know, label it or pay up, you know.
RONNIE: Because Ralph Nader didn't get to them yet, that's why.
PAUL: You know, I never understood why these people who are trying to sell health foods which say "no additives," all they have to do to sell it is to say "no poisons." Why don't they just say "no poisons in this food," and they would get much more attention.
ANDY: Well, liquor doesn't have any additives.
PAUL: You know what does have additives? I'm just looking at this, is all these beers they're writing about.
ANDY: All of them?
PAUL: They have acids and all sorts of additives in these beers which are very bad. And they don't talk about it at all in this stupid article. All these beers have additives.
ANDY: But not whiskeys, whiskeys don't.
ROB: Sure they do.
RONNIE: Champagne does.
ANDY: Champagne does, nothing is. I always . . .
RONNIE: Champagnes use vitamin C.
ANDY: I don't think they do.
ROB: But apparently the coloring in whiskey is really bad for you?
ANDY: It's just sugar.

11

PAUL: The big, I think the biggest thing is junk food movies. Movies that look like movies, but have no story, no characters, no nothing, and there's nothing there. It's like you saw a movie. It's like *Animal House,* or this thing *Days of Heaven.*
ROB: Did you see *Animal House?*
PAUL: Yeh. And it has the appearance and it looks like, it was a comedy.
ANDY: You should have thought of it.
PAUL: It's just, you know . . .
ANDY: You should have said, "Now, movies that look like movies."
PAUL: I don't think it was thought of. It just sort of evolved when they realized they don't have to give the public anything, just the appearance. That's what these things are, just the appearance of movies. I mean, how can you have movies without a script at all, without any story, and have enormous success! Oh gosh!
RONNIE: Why, you did it for years!
PAUL: We always had a script. Or if we didn't have a story, we said we have no story and that was obvious. And that was a story in itself. But—
ETRA: In summer, people just want a cool place to go to for two hours.

12

ANDY: It's funny to see the, ah, White Towers. They are really white towers. I saw two yesterday.
BRIDGET: Remember the little hamburgers?
PAUL: They still exist? Where? In the Bronx?
ROB: Yeh, they're in the worst neighbor-hoods. Yeh, you see 'em, it's all jigs, you see a White Tower.
ANDY: O I know.
BRIDGET: Are they still edible? The little things that they bring to your car? Are those awful!
PAUL: I remember when they were seven cents, and then if you brought in a coupon . . .
BRIDGET: So romantic.
PAUL: You could get two for eight cents. But they were only that big.
ANDY: They're all in Long Island.
PAUL: Still in Long Island?
ANDY: Yeh, beautiful new white buildings. They're all white.
PAUL: O, they're new? There's White Tower and White Castle. They came in the '30s. One was a copy of the other.
ANDY: No, White Tower is White Castle.
PAUL: No, one was a copy of the other.

13

PAUL: The big, the big, the first big junk food success was Chock Full O' Nuts. And they had, they had their famous slogan, ah, hands, hands never touch the food. We employ . . .

Much laughter.

RONNIE: Dogs, we only have play animals here.
PAUL: You don't remember but that was their slogan. They used to have little people pick, the people always picked up everything with pincers. I don't think they still do any-more, they used to pick up everything and they used to show you making the sandwiches with ah, spatulas. And the bread was picked up and you were supposed to watch them make the sandwich without ever touching. You didn't see them make the stuff that goes into the sandwich, but in front of the counter, the big attraction at Chock Full O' Nuts initially, was you saw them do it right in front of you. All that's gone by the wayside. All the tradition, all the big traditions are gone. But Chock Full O' Nuts still does business.
ROB: Chock Full O' Nuts is still good.
PAUL: They sort of adapt. They keep putting in tacos and, ah, whatever.
RONNIE: I always liked their cream cheese and, ah, date nut bread.
PAUL: That was their original thing, they still have that?
RONNIE: I think so.
PAUL: That was the thing they built their for-tune on.
ROB: Mom always called it chock full o' creams.
PAUL: It was, ah, you know, it was some-thing.
ETRA: Well, what happened to your restau-rant? Is that gone with the wind?
ANDY: No, the Japanese might be doing it.
ETRA: Are there designs and things? Were there tablecloths. . . .
ANDY: Yeh, O yeh, there were.
ETRA: Must have been lovely.
ROB: What, Madison Avenue?
PAUL: But it was all pure, wasn't it?
ROB: Was that where you were going to put it, Madison Avenue?
ANDY: Pure frozen.
PAUL: Pure frozen, right. But no additives.
ANDY: No.

Catherine Guiness stops by.

PAUL: What about the art food of Les Levine? The Irish-Jewish food? That's a big thing, he put out food that was art. Cause he was Jewish-Irish, right?
ANDY: Yeh.
PAUL: Is that what made it art?
ANDY: Yeh.
PAUL: Yeh, it was Jewish-Irish art and was just around the corner. Because he was Jewish-Irish, he called it art food. Which was it? I never had it. Did you ever have it?
ROB: Uh-um.
PAUL: You must have had it?
ANDY: Yeh, everyone did.
RONNIE: He used to own the place . . .
PAUL: The Chock Full O' Nuts.
RONNIE: No, up top of Max's.
PAUL: Yes.
RONNIE: Levine's, Levine's. . . .
PAUL: Isn't that now Chock Full O' Nuts?
RONNIE and others: Yeh, yeh. It is. You're right. Yeh.
PAUL: So he went from art to Chock Full O' Nuts.
RONNIE: What would you call that?
ETRA: It's condensation. Do you ever go to the Belmore?
ANDY: Yeh, years ago, by taxi.
PAUL: On Madison?
ETRA: On Park.
ANDY: No, on Park. You know, where the taxicabs go.
PAUL: On Park, yeh, yeh, with the free selt-zer. They still have free seltzer?
ETRA: Still have free seltzer.
PAUL: Still exist. You know what? They put additives in Perrier.

14

ANDY: They do! No! They. . . . Who told you?
PAUL: Somebody told me they put lithium in it.
ANDY: No, lithium is a—
PAUL: Salt or something, no?
RONNIE: Lithium is natural. I don't know what it is. I can't tell you. . . .
PAUL: O yeh, a lot of things are natural, but in quantities they're killers. I mean it, they're toxic.
RONNIE: Well, tonic water also. Did you ever think—
PAUL: All Schweppes has got saccharine. Schweppes has no sugar; maybe strictly in America, but in Europe Schweppes can't af-ford it and everything that Schweppes puts out is saccharine.
RONNIE: Even the carbonation is bad. I mean, just think—
PAUL: Is that bad?
ANDY: Why?
RONNIE: Because it's artificially induced.
PAUL: But it might be the gas.
RONNIE: Right.
PAUL: And that goes into the water.
RONNIE: Right. All those bubbles.
PAUL: If you boil water and then drink it, is that any good?
ANDY: What keeps you so thin?
ETRA: I get sick every week.
ANDY: O, you do?
ETRA: Yeh, every week something makes me ill.
ANDY: O.
PAUL: You eat a lot of junk food?
ETRA: I don't eat too much junk food. I eat an occasional junk food tidbit. And then, I think, it's the company I keep.

ANDY: What kind of loose company do you keep?

ETRA: *I don't know. I keep the company of either frantic intellectuals or, sort of, lethargic businessmen, or just dangerous shysters.*

Discussion of Sid.

15

ETRA: *The people who fill the refrigerator and the people who empty the refrigerator are different sorts of people. Is that true in your world?*

ANDY: A lot of them are looking *for* a refrigerator. We get to look at the real porkers.

ROB: Last night I had dutch loaf at the delicatessen.

ANDY: Really?

ROB: And Lex had ham and cheese. And Lex looked at it and he thought, he said I was a pervert.

ANDY: Why?

ROB: For having dutch loaf. It's really good. It's like meatloaf.

ETRA: *Is there an egg in it?*

ROB: Uh-uh, dutch loaf. This is, uh, delicatessen food. You know, seasoned delicatessen.

PAUL: You mean they make it in the back of the deli?

ROB: You know, Brunckhorst, or Boar's Head brands from Brooklyn, deli meat.

RONNIE: Deli meat?

ROB: You know, sandwich meat.

PAUL: Sandwich meat, that's another funny kind. That's another junk food, too, luncheon meat.

RONNIE: Luncheon meat!

ROB: Some guy in college used to call me Lunchmeat. He said, he said, this guy Whitney. . . .

ANDY: He'd always meet you after lunch, right?

ROB: No, he'd go, he'd go, "I look at you." You know and he'd come to the meals during the day, "And I look down at the lunch meat and that's what you look like." So I was just Lunchmeat from there on in.

PAUL: You mean you ate this thing for school? You ate this kind of food at school?

ROB: He just called me Lunchmeat all the time.

ETRA: *I think one is always punished by what one is called in high school. I think high school is prepunishment for something. Did you ever get revenge?*

ROB: Ah no. He. No, no, you know the way I got revenge? His name was Whitney Tilt. We always used to call him Wilky Tit.

ETRA: *There you are.*

ROB: Which I thought was revenge.

ANDY: Whitney Tilt! It's like Whitney Tower, isn't it?

PAUL: Whitney Tilt! That's a funny name, Tilt.

16

ROB: I worked as a headwaiter at this really nice hotel-restaurant in the North Shore. And I used to get, ah, you know, the cook was a good buddy of mine. And he'd go, "Hey, Rob, come 'ere. Ah, here, I couldn't make it over to Lawbry's to pick up a bottle of Black Velvet. Here's five bucks, could you get me a bottle?" I'd go over, bring it back, hide it in this little corner. And every night before I went back to school, he would cook me up a big steak on a hero with mushroom sauce or something. So think, a very good restaurant goes for anything I wanted, lobster. . . .

PAUL: People who work in restaurants are so horrible-looking, you can't imagine they have any respect for the food.

Special Sauce

photographs by Shig Ikeda

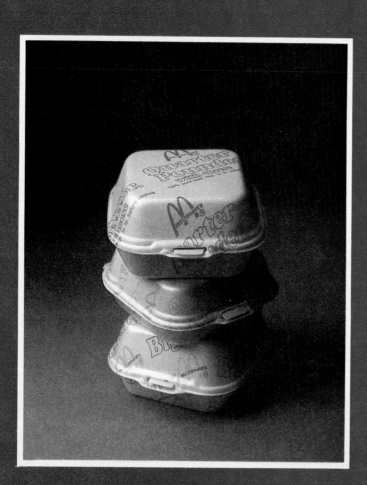

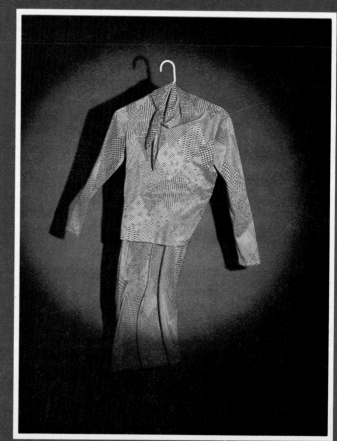

17

SECRETARY: There's a girl on the phone who wants to know about film producing.
ANDY: What's her name?
SEC.: She says she has a degree in filmmaking.
PAUL: And . . . ?
ROB: Don't we all.
PAUL: Tell her to get a degree in film producing.

Rob leaves.

ANDY: What's a natural sweetener?
ETRA: *A natural sweetener? That could be anything from what they get out of a sweet potato. . . .*
PAUL: You know about ketchup?
ETRA: *What?*
PAUL: You know what's in ketchup? American ketchup?
ANDY: Yeh?
PAUL: Ketchup is 30% sugar.
ETRA: *There's sugar in everything.*
BRIDGET: Did that just come out? How come everybody knows it?

ANDY: It just came out on TV.
PAUL: Somebody told it to me. I haven't seen it.
ETRA: *There's sugar in everything. My final theory is that there's a little bit of everything in everything. And it's just what's gonna hurt me tomorrow. I've become very concerned with, I don't know, do you find food menacing?*
ANDY: Food what?
ETRA: *Menacing. I feel very menaced by food of late. I feel it knows I'm coming. And I think it also knows when I go away.*
PAUL: You mean you don't eat everything?
ETRA: *Why no, I think certain foods know when they're being approached, and they know when they've been rescued.*
ANDY: You're talking like Czechoslovakian movies, and they always, they play with the foods. And all those film festivals where they do food cartoons and stuff where all the food would run around and eat everybody up. Remember that one?
ETRA: *Um-hum.*

18

ETRA: *So when did you realize you were addicted to junk food?*

Ronnie goes to the men's room.

ANDY: Junk food?
ETRA: *Fast food. Hamburgers, chocolate bars.*
ANDY: I don't know. When, when . . . how old were you?
ETRA: *I think I realized. . . .*
ANDY: You learn this at Harvard or Yale?
ETRA: *No, I learned nothing there. If I could possibly write that I learned. . . .*
PAUL: You know what you should write about? It's an interesting issue, how McDonald's definitely, you know, purposely, stayed out of New York City for so many years until the court ordered them to allow them in New York City.
ETRA: *You mean that's true?*
PAUL: Cause you know why? They were right. They knew exactly what would happen is. They didn't want to go into New York City or any of the cities because they realized that their low-priced hamburgers, they were selling hamburgers to Americans on the road as healthy, American-style, you know, intelligent food. And they realized, once they went into the city, it would be monopolized by Negroes

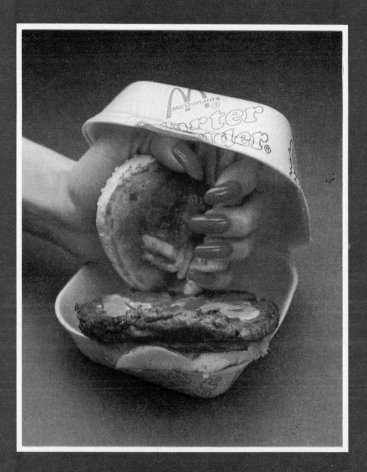

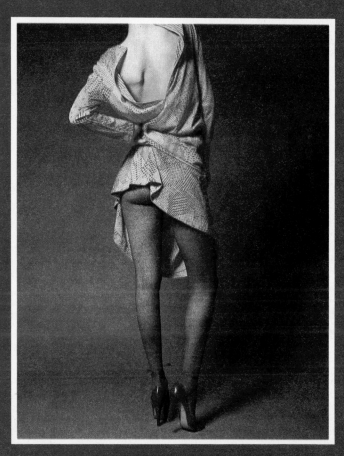

and drug addicts. And so it's true. And so McDonald's has become the food of the Negro and the welfare, the drug addict. And the white people now disdain it on the highways where the big money was because they think it's Negro food. And it's true, and it's interesting that they knew enough.
ANDY: Is that true?
PAUL: Um, they tried to keep out of New York City for years.
ANDY: But. O, that's not true.
PAUL: Yes it is. McDonald's had been a big success for years, and it was only because someone took them to court, because they wouldn't allow a franchise in New York City. That's true. 'Cause the said, "No, we don't want our food connected with the Negroes." They didn't say that but that was their logic, and that's what happened. Now it's the food of the colored people.
ETRA: But you know where they're making inroads? With kids.
PAUL: Well, kids like McDonald's because they go and buy it themselves. They're not stranded at a table.
ETRA: But it's all their own environment. It's sort of a kid's world.
PAUL: Well, the kids are being raised to become Negroes in America. The noise, the music, it's true. Negroes have won the game. They don't have to assimilate to be whites, the whites are changing into Negroes. The kids bop to the Negro bop. You know, boom, boom, boom, boom, whatever that sound is that they like. They're raised on it and they think the Negroes are great, and they're indistinguishable from the Negro now, the American kids, the white kids.
ANDY: But I don't understand the leukemia thing. You know, they do this artificial bananas. There's no banana in it, and then they give 25¢ to leukemia, young leukemia victims?
PAUL: It's really, you know, for murders.
ANDY: Well, I mean, isn't that artificial stuff additive? I mean—
PAUL: Well, they can't say leukemia is caused by that entirely. Additives certainly cause some type of cancer. Leukemia is a type of cancer.

Side Two

ANDY: You know, really, Bridget went up ten pounds because of you last week.
ETRA: Is that my fault?
ANDY: Yeh, your fault.
ETRA: Well, I take responsibility.
BRIDGET: I lost ten pounds this week.
PAUL: Remember how everyone wanted a McDonald's on their block? Now they say it'll bring Negroes onto the block.
ETRA: I know of neighborhoods that don't want bookstores.

19

PAUL: How about the Rockefellers, they could have done something about not abandoning the city to high rises, but they didn't care. Rockefellers don't seem to care about anything anymore. I think they're Communists. They don't care about Radio City Music Hall. They don't care about anything. I think they've gone totally Bolshevik.
ETRA: And they did kill that little kid.
PAUL: He killed them.
ETRA: He killed him? That little kid who col-

lided with the senior Rockefeller?
ANDY: O, you think it was the Rockefeller that killed him?
ETRA: Yeh.
ANDY: Why? They said so?
ETRA: Well, it's just a surmise. I can't really back it up, but it really seems like, you know, that old man probably had—

20

ANDY: You know, isn't that very funny. They just came out and said the little boy did it, and we just believed it. We didn't think anything of it.
ETRA: I just see that big limousine with—

21

ANDY: He didn't have a limousine.
ETRA: O, what was it?
PAUL: It was a Ford Mustang, a '65 Ford Mustang.
ANDY: It was his own car. It was a Ford Mustang GT. You know, once you get a limousine, you get someone else who's a moron. . . .
ETRA: Well, you just see his little car with little bodies on—
ANDY: His car was smaller.
PAUL: No, there was something wrong with him. I hear he was either blind or he had no driver's license.
ANDY: No, he was 16.
PAUL: There was something wrong with him, I read in the paper, that they felt was the cause of the accident. I forget. He probably wasn't blind in a car.
ETRA: I see that little car with, you know, like in World War II you have the bodies on your tank or something? I just see that car, that old man just knockin' 'em off as he goes driving. . . .
ANDY: His secretary was driving.
ETRA: His secretary? You know, I distrust those people.
PAUL: You can't trust a Rockefeller, you can't trust anybody.
ETRA: I always feel the Rockefellers have too much.
PAUL: Some of the people who think that, they get upset if the cook just tries to get some.
ETRA: I heard stories of Pocantico. You must have been there? It's supposed to be unbelievable.
ANDY: It's unbelievable.
ETRA: Absolutely unbelievable. I'm no Democrat, God knows, but it would make a nice park or a nice housing development. I don't know, I think if you've got to have people live in that kind of environment, I think it should be given randomly by lottery, maybe rotated.
ANDY: Huh?

22

ETRA: You know, that every year somebody else gets to live in Pocantico and they put all the stuff in a museum.

Peter Beard

ANDY: He'll probably never come back from Africa. He's over there right now.
ETRA: Is he over there for a long time?
ANDY: Might be. Yeh, I don't know.
PAUL: Cheryl Tiegs. He should get her away from her husband.

ANDY: Who?
PAUL: Peter. He should get that Cheryl Tiegs away from her husband.
ANDY: He's going to?
PAUL: I don't know, but he's going to try.
ANDY: Do you know Fran Lebowitz at all?
ETRA: I've spoken to Fran.
ANDY: O really? Is she doing something for you?
ETRA: We talked. She just seemed too busy.
ANDY: Really?
PAUL: Doing what?
ETRA: Well, when I talked, she was going to replace Russell Baker.
ANDY: O no, the newspaper strike is on, her big career is over.
PAUL: What do you mean, Russell Baker? Has he quit?
ETRA: No, she was going to replace him.
ANDY: He's on vacation.
PAUL: O, is that?
ANDY: Yeh.
PAUL: She was going to be the vacation Russell Baker?
ANDY: Yeh.
PAUL: I find him unreadable.
ETRA: He's an acquired taste.
PAUL: O yeh, must be. And Art Buchwald also is awful and he would be a step up. You know I just read a great book by, Fran Lebowitz doesn't hold a candle to, Oscar Levant, who she's very much like. But Oscar is so brilliant. He's much funnier.
ANDY: O yeh.
PAUL: He also, he directed—
ANDY: Is he still alive?
PAUL: No, no, he's dead a long time now, but he directed most, see, what was great about him, he directed his humor at himself, which Fran doesn't do. She's too immature.
ETRA: And he also played the piano.
PAUL: O, he was, ah, he was very artistic. He had a piano, he had a beautiful house and things, and his books are pretty funny but they're mostly about how hideous he himself is. He said somebody came up to him at a party and says, "I always wanted to meet you. People always tell me I look like you." And he said, "We both recoiled in mutual horror." But he was very funny.
ETRA: He was one of the great hangers-on.
PAUL: He was a friend of everybody. Everybody liked him because he was always funny.
ETRA: There really are no more professional hangers-on on a major scale, are there?
PAUL: Yes, I'm sure there are.
ETRA: Who?
PAUL: I'm sure there are.

23

ETRA: It's such an odd day. It's not like the fall. I brought you a kite.
ANDY: You did?
ETRA: O absolutely.
ANDY: Why?
ETRA: Because it's almost the fall.
ANDY: It is? O, what kind of kite?
ETRA: I don't know. You want to unwrap it?
ANDY: O yeh.
ETRA: Let's unwrap it. I hope these things work. [Tape recorder] I was brought up, I confess, on foolscap and ink.
ANDY: What's that?
ETRA: I brought paper.
ANDY: O really.
ETRA: But we must change, we must change. No one uses paper anymore in publishing.

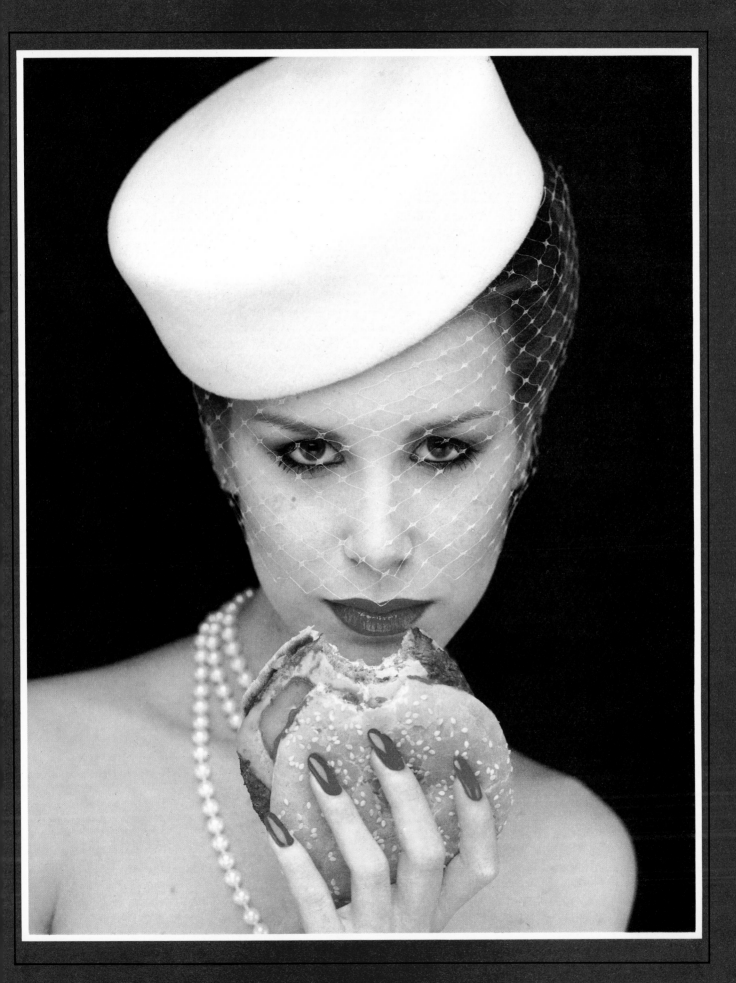

Doll Food

by Anne Beatts

Editors' note: Anne Beatts currently shares her Greenwich Village apartment with 27 dolls, having received one doll on every birthday and every Christmas Day from age three through thirteen, and others on the occasion of her contracting mumps, strep throat, whooping cough, or the like. Although she modestly declines a reputation as the Elsa Maxwell or Perle Mesta of the doll world, she has certainly tossed a few memorable fetes, such as her semiannual Mouse Ball. Nor will doll society soon forget her Spring Regatta, held in the Plaza Fountain, where one of Milos Forman's dolls, Jack, unfortunately became involved in a nasty squabble with one of Irving "Swifty" Lazar's over the attentions of a doll belonging to Viveca Lindfors. (The following year, the Regatta's location was shifted to the Pets' Drinking Fountain near Saks Fifth Avenue, the festivities somewhat abridged, and the guest list pared down considerably to avoid further such regrettable incidents.) Herewith, then, are a few notes on entertaining dolls set forth at the request of the editors by Ms. Beatts, who trusts that they may prove both amusing and informative. Ms. Beatts says that the dolls' party she herself would most like to have attended was the famous Parisian soirée at which Nijinsky's dolls met Jean Cocteau's dolls for the first time, much to the dismay of the only doll ever owned by Carl Van Vechten, who prophesied, perhaps rightly, that no good would come of it. If contemporary press accounts are to be trusted, the menu, in honor of the many White Russians present, consisted entirely of "les petits aliments blancs" such as breast of ortolan and tips of white asparagus.

Dolls are not "little people." Despite their apparently human characteristics, such as two arms, two legs, eyes that open and close, naturally-rooted hair, and so on; and despite the love that may be lavished on them by their human mothers, they are not human. In fact, there is some evidence to support the theory that children themselves are not human, but some genetic way-station between human beings and dolls.

For instance, parties. While adult human beings are often afraid of parties, or uncertain what to wear to them, dolls and children both love parties. And a party means food, appetizingly and attractively arranged.

Dolls don't eat, but they are great appreciators of food, and sometimes quite fussy. You may have noticed that many dolls have uptilted noses, and seem to have been born looking down them. On the other hand, dolls are often the willing recipients of foods you yourself detest, such as Brussels sprouts, often called the queen of doll food for its close resemblance to tiny cabbages.

The essential thing about doll food, then, is not so much cooking method, speed of preparation, or taste, but how it looks. Incidentally, this is also true of the fare provided by many well-known restaurants.

Dolls do not want to be embarrassed by foods that are messy, drippy, or worst of all, too big. All doll foods should either be made small, or bought small. However, the doll food enthusiast should be careful not to go overboard in the cause of miniaturization, and seize on, say, packaged prepared breadcrumbs, simply because a teaspoonful of commercially ground breadcrumbs looks much the same as a tablespoonful. Remember that breadcrumbs are merely an ingredient, and should not be offered as a food by themselves.

The easiest and often the most enjoyable way to reduce the size of food is to eat it yourself. For example, eating all around the edges of your own, normal-sized hamburger will eventually transform it into a tiny burger, just right for dolly. Finger sandwiches can be made small enough for the smallest fingers by the same method. Ice cream cones can be deftly nibbled down so that some ice cream remains in the very tip, to create a tiny and extremely realistic treat, but remember that this only works with sugar cones.

This system could theoretically be applied to a wide variety of foodstuffs, but the age and relative autonomy of the doll owner must be taken into account. It is a rare parent who will permit a child to reduce everything on his or her dinner plate to doll-sized morsels and then cart the morsels off to the playroom for the dolls' delectation.

For the youthful doll owner, however, after-school snacks may be a valuable resource. A single Mallomar makes an excellent substitute for Sacher Torte on any doll's dessert cart, and one Sara Lee chocolate brownie, whether licked round or left square, is a perfect stand-in for chocolate layer cake.

Sunkist raisins are perhaps the most easily obtainable of all doll foods. They may be served as raisins or as prunes, depending on the size of the doll. Any doll food fancier who is not able to score a few packs of raisins is a poor chef indeed.

Those little balls of colored sugar used in cake decorating and known as "hundreds and thousands" are also readily available, and although there is no equivalent in human food for a round ball of hard sugar as big as your fist, dolls seem to enjoy them. The Hershey company makes miniature Hershey bars and Hershey minichips, which are chocolaty and delicious, although during the war in Vietnam they were boycotted by some politically conscious dolls.

Those same dolls are now liable to decline hearts of lettuce, especially in California. However, with miniature carrots, tiny button mushrooms, cherry tomatoes, and petit pois on every grocer's shelf, vegetarian dolls, who are usually soft or cloth-bodied, do seem to have a slight advantage over hard-molded plastic dolls like Barbie or Ken, who prefer red meat. Filet mignon may of course be disguised as rib steak, in reverse of the usual practice of unscrupulous butchers.

In planning a fish course, sardines and tiny shrimp are invaluable. But it is best to stay away from lobster bisque:

Back cover, 1939 New York World's Fair guidebook.

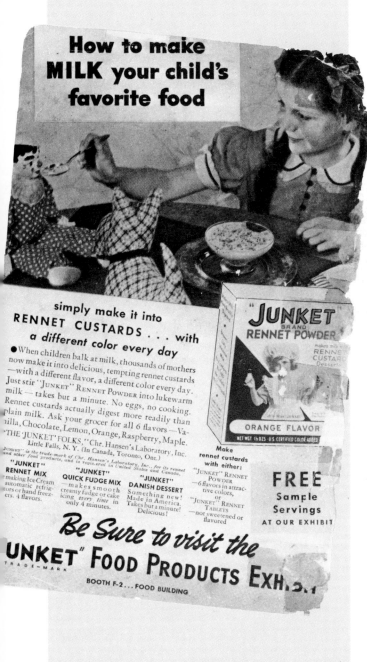

How to make MILK your child's favorite food

simply make it into
RENNET CUSTARDS . . . with
a different color every day

● When children balk at milk, thousands of mothers now make it into delicious, tempting rennet custards —with a different flavor, a different color every day. Just stir "JUNKET" Rennet Powder into lukewarm milk — takes but a minute. No eggs, no cooking. Rennet custards actually digest more readily than plain milk. Ask your grocer for all 6 flavors — Vanilla, Chocolate, Lemon, Orange, Raspberry, Maple. "THE JUNKET FOLKS," Chr. Hansen's Laboratory, Inc. Little Falls, N. Y. (In Canada, Toronto, Ont.)

JUNKET is the trade-mark of Chr. Hansen's Laboratory, Inc., for its rennet and other food products, and is registered in United States and Canada.

"JUNKET" RENNET MIX —making Ice Cream automatic refrigerators or hand freezers. 4 flavors.

"JUNKET" QUICK FUDGE MIX —makes smooth creamy fudge or cake icing every time in only 4 minutes.

"JUNKET" DANISH DESSERT Something new! Made in America. Takes but a minute! Delicious!

"JUNKET" RENNET POWDER

Make rennet custards with either:
"JUNKET" RENNET POWDER —6 flavors in attractive colors,
or
"JUNKET" RENNET TABLETS —not sweetened or flavored

ORANGE FLAVOR
NET WGT 1½ OZS. U.S. CERTIFIED COLOR ADDED

FREE Sample Servings AT OUR EXHIBIT

Be Sure to visit the
UNKET" FOOD PRODUCTS EXHIBIT
TRADE-MARK
BOOTH F-2 . . . FOOD BUILDING

the word "bisque" on the menu may be painfully reminiscent, for some dolls, of the composition of their heads and torsos.

"Tidbits" created for human cocktail parties can make an excellent main course for your dolls. Cocktail sausages can be served as knockwurst, accompanied by cocktail onions, tiny pickled ears of miniature corn, and boiled new potatoes. A miniature *cornichon* makes an excellent giant dill pickle.

Although I would normally avoid food products with "z's" in their names, it is hard to pass up La Vache Qui Rit Cheezbits, small cubes of soft white imported cheese, or cheez, wrapped in aluminum foil, each, with its tiny red laughing cow's head, a perfect doll-sized replica of the original La Vache Qui Rit product.

Or one might select a small, round, soft French cheese, of the right proportion and ripeness to represent one of those enormous wheels of runny Brie or Camembert sold at open-air markets in the South of France. To accompany it: a section of freshly baked baguette. The combination of flavors recalls the many long, leisurely picnics on the banks of the Loire my dolls and I have enjoyed *ensemble*. And here it might be added that good wine, like love, knows no dimension. Simply decant it and serve in tiny paper cups.

You might further educate your dolls' palates with such delicacies as quail, caviar, whitebait, or periwinkles. The more adventurous among them may even wish to experiment with bite-size chocolate-covered ants and grasshoppers, which, everyone says, taste just like chicken.

There is an entire range of miniature plaster food for dolls, some of it very cunningly executed. This food is costly but reusable. The same dishes may be placed before your doll family again and again, and, no matter how tired they grow of this repetitive fare, they are not likely to complain about it. A word of warning, however—real and plaster food don't mix. If both are served at the same meal, nasty accidents could occur, and it is most likely you and not your dolls who will be the victim. (Despite inflation, most people will not care to feed their dolls mud pies. But if you must serve actual dirt, be sure to do so in acorn cups.)

Whatever it takes to set out a balanced meal in front of your dolls, isn't it worth it? Think about it. Your dolls may be the best friends you have. Dolls are never critical, they never disagree with your opinions, and they don't interrupt. Although bad at returning phone calls, they're great listeners. They put up with all your little moods without inflicting theirs on you. You can cuddle them whenever you like, but they never embarrass you by being demonstrative in public. They never get drunk and have to be sent home in taxis. They don't ask hard questions like "Do you still love me as much as you used to?" or "Are you picking that scab again?"

Dolls may be hard to feed, but they're easy to love. And for me, that's what makes the extra effort and imagination that go into the preparation of doll food worthwhile.

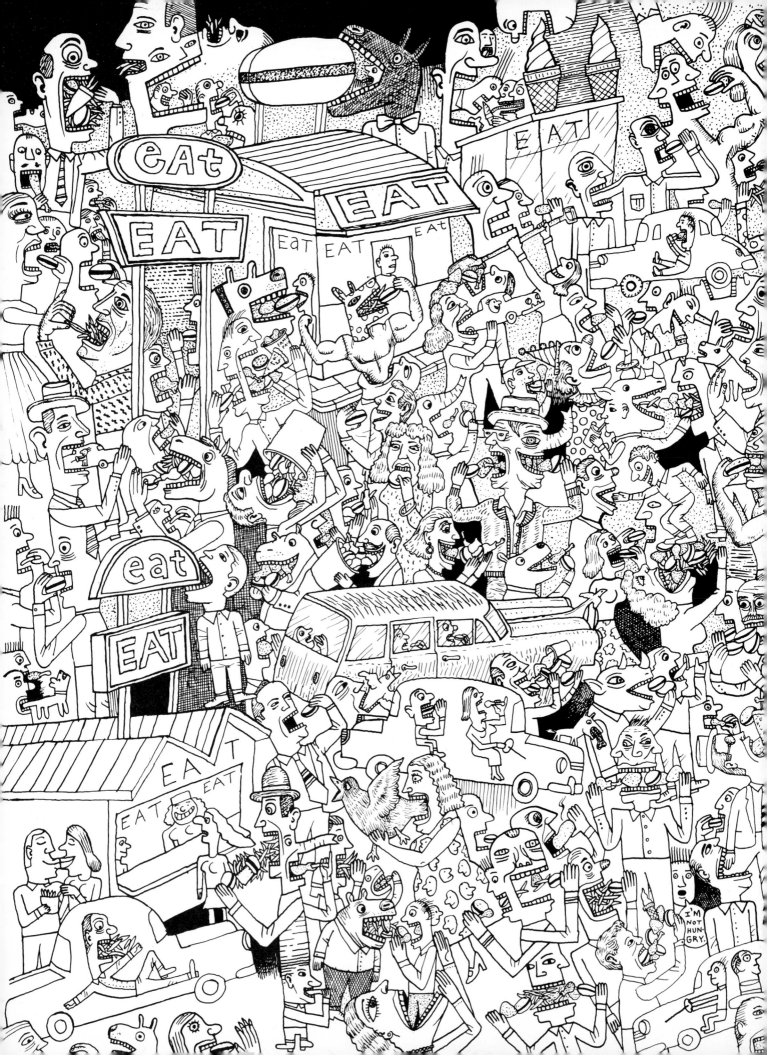

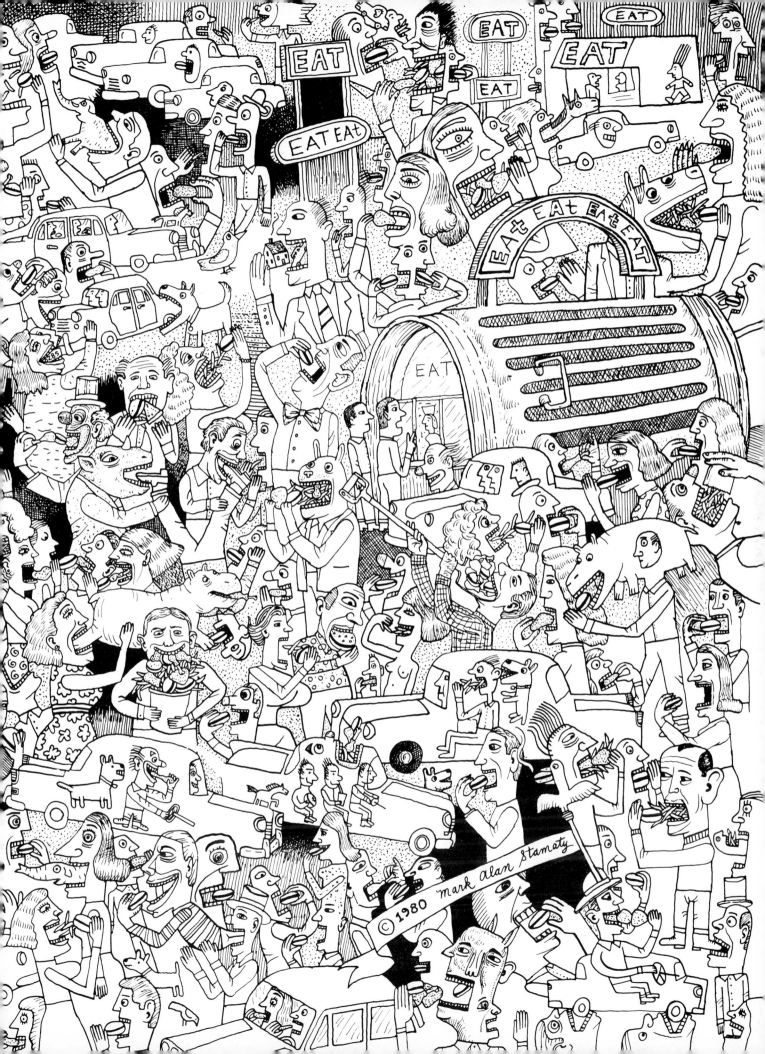

© 1980 mark alan stamaty

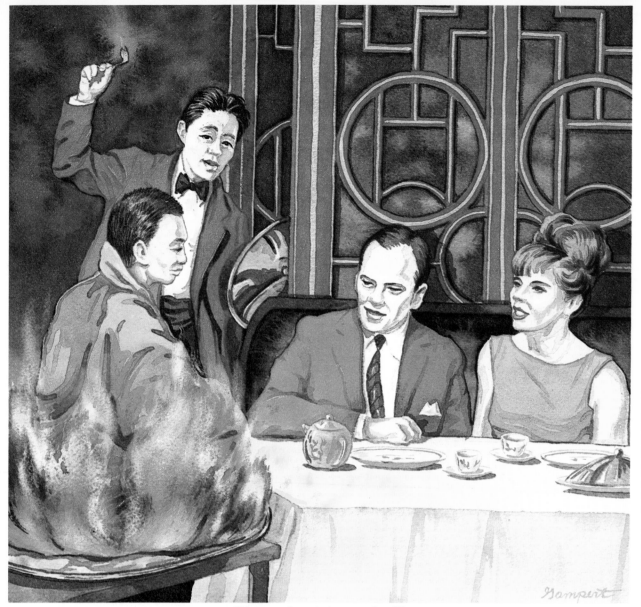

"Not too hot, it is promised"

SHU KU SHIYA RESTAURANT
& RELATED TEA HOUSE & PARLOR DING

שו קו שייה

In the heart of Chinatown
Andover, Mass.
"Look for spire of prep school"

"Copy Dynasty bell
over door
reveals you are here"

TV Guide says: "The increasing popularity of Chinese food..."

March 28, 1980

OCTOBER 1983

SUNDAY	MONDAY	TUESDAY	WEDNESDAY	THURSDAY	FRIDAY	SATURDAY
I cried because...	I had no R's.	And then I met a man...	Who had no Rice.			1
2	3	4	5	6	7 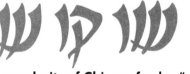	8
9	10	11	12	13	14	15
16	17	18	19	20	21	22
23 / 30	24 / 31	25	26	27	28	29

The Chinese Restaurant

by Alexander Theroux

There are absolutes here, right off. The urge for Chinese food is always unpredictable: famous for no occasion, standard fare for no holiday, the demand usually generated by little more than whim, pregnancy, or the inexplicable craving that follows hard upon a night of boisterous drinking. Any supply/demand ratio, born of such flux, can do nothing but create, even in the genetically silent, a terrible apprehension, suspicion, and despair. Why is there always such a pronounced mood of *suffering* in those shadowy emporia that otherwise serve up such joyful, toyful food?

The Chinatown—of movie, of myth, of mood—is of course the locale that primarily comes to mind when we think of such restaurants, an area, as one wanders into it, that turns darker, more dismal, than other parts of the city. The frail buildings on each side rise to great but narrow heights, their lowest stories forming a double line of insignificant shops and restaurants into which for some reason the sun never seems to enter, and from the dark recesses of which—or am I being cruel?—water-rat-featured dinks and xyy-chromosome types with faces like sudden night always come flashing out in black slippers and pigtails only to *disappear!* Why does one feel they are always up to terrible—*terrible*—things? The calm, probably. It's an *awful* calm, a looming, a preamble, it seems, to some sort of unnamed disaster. I mean, even in a moment of interior peace they look like they could piss their eyes out from anger. And we know what that can mean, right? Tong wars! Beheadings! Scarfing parties!

There is a mood of melancholy, within those intersecting streets, adhibiting to the very nature of Chinatown, a closed-circuit world of butteries and live poultry places, provision companies, and jade-shops with their windows full of Asian whimsies: teak boscages, compacts of balm, Mao hats, wind-up toy chickens, lacquered bowls, jewelry boxes, harmonicas, silk sheaths. Little boys run—and their hair swings! Teen-age girls, looking like they are made of bisque, wear immaculate Catholic school blazers and walk hand in hand with perfect custody of the eyes. Old ladies are always bushing around like little wish-niks and carrying net bags, while their husbands, wearing Borsalinos straight-up like

Hassids and puffing Chung-hwas, are standing under the street lamps reading incomprehensible newspapers from left to right or back to front or down to up, who the hell knows? A metal door is always opening up out of the sidewalk and at the bottom of a wheel-castered chute an angry little potato cask of a fellow is barking for the truckman to hurry unloading his boxes of produce, an olla podrida of leeks, lettuces, and legumes.

The restaurants—you know them, usually, by those exquisite bits of registration, three golden ideographs, all slivers and wings, and the unavoidable stairway (going up in shadow, going down in shim)—almost all have the characteristic red and gold porte-cochère, swirking up in diminishing stages and prinked out at the sides like a Dutch girl's cap. They are, invariably, a cross between a brothel, a miniature golf ziggurat, and a Cambodian doss house. Balconies protrude. Stucco's a favorite, with shell slate roofs. There is an Old World quality to these places, creating, what with the fading pictures of Sun Yat-sen or the Empress Dowager-surrounded-by-eunuchs, a kind of nostalgia for Pearl Buck's novels and '30's movies set in Shanghai or Shantung; and the endlessly munching ungulates within?—at least they care enough to hunt out the right place, give them that. The trouble, you see, is that a good many of these old places, hunched together and secretive and rich in lore, have become as obsolete as buggies. The Chinese restaurant is, alas, no longer limited to the confines of Chinatown, and much of that magic, mysterious world has shifted or spread out or just plain sallied away, moving out to the suburbs, to the plazas, to the malls, sprouting up in the form of fast-food places like Wok-In, Fortune Quickie, and The Pork Strip, where, tray in hand, you can now walk the arches in deli-fashion and point to whatever redi-made choke or chow you want and within this side of a minute be sitting at a table plain as the way to market and eating from a paper plate with a plastic fork pathetic dollops of things that never touch each other, taste like mouthfeel, and digest like a bump in a trash bin. And yet, whether in Chinatown or in any one of its million closet clones, you can somehow still experience those strange and dreadful frissons curiously apposite to the Chinese restaurant alone. . . . What, you wonder, for instance, has happened since your last visit? Or worse: you're happily noshing away when you glance up and—*you're the only one there!* The other customers have gone! Where have they gone? Why didn't you hear them go? It's weird. It's off-putting. It creates a *whingeing* feeling.

I am thinking, right away, of the scowl on the owner of the Chinese restaurant. The owner, always the manager, is that tiny fellow with the monstrously thick glasses and water-parted hair who is found either sitting up behind the cash register, with only his eyes visible, or who stands, hands locked behind him, glowering out the front window for hours upon end. Why is he never happy? Why do you have the feeling, upon entering, you've just interrupted him? Why do you just then feel that trying to keep a secret from him would be like trying to sneak daybreak past a rooster? Why are you convinced that, not ten minutes ago, he's just flayed his children, vivisepulted his wife, or howled a mouthful of bloody execrations at the underlings in the kitchen who weren't working frantically enough?

The place is called The Suffering Duck—it could just as readily be called The Egg and Roll, Cathay House, Kowloon, Inn of the Magic Dork, Wak-Wak Palace, or any of a thousand other names evocative of eastern mystery and splendor—and you're ravenous. The owner bawls at the maitresse d' (always an ice-cold beauty in black) who meets you without emotion in the sudden darkness with an armful of red menus the size of craft paper and imperiously nods for you to follow her through a maze of black lacquer-work partitions, the filigree work of which actually hurts your eyes. A waiter with teeth like a crossword puzzle is whipping a dirty tablecloth out of a booth. You sit down. He screeches. Your table is *there!*

This fellow, humorless no doubt for the floral multi-colored Hawaii Five-O shirt he's forced to wear, fills your water glasses and removes the two plates sitting there. There they are—but he *removes* them! Your wife decides she wants a drink before she eats, you'll join her, and after you're brought the two over-befruited brutes in anthropomorphic glasses (Aku-Aku's the favorite), you sit back to listen to the Hawaiian music—has anyone ever figured that one out?—and turn to look at the decor: the green figurines, red-gold dragons with tongues barbed at the end like arrows, and the dime-store murals and sea-scapes showing Samoans-under-palms or Pago-Pagoans shoving out to trawl in the moonlight. There is a cute bridge by the dance floor (ca. 6′ × 8′) over which, to the pee-like tinkle of a waterfall, lit by blue light, you can pretend on your way to the toilet you're crossing into Peking. The three gold ideographs on the wall? What do they mean? Your wife turns to look, slurping the last sip out of her ceramic coconut, and shoves your arm with obvious exasperation. "The Suffering Duck," she says simply. Probably. And that's probably why there's that little animated logo on each menu. A Peking Duck. Frowning. Get it?

And then the waiter, a phantom whose footfall has attained the highest perfection of noiselessness, is standing there again. Your wife smiles at him to be friendly but nothing registers on his face, only a twitch of anger—an imperceptible nictitation in the eyes—when you tell him you can't decide what to order—*it all looks so good,* he thinks, murderously, *right?*—because it all looks so good. "What's this here Yee Hon Su Su Twee?" asks your wife, sucking a finger. "I mean, the Moo Goo Gai Pan?"

The waiter shouts two glottal-stopped words—ferocious snaps—something like, *"Be Boh!"*

You both confidentially lean toward each other, biting your lips not to laugh, and whisper, "Bean sprouts?"

But, looking up, you find he's gone. I mean, he's heard it all before, the flied lice jokes, the dumb questions, the "it all looks so good" bit, and for years, at least fifty times a night, he's been having to identify, rectify, and clarify the words Moo Goo Gai Pan to dunces, brainless occidentals, banqueters, groups of teenagers ready to pig it, huge horrible families, and, always, table after table of fat, friendly ladies in white pillbox hats who, reviewing the menu, can spend hours swallowing in hunger, changing their minds, and giggling at each other. Can't they all see? The waiter's suffering. The owner's suffering. The place has to *do* with suffering!

The ruby menu, tasseled—sometimes in the poorer places it's only a sad single sheet—is always too vast of subject, the categories recapitulating the membral, submembral, subsubmembral headings of a federal tax-form. Your eyes run from the Beef Group to the Pork Group to the Chicken Group, range down through the appetizers, vegetables, soups and sueys, mings and meins, and cross over into a thousand unpronounceables — you're not in a rush and, after all, reviewing this dress parade is a part of your gluttony — and while you're looking, you talk, inevitably, about the subject at hand, you know, the old rumors that they once found a dead cat in the restaurant kitchen, that Chinese food shrinks in one's stomach an hour after eating, that monosodium glutamate can sterilize you, chat, chat, mumble, mumble. The waiter, meanwhile, is almost biting his fingers off from the delay, suffering like a bitch.

You take one last long look at those monosyllabic names, dishes pronounced like a choo-choo train getting up steam, inviting mockery, and then you decide. You'll both start with Won Ton soup, then you'll have Sub Gum Suey—no, Low Hung Mein with a side order of chicken fingers, OK? And your wife will have the Yum Poo Sung, but instead of pork strips she'll have the beaver-ball chestnuts and—

The waiter snorts in exasperation, reaches over, and pulls the ears of the menu. "Specew combinations? No!" His eyes roll skyward and he grabs his groin. "No!"

After a long scrum, you both settle on the several dishes you want, uneasy for the frosty silence and suddenly diffident as you tick off the long list you've decided on to find the waiter's writing *nothing down!*—a particular enigma that is solved for you seconds later, through delayed revelation, when he steps over and maniacally hoots through a peephole in the kitchen door, *"Num-mah doo! Num-mah twee!"*

Well, the soup's too pale, the tea weak, the dermata on the pork strips a wee too neon-red for nature to have had much to do with it. But the food has that wonderful, discernible, gum-smacking macedoine of sweet-sour-crunchy-munchy poo poo, overabused only slightly with

MSG and salt and its rather strange capacity to squelch. It's soft, rich mouthfeel, every good bit of it, and not even the Arctic breezes of other waiters flying by with tureens and plates all the way up and down their arms can bother you now. They wouldn't serve you any bread, true. There's not enough mustard, and too much duck sauce. And your water glasses have been empty long enough to make you feel like Lot's wife on vacation in Utah. But it doesn't matter. You've been looking forward to this all week. No, nothing can really bother—

But wait, that's not strictly true. What does bother you—I mean, what is in fact driving you right out of your *rubbers*—are the other patrons in the goddamned place! Right? You're always seated directly next to a couple—he's fatter than she, and she's a blimp—sucking wings and ribs, their faces buried in an explosion of grease and perspiration, and the bones they've gnawed white are always being dispatched sideways with a *clonk!* A nasty little bluto in short pants diagonally across the way is screeching mercilessly at his mother who put soy sauce on his teriyaki—he didn't WANT soy sauce on his teriyaki! And behind you is a group of ladies—they look like the Gang of Four—all mousing through the wilted vegetables for the last little pieces of steamed bass, delaying in a kind of displacement activity before wasting away half the night trying to balance the check, reworking the figures, each by each, as a make-weight to a scale adjusts a gain. ("I'm the Pu Pu platter," says one. "Yes, and Doris had the mumpie beans with the goolies." "No, *you* had the Lung Lung rice, I ordered—") That's bad enough. But what about the six guys over there? There is nothing in life as revolting as watching someone, *anyone*, chewing a rib — not only a primordially indecent posture, but in the very hunch of which can be detected the starkest, most immemorial fears one has of

out-and-out cannibalism. And then look around, there is always that giant Chinese family sitting over in a corner — and they're always eating something bigger, better, and entirely different! Why? Why?

After dessert—the five pineapple chunks-cum-toothpicks and the two stale fortune cookies with those sententious squibs guaranteed either to embarrass a couple ("The lady with you is a wonk"), provoke ("You will find a happy excuse tonight to see your neighbor"), or bewilder ("It's a vice of distinctiveness to become queer")—you go over to pay your check at the cash register, beside which you note the familiar glass case offering paper umbrellas, leechee nuts, chopsticks, real replicas of Buddha, jade ashtrays, and back-scratchers, and topped invariably by a Woolworth-framed photograph of the current proprietor and six dozen of his clan, all engulfed in sleeves and staring bewilderedly out into the world.

"*No Sha!*" barks the owner, growling at you xenophobically. You look up staggered. He blinks maliciously through his glasses and points to a sign behind him: No Checks. You hold up your license. He munches angrily, shutting his little face to explanation. You look over at the dragon lady, a.k.a. the maitresse d'—she refrigerates you with a blank stare. You look back at the waiter; he's not been tipped yet and is standing there rubbing his arms up and down as if in preparation of frightful attack. You pay and leave.

"We'll have to remember this place," your wife says, wobbling her full belly into the car.

You look back at the restaurant, only to see the little face of the owner again glaring at you through the painted letters on the front window: The Suffering Duck.

"Don't worry," you reply. "It'll be easy."

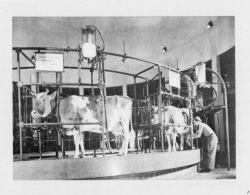

Exposition Extradition

The recent mass extradition of Illinois refugees has raised a host of disturbing questions which call for responsible and reasoned inquiry. Nevertheless, we think certain self-appointed investigators' premature and tendentious allegations of conspiracy are just that: tendentious and premature.

For example, these parties point to the fact that the cattle cars that transported these citizens back to Illinois were operated by the CO'P Development Authority. However, it should be noted that some 95% of all rolling stock in Illinois has been assigned to this same organization. So it may well have been impracticable for Illinois to have transported these 2,000,000 passengers unaided.

Frankly, the extradition itself confronts us with more troubling considerations. It does appear that by ignoring court injunctions for delay, officials of the states neighboring the Illinois-CO'P complex may have infringed upon the civil liberties of the extraditees. Still, it could be argued that the mass exodus beginning in October of 1980 was endangering that region's economy, persistently. And most reputable historians and qualified thinkers agree that the continued enjoyment of our civil liberties depends, in part, on economic opportunity.

Granted that the officials responsible for carrying out the extradition should not have accepted convenience store franchises from the CO'P—or, in two especially flagrant abuses, personal pavilions at the much-vaunted Great Fair in preparaion. Moreover, having accepted them, they probably should have made knowledge of these gifts public. The gifts only serve to undermine these officials' authority, though it should be mentioned that the pavilions, at least, are attractive.

Still, just as the CO'P Development Authority represents a different and novel kind of enterprise, so what has been facilely construed as an old-fashioned bribe or "sugar" may, in fact, be open to a different and more sympathetic interpretation. Nonetheless, these actions and transactions do warrant investigation.

Therefore, we call on the present Administration to create an impartial, investigative, blue-ribbon panel composed of responsible labor, industry, and government leaders. It should be given an absolutely adequate mandate to examine all aspects of the Development Authority's activities.

Ironically, we do not expect, nor indeed wish, that the panel members come up with any quick or easy answers. The issue is too complicated for that. It would well behoove them to recall the words of Abraham Lincoln, Illinois' most famous son: "Given time, a man can thread a needle as well as any woman—but not with rope." Those words are no less relevant today than they were 100 years ago.

Tabula Race-A

The 113th Anniversary today of the laying of the Golden Spike—the linchpin welding the eastern and western halves of the Transcontinental Railroad—seems a fitting time to honor the Irish and Chinese Americans whose ancestors labored to make possible that endeavor. Despite grueling, hazardous working conditions, and low pay, they persisted in their efforts until the Union Pacific kissed the Central Pacific at Promontory Point, Utah, and were joined as one.

In that collaborative respect, they and their descendants have much in common. The Irish Americans, however, endured more than a century of harassment and blame for starting the Great Chicago Fire of 1871. Though recent advances in historiography prove that the blame was justified, the result—the birth of modern Chicago—was ultimately beneficent; yet these findings did little to ameliorate what might be called "the lot of the Irish," as the Irish did not know to expect them. To many unforgettably, at the height of the Depression the Irish were held responsible for the entire year of 1931.

The Chinese Americans, for their part, remember 1941. Victims of a wave of fear-mongering and jingoistic hegemony sweeping this nation in the aftersmoke of Pearl Harbor, Chinese living in Western states were herded into detention camps and deprived of their chopsticks: then suspected of containing wireless receivers. Few were uncovered. Yet, until quite recently, this, one of the silliest civil-liberty denying episodes in American history, was misrepresented in high school textbooks under the euphemism "Rice Clubs."

Other bad years for the Chinese were 1880, 1882, 1894, 1902, 1921–23, 1926–28, 1932, 1936–39, 1942–43, 1947, 1949–53, 1955–58, 1960–64, 1976–78. 1931 was not so hot for them, either. And in 1954 the Indians won.

Thankfully, these eras of insalubriousness now appear behind us, as a nation, like a worn-out pair of knickerbockers. Today, though Irish Americans tend to do their good work in public, whereas Chinese Americans toil behind the scenes, the zeal of both groups for bringing us all closer together burns as brightly as ever. Witness their unflagging promotion of the much-anticipated Century O'Progress. On this newspaper alone, the Sino Fein Joint Interracial Council is sponsoring daily, two-page public service ads about the CO'P, and they have sworn to continue this practice for the Fair's duration.

Upon reflection, we see this boostership as being entirely fitting. Located in the heartland of America, the Fair should unite our country in the "Emergent Eighties" just as the Irish, the Chinese and the Golden Spike did 113 years ago.

The Moral Equivalent of Ten Percent

Unspeakable as it may seem, it is time to pipe up against flagrant abuses of the agenting system by which talented foreign correspondents with in-depth proposals for a you-are-there style treatment of life among the Saudis find themselves unable to get even the humblest of agents on the phone for purposes of perhaps arranging a lunchtime meet and discussion, or, at the very, very least, the ironing out of a talking agreement to read through an outline, which if

will she be in, then? Hello? Hel—?" I said. "May I leave my name? And I want you to put down who told me to call. All right? Because I think it's important!

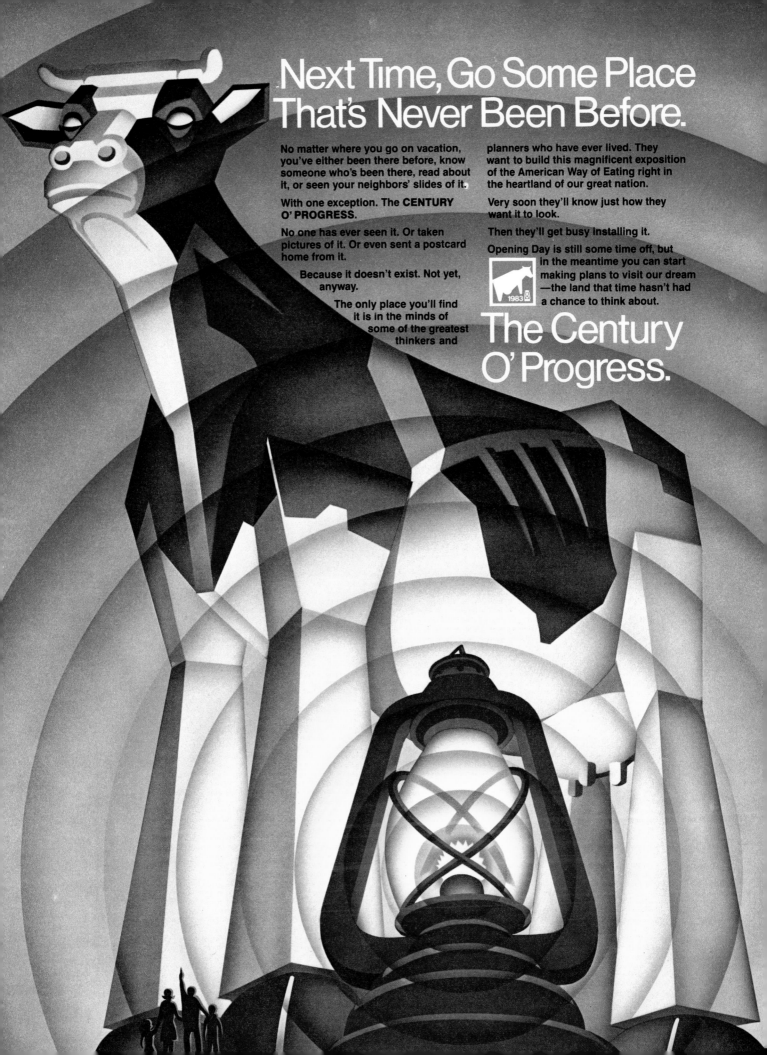

Next Time, Go Some Place That's Never Been Before.

No matter where you go on vacation, you've either been there before, know someone who's been there, read about it, or seen your neighbors' slides of it.

With one exception. The CENTURY O' PROGRESS.

No one has ever seen it. Or taken pictures of it. Or even sent a postcard home from it.

Because it doesn't exist. Not yet, anyway.

The only place you'll find it is in the minds of some of the greatest thinkers and planners who have ever lived. They want to build this magnificent exposition of the American Way of Eating right in the heartland of our great nation.

Very soon they'll know just how they want it to look.

Then they'll get busy installing it.

Opening Day is still some time off, but in the meantime you can start making plans to visit our dream —the land that time hasn't had a chance to think about.

The Century O' Progress.

Mike "Jedediah" Stone, 1842-1893

Another World's Fair teeters on the horizon. Therefore, this might be a fine time to examine the legacy of Mike Stone, this paper's founder, and what he left for future generations.

Old Mike—if one is to believe the stories handed down through correspondence, word-of-mouth, and court proceedings; and which would be the alternative?—was never afraid to admit if he was wrong.

Take the naming of this newspaper, the 104-year old Carbondale *Atom*.

Everyone in the Nineteenth Century (and oh, if we could just turn back the clock. But we can't) was deadly afraid of "Microbes." Today we call them germs. They were a bane to the existence of Nineteenth Centurarians.

But Mike thought "Atoms" were their cure! He claimed he'd read this "new Theory" "somewheres," and with typical feistiness, that we'd better believe him! His very first editorial stressed "Our need for Good microbes to ward off the Bad."

Well, after a while, people just began telling Mike that he was wrong, or asking to see his "source." "I don't have to show you anything," he'd say. And later: "Nobody got hurt. *Did* they?"

And then one day he just laughed. That was Mike Stone's way of admitting he was wrong.

But—

Wait (Mike "Jedediah" Stone, II)

So about Mike it was always said after that, "He Was Wrong, But He Was Right." A fitting epitaph for the body of his lifetime!

Then Carbondalers began telling Mike that atoms were in everything, too, just like microbes ("Germs"). They were "in" every sheet of his newspaper, just like the filth!

Now,

One thing Old Mike was never wrong about: World's Fairs. He knew they were the "*Herald*" of the future, like seeing newspaper headlines in a crystal ball.

From the start, Mike was an ardent adherent of the World's Columbian Exposition, held in Chicago in 1893. It was doubly ironic that he was fated to die there, in a stupid accident.

If Old Mike was alive today, he'd get this newspaper and *all* its staff behind the coming Century O' Progress. Upon reflection, we see this boostership as being entirely fitting.

Then he'd see to it that the Carbondale CO'P Action Men—the ones in the tan VIGILANTE t-shirts—got off their "duffs," and began dreaming up ways for the Fair and Carbondale to mutually respect—and affect—each other.

Ironically, we do not expect, nor indeed, wish that the panel members come up with any quick or easy answers. The issue is too complicated for that. It would well behoove them to recall the words of Illinois' most famous son, Abraham Lincoln: "Given time, a man can thread a needle as well as any woman—but not with rope." Those words are no less relevant today than they were more than 104 years ago.

THE Historical CARBONDALE ATⓄM

"Prairie Avenger—Mountain Lion"

Founded in 1879 by
Michael "Jedediah" Stone

Editor-in-Chief
George Lincohen-Rockwell

Managing Editor
Vida "True" Wu

Roving Editors
Aaron Buckley, Christopher Latham,
Barney Stone

Verse Corner

Food
Pretty
  damn good
Look at the students
Studiously studying their studies
Is also clever.
                    Wanda Dupree
                    Johnson City, Ill.

Today's Chuckle
All the World's a Triage!

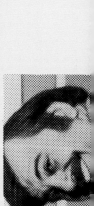

I'M YOUR "FAIR"-HAIRED BOY

Barney Stone

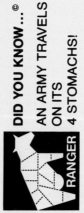

This is an expanded version of Barney Stone's regular Monday-Thursday column. It does not represent the views of this journal and when we got a load of it, we were pretty irritated. Our paper is justifiably proud of its long tradition of granting "equal time to all," however. We print his unsubstantiations with only a remainder to the reader to read the editorial on this page, and that Mr. Stone is quite generally known as a barfly.

I never get it right. Ingenuous—or ingenious? Everybody blocks on something, this one's mine. Pumping along on a story, I get mixed up. So what I do is, I just stay away from those words. Let me tell you. It's easy. Damn little in this world's surprising enough—or right enough, or clean enough—to call itself ingenuous. And ingenuous: I always forget what it means.

I never said I was a great writer. Never said I could stick my hand in the blue flame and bring back silk from China. I just promised Carbondale—brawling city of farmers and near-farmers with a driving energy in its fine dark engines, yet somehow, sometimes, like a wounded deer—the best I had in me on any given occasion. That's what art is, a kind of professionalism. I said I'd go beyond the who-what-where-whens, the sacred 4W's of journalism, and supply you with *mood*... the story beneath the story. Did he smile when he said it? Or frown? Cross his legs? Pick up a pen? And all captured on my Sony TC-55 Cassette-Corder. They call that "Creative Journalism"— the story you don't get in the newspapers.

That's why I'm your boy. And I'm telling you this: There's something rotten in the State of O'Progress.

*

But I better come clean first, before I start in mugging the Fair. World's Fairs have always been a plague on my family's house. My great-grandfather, Mike Stone, who founded this paper, died at Chicago's Columbian Expo. He was apparently paranoid about being short-changed, and when he came up a nickel short at the Extremely Rapid Consumables booth, he blew his brains all over the Midway. That was 1893. The grandfather, Seumas "Joke Parnell" Stone became editor and publisher of the then-weekly at the age of 24. Eight years later, he arranged his first exclusive: a Sunday stroll with President McKinley as he toured the Pan-American Exposition in Buffalo. Seumas turned up just in time to see McKinley assassinated by a crazed anarchist—a story he was forced to share with the rest of the press corps. Predictably, Seumas demanded to break the item in Thursday's *Atom*. Rebuffed, he never had a kind word for Teddy Roosevelt after that. He called him "Hasty Teddy," in his editorials. No one understood why, except Seumas. And maybe Teddy.

That's how the Fairs soured my grandfather, the plague on my family's house. (Tip: You should drink it up before you start.) Despised by his staff and town, Seumas disappeared in 1933 at the Century of Progress Expo, in Chicago again. They found part of his topcoat lodged in the door of the Time Capsule as they were lowering it into the ground. F.D.R. himself, ruling that the Time Capsule would remain sealed, said "They'll give him a nice funeral in 4933. I just hope he doesn't cr— up the Chippendale."

Back in the Roaring 20's, a Classics professor asked Seumas if he had a Philosophy of Life. Yes, he replied. "All it is," he said, "is stinkums."

My father, Hughie "Baby" Stone, inherited a town full of enemies and a paper full of debt. Though they kept him on as editor, pretty soon he had to sell out to the Chalmers syndicate. He tried laughing it off, but I remember, even as a very young child, looking up from my crib at his great ruined face. Years later he'd tell us kids, "I'm just a working stiff. And, you know? I've never been happier." I remember thinking: He looks like a wounded deer.

Then the World's Fairs came and they broke him. Late 50's, early 60's: boom times. I was just

CREATIVE JOURNALIST

out of the army. One day I stopped down at the paper. Dad said, "Those Kennedys—pushing each other in swimming pools. Boy, it's hot around here." It sure was hot, for my Dad—local businesses pressing him to write the editorials, set up the Benevolence Committees, attract a World's Fair to Carbondale. It seemed like every place was having these Fairs, in those days. Brussels '58. Paree '59. Guatemala '60. Hyannis Port '61. Rye, N.Y. (Sally Suburbia Festival) '62. Space Needle, also '62.

They pressed him for special supplements, colorotos. He died in Springfield, in 1966. Lobbying for the King Carb Extravaganza on the Capitol floor. He was a good man in a bad time pushing a worse idea. There ought to be a monument there, saying that. Last time I looked, there was a giant cow and lantern.

This column's for my Dad.

*

There is this guy, Dr. Gus Cinquemani, and he's probably about forty-two years old. He's one of the New Carbondalers, I could tell by his voice because that's his trade. He said he was a vet and when I said, "Did you have your breakfast grits this morning?" he said, "What?" and I knew I was right—New Carbondale. "What about you?" said Cinquemani. "You eat you grits?" His thick accent flashed a mirthless grin across the cables and into the receiver. "They make me whoops," I said, and shook my head like a stallion. Besides, I'm no farmer.

Maybe this town is changing. People used to let their eyes speak for them. Now their mouth does all the talking. But is the land of Illinois changing the way Doc Cinquemani says, puffing up and losing its hair, America growing old? "Let me tell you what I saw this weekend," said the Doc. I looked down at the TC-55. The cassette was turning smoothly. My "Li'l Listener's Loop" was taut around the phone. My pants were brown. "Turn down your radio," I asked. "I saw tractor trailers," said the Doc. "Miles and miles of tractor trailers. And carrying you know what?" I didn't know, and told him so. "*Houses.* All carrying houses. They're busting up the state for this Century O' Progress!" "Yeah?" I rejoined, my reporter's instincts thick and matted, like a brilliant setter when it comes in from the rain, all stinkums. "How come I don't know about this?"

Cinquemani swore. "They're leaving Carbondale *alone,* for some reason, but—" "You know what this sounds like to me?" I said. "No offense, but it just sounds like funny upstate stuff. I bet you Daley's behind it. Mayor Daley?" "Daley's *dead,*" howled Cinquemani. "For six years!" Now I knew I had a real cookie on my hands. "No offense," I said gently, crossing my legs and frowning. "How come nobody else knows this?" Then I slammed the phone down. His line had gone dead.

*

But I couldn't shake that Daley thing. Could they be hushing it up around here? I remember when Vince Lombardi died and they didn't want the football players knowing, so they just propped him up on the sidelines all season. That was a big story. A guy down in government, Challenger Wu, said he'd see me, if I made it quick.

Then a funny thing happened. On my way over to City Hall, a guy tried pulling a fast one on me. "Hey, buddyroo," I confronted the newsdealer, a red-bearded old man with foul yellow breath. "That's a quarter light." He felt the coins in my hand. His menacing dog snarled, baring yellow fangs. "Twenty-five. Five. Ten. Another nickel," he blushed crimson. "Sorry." He forked it over.

...And it's Mike "Jedediah" Stone and the Extremely Rapid Consumables booth at the World's Columbian Exposition, all over again, that's all I could think...

*

You know, there *had* **been some funny stuff** about this Century O' Progress, starting after Chicago burned a year ago. A lot of folks thought the rebuilt city was smaller, almost 7/8 scale. "It's not smaller," you, kept hearing all over the state. "You've grown!" Then the buttons started appearing: I'VE GROWN, TOO! And later, FROM A GREAT FIRE, A GREAT FAIR.

Wu was willing to talk CO'P, but off-the-record. I agreed. Tape recorders scare some people, and you've got to honor that. I switched over to my reporter's notepad. The *Front Page* wasn't all that long ago. The beardless Wu crossed his legs and smiled. His eyes were blue, like Imperial jade must be. He picked up a cup. Nervous.

"...are the ones behind the Fair. Because America was dying. Is dying," Wu said. "I know, I replied, America is old. It's got foul yellow breath. "It needed another Frontier," he said. It had retired, I put in. "Okay," he said, playing with his hands. "Another West—with its endless possibilities for human enterprise. That's Illinois. And that, we like to say, is Fair."

I shut my notepad to talk turkey. Let's go not-for-attribution, I said.

Are there going to be those change machines at this Fair? I queried.

"What?" asked Wu.

You heard me. Where you put in a dollar bill, turn the handle—

"Oh, sure. You like? We get you plenty change machine."

I stood up tall, dusted my shoes with my eyes. "They never work," I said, and stalked out. Right at the door I added, "Save it for the suckers in the seersucker sportcoats." He heard me.

*

Men and ladies of Carbondale, heed my col- umn. This is a good town, an imperfect town, but cleaving to the good, imperfect vision of the men in buckets and skows who landed so many centuries ago on our Eastern shores and said not "This is Fair" but "This is our dream." We must stand up to this exposition, which wants to swindle us of our birthright. Old we may be, but have we lost our innocence? Too? Lost it—or been cheated, rooked, flimflammed, plucked, fleeced, or shaved? Stand up, Carb Town, impossibly innocent, city of farmers and near-farmers whose overalls can't cover all: the hunger and desperation, the tainted meat bellies, the mortgage coming due, the abused, and diseased, piecemeal and pennyante ... the children of our town.

*

I was crossing through the nine o'clock sidewalk traffic in the Carb Town. Almost ten o'clock: newspaper hours, all the grey suits gone to work already, and the truckers and mechanics. Only newspapermen going to work now, and whores, who never sleep.

And the Creative Journalist, who also never sleeps. And when he goes, who leaves his tape recorder on. I'm your boy.

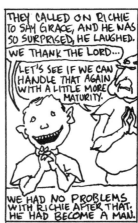
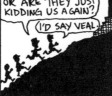
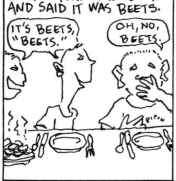
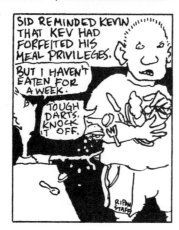
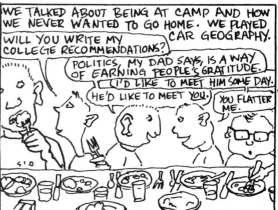
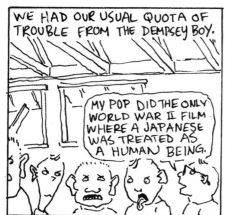
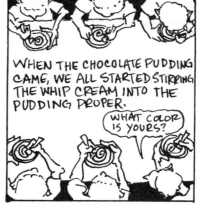
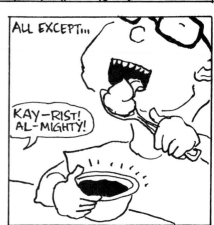
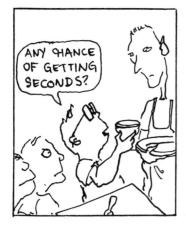
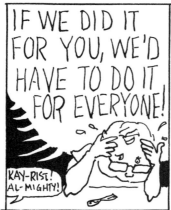
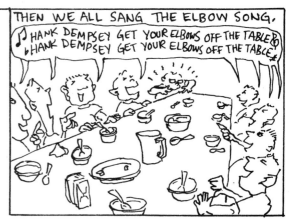

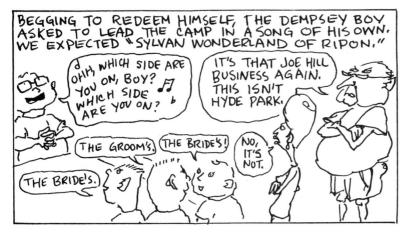

BEGGING TO REDEEM HIMSELF, THE DEMPSEY BOY ASKED TO LEAD THE CAMP IN A SONG OF HIS OWN. WE EXPECTED "SYLVAN WONDERLAND OF RIPON."

OH, WHICH SIDE ARE YOU ON, BOY? WHICH SIDE ARE YOU ON?

IT'S THAT JOE HILL BUSINESS AGAIN. THIS ISN'T HYDE PARK.

THE GROOM'S

THE BRIDE'S!

NO, IT'S NOT.

THE BRIDE'S.

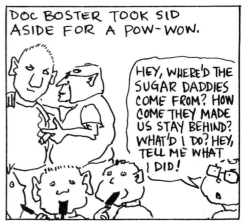

DOC BOSTER TOOK SID ASIDE FOR A POW-WOW.

HEY, WHERE'D THE SUGAR DADDIES COME FROM? HOW COME THEY MADE US STAY BEHIND? WHAT'D I DO? HEY, TELL ME WHAT I DID!

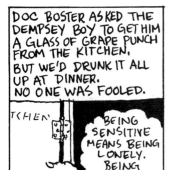

DOC BOSTER ASKED THE DEMPSEY BOY TO GET HIM A GLASS OF GRAPE PUNCH FROM THE KITCHEN, BUT WE'D DRUNK IT ALL UP AT DINNER. NO ONE WAS FOOLED.

TCHEN

BEING SENSITIVE MEANS BEING LONELY. BEING SENSITIVE MEANS...

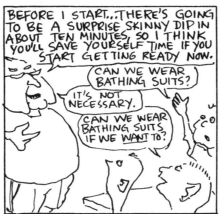

BEFORE I START... THERE'S GOING TO BE A SURPRISE SKINNY DIP IN ABOUT TEN MINUTES, SO I THINK YOU'LL SAVE YOURSELF TIME IF YOU START GETTING READY NOW.

CAN WE WEAR BATHING SUITS?

IT'S NOT NECESSARY.

CAN WE WEAR BATHING SUITS IF WE WANT TO?

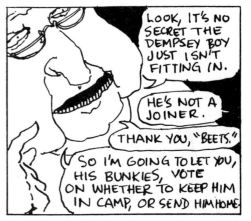

LOOK, IT'S NO SECRET THE DEMPSEY BOY JUST ISN'T FITTING IN.

HE'S NOT A JOINER.

THANK YOU, "BEETS."

SO I'M GOING TO LET YOU, HIS BUNKIES, VOTE ON WHETHER TO KEEP HIM IN CAMP, OR SEND HIM HOME.

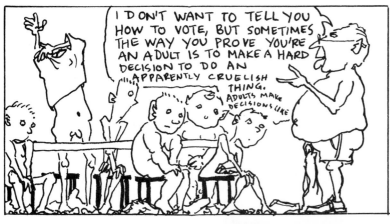

I DON'T WANT TO TELL YOU HOW TO VOTE, BUT SOMETIMES THE WAY YOU PROVE YOU'RE AN ADULT IS TO MAKE A HARD DECISION TO DO AN APPARENTLY CRUELISH THING. ADULTS MAKE DECISIONS LIKE

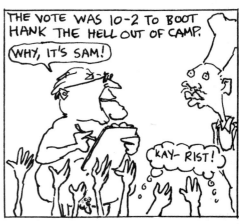

THE VOTE WAS 10-2 TO BOOT HANK THE HELL OUT OF CAMP.

WHY, IT'S SAM!

KAY-RIST!

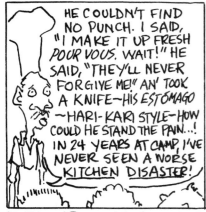

HE COULDN'T FIND NO PUNCH. I SAID, "I MAKE IT UP FRESH POUR VOUS. WAIT!" HE SAID, "THEY'LL NEVER FORGIVE ME!" AN' TOOK A KNIFE~HIS ESTÓMAGO ~HARI-KARI STYLE~HOW COULD HE STAND THE PAIN...! IN 24 YEARS AT CAMP, I'VE NEVER SEEN A WORSE KITCHEN DISASTER!

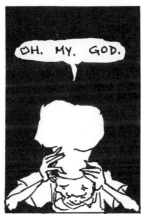

OH. MY. GOD.

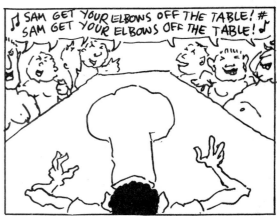

SAM GET YOUR ELBOWS OFF THE TABLE! SAM GET YOUR ELBOWS OFF THE TABLE!

MORAL= IF YOU CAN'T STAND THE HEAT, STAY OUT OF THE CRUCIBLE. RIP-RIP-HOOORAYYYYY!!!

The Glutton's Guide to Eating Out

**Or, how to come up a winner
in the all-you-can-eat league**

by Paul Zimmerman

When I was nine I went with my parents to the Gripsholm, the famous smorgasbord restaurant in New York. I saw people circling a big table with food on it, helping themselves. My eyes popped open. My father read the look correctly.

"You get three plates and that's it," he said. I was a novice, I made some crucial errors. I grabbed the medium-sized plate, not the big one. I stacked according to engineering principles, laying the large, flat objects, such as cheeses and cold cuts, on the bottom, and built vertically to an upper stratum of Swedish meatballs, which kept rolling off the pile onto the floor.

This caused stares and some laughter, hence embarrassment, as I hadn't learned to shut off crowd noises yet, so my second plate showed definite inhibited tendencies. Plate three was built in panic, since I realized I'd reached the end of the line, i.e., a circular wall of potato salad around the perimeter of the plate, to act as a fortress against landslides. Naturally I gulped everything nonstop.

Next day I tried to analyze what had gone wrong. I hadn't reached capacity—I could have gone another two or three plates easy—but I wound up with a monumental bellyache that night, anyway. Half the stuff I ate I never wanted in the first place. I had no game plan. I let the crowd distract me. I drank milk, a cardinal sin in all-you-can-eat dining. Plain water would have been better, or even better still, club soda with a little lime.

Over the next 35 years I have honed and perfected if not a brilliance, then a technical competency that has conquered all but the most overpowering of buffet tables. I was part of a combine that broke the bank at the Krebs in Skaneateles, N.Y., and Albert's French Restaurant in Greenwich Village, and Simpson's In The Strand in London—in fact most of the famous restaurants that claim to give you all you can eat for a set price. We brought The Old Mill Inn in Bernardsville, N.J., to its knees, drove them to physical threats at Ken's Chuck Wagon on Highway 101, south of L.A.

I don't consider myself a competitive eater. I'm more of a dedicated minor leaguer, able to hit Triple-A pitching at a .300 clip, but hamstrung by Major League sliders and spitters. I've had one crack at competitive eating, and I know what the big boys are like, and I'm not in that league.

When I was stationed in Germany in 1957, the S-2 office of our Company had a pie-eating contest as the topper to Armed Forces Day. The pie was lemon meringue, which played right into my hands, because (1) it's my favorite, and (2) it's built for absolute speed, because of the fluff content. You can go much faster than you'd ever dream. I knocked off two pies in less time than it took to call the Company Commander and tell him about it. It was a clear win without any serious challenges, and a few people in my outfit made the mistake of equating speed with capacity and entered me in a professional eating contest in the village, which was called Landstuhl.

I was the only American. The contest attracted famous fressers from the Black Forest to the Ruhr Valley. There were about 50. I didn't finish dead last, but third from last. I beat two guys who got sick and collapsed. There were fat guys and thin guys, the thins being scarier because of the fear of the unknown—you didn't know where they put it. The psyching was fantastic. They ate things they didn't even have to eat, as a psychological ploy. It worked on me. I was full before I tackled the first course, a pail of leber knodel—liver dumplings. From there on it was just survival. How to avoid embarrassment. Nobody talked to me. Nobody even looked at me. I was the kid from the Three-I League, up to the bigs for a cup of coffee.

I'm trying to say that I'm not a freak eater, just a serious one, but few of the restaurants that offer all you can eat are equipped to handle serious eaters.

There are a few things you have to know before you take on one of these establishments. The first is: **Why are they giving you all the food you want?** If a prestigious restaurant is running it as a once-a-week gimmick, as a hook, then you're in good shape, because the quality of the food will generally be top grade. Even better, they'll probably attract women—dates, wives, ladies in pairs, etc.

Women are the glutton's best friends, because they kill off the competition—a guy doesn't want to embarrass himself in front of his date—and women also don't eat much, which holds down the per capita consumption rate, and keeps the restaurant fairly friendly and willing to tolerate the occasional serious eater.

Hotels, particularly in resort areas, run buffets all the time, and trial and error will lead you to the better ones. They do it because the competition does it. They're willing to absorb the loss to get you into the hotel.

RULE: Be ready to assert yourself, if you have to.

There are places that are regularly attacked by the big eaters, and they have developed a subtle, or sometimes not-so-subtle, line of defense. The standard one, in the sit-down places, is simply to ignore you if they read you as trouble. You'll find your area suddenly barren of waiters, or if you do spot one, you won't be able to catch his eye. The easiest way to combat this is through noise. Make yourself impossible to overlook. Force them to choose between absorbing the loss on one table, or risking a disturbance, thereby driving away business.

Too crude? Well, sometimes it's a war—and I assume you're serious about this. London's famous roast beef house, Simpson's In The Strand, used to claim (not too loudly, though) that they would give you as much beef as you wanted. I tested them. Fresh in my memory was that disastrous eating contest in Landstuhl. I needed a win real bad, and besides, I was hungry. After two extra slices of thin, gray roast beef they rang down the curtain. I couldn't find a waiter. I was young, a GI in London for the first time. I bowed out.

I have since erased that blot on my record. Weight of numbers helps. The Old Mill Inn in Bernardsville, N.J., had, and still has, something called a Monday Bountiful Beef and Champagne Night. This is a deadly combination—for them—which leads us to this **RULE: Champagne is absolutely the best thing to accompany serious eating,** the effervescence of the wine acting to lighten the food.

We were six stout fellas. The first round of roast beef disappeared and we hollered for more. "Make 'em thick!" The chef decided to shame us and nip our act in the bud. He cut the second round embarrassingly thick, figuring to put down the insurrection before it got serious. He didn't understand that the argument was just beginning. The waitresses tried to hide. We caught them as they came out of the kitchen. The lady serving the champagne retreated to the bar. We tracked her down.

Finally a sad-looking man in a tuxedo waved the white flag. The battle was over. They were running out of roast beef. They had another seating to serve. Gimme a break, fellas. We accepted his sword.

The Krebs showed no such class. For many years this was the most famous all-you-can-eat in the Northeastern United States. But who ever went up to Skaneateles, stuck up there in the Finger Lakes? Then one night we played Freddy Mautino's Mohawk Valley Falcons in Herkimer, N.Y. This was in the days of the old Atlantic Coast Football League. We were playing for the Westchester Crusaders, $40 a game and gas money. We lost the game on home-town officiating. Ron Luciano, the 300-pound baseball umpire, had a big night for the Falcons, if I remember right. Driving back to the motel we nearly got run down by a train. A tough night, and we decided to take it out on The Krebs the next day.

It was me and a back-up defensive end named Bob Baden and Freddy Hovasapian, our 265-pound offensive right tackle who made national headlines a month later by assaulting a ref and getting thrown out of the league in a game in Utica. We were accompanied by our respective wives and dates.

The Krebs was famous for its Big Three, a platter of lobster, followed by a platter of chicken, followed by a platter of roast beef. Finish one platter and you get another, the sign said. This was called Family Style. We had a hungry family.

We paced ourselves through the lobster and chicken, tapping them for only one extra platter of each, and then sent it all in on the roast beef. After three platters they quit cold. Go on, do something. Now, the first thing you do in a situation like that is to argue logic, then to demand your rights, and then, crazed and hungry, you look to get even— you look for things to break. The Krebs had been over the course before. They anticipated each phase, and when Phase III arrived so did two New York State Troopers. Case closed. City folk don't argue with the upstate boys.

On the way home Freddy got so frustrated he pulled into a diner and knocked off three cheeseburgers. Well, The Krebs is now defunct, and so is Freddy's marriage. I think that set of cheeseburgers was the straw that broke it. This isn't a story I'm proud of.

For me the Golden Age of all-you-can-eatery was in the late 1950's in Sacramento, my first newspaper town: Sam Gordon and the two lovely restaurants which bore his name, Sam's Rancho Villa and Sam's Chuck Wagon—lobster newburg, and crackling fresh salad, and huge sides of beef, all for $2.95—and the little Filipino who'd giggle hysterically and carve you those big end cuts after you'd slipped him a buck....

One day my buddy, Al Ginepra—he's president of the Southern California Rugby Association now—and I drove down the old Coast Highway to San Diego, and we stopped

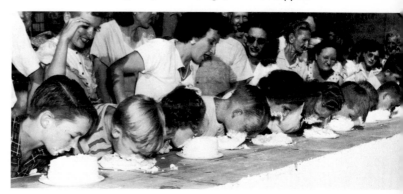

off at Ken's Chuck Wagon, which used to throw a mean salisbury steak and gravy onto their all-you-can-eat table. There was no messing around at Ken's. You just loaded up on the salisbury steak and absolutely shunned the window dressing, the vegetables and cole slaw and soup and Jell-O and all the other meaningless stuff they dress up a buffet table with. That's a cardinal rule of serious buffet dinery. Don't waste time with trifles. Go right for the jugular.

Ken's must have fallen on hard times because that day the lady told us right away, "You've got to take vegetables along with the salisbury steak." No problem. When we got back to the table, we just slid the booth aside, dumped the vegetables, and ate the steak. After about half an hour of that, they told us what they meant by all you can eat was all THEY wanted you to eat, and they wanted us to eat vegetables. So we started working on the vegetables. Three trips later there was a big guy standing there with a cleaver.

"Party's over," he said. Al gave him some story about how we played for the L.A. Rams and had to keep our weight up, and the story had about as much chance as a soufflé on a handball court. I didn't have fond memories of Ken's Chuck Wagon.

RULE: Be wary of the restaurant whose all-you-can-eat price is too low. They're unloading bad stuff on you.

Maybe if you're young and of naturally strong constitution you can cover it. In our college days we used to eat a lot of bad food at Albert's French Restaurant in the Village—all we wanted for $2.79. Steak, ham, or jumbo shrimps, all you can eat. Pick one. No mixing. After the first round, they'd stall and it took 40 minutes to get any action from the kitchen. You had to wait 'em out. One night five of us knocked off 32 steaks (one guy only ate two), but it was no great achievement, because after the first set they were little and rubbery, and the waiter would laugh when he brought them out. "You really gonna eat these things?"

I asked him what the record was. "You'll never set it," he said. He told me a little old man, a cab driver, walked in one night, ate 14 steaks, and passed out. They took him away in an ambulance.

"We never even got a dime out of him," the waiter said. Shock therapy. Nice try. Albert's is now defunct.

RULE: Always get the finances straight.

In Germany I came across a new one. My first day in Munich in '72—I was there to cover the Olympics—they touted me onto the famous Hotel Zum-something . . . I've blocked on the name . . . which had one of the great buffets in Europe. A little head waiter accompanied me to the table, which was unusual, but not at all inhibiting.

"Will you have a bit of our herring, sir?" So I had some herring. "How about some of the weisswurst?" So I had some weisswurst. After it was all over he presented me with a bill for $58. They charged you for absolutely everything you ate. I sat there stunned. They had never claimed otherwise, you see. A new one, boy.

SOME QUICK RULES:

Buffet Dining—Pick the desserts early and store them. Desserts go quickly. They are the most underrated items on buffet tables. Those jellied aspic things are the most overrated, but people always go for them, for some reason. A good way to separate the pros from the amateurs on buffet lines is to see who dawdles over the aspics.

On Plates—Always pick up two at the beginning, one for hot food, one for cold. Who the hell wants the Newburg running into the cole slaw?

Check the Competition—We're still talking about the buffet line. The aspic-dawdlers are usually trouble. They slow the show. Ladies, especially of older vintages, also slow the lines. They can never decide. Sometimes you can put a move on them, though, and cut corners by hitting the hot food section first. Traffic tends to bunch up less in that area.

Fat Guys—Fat guys are generally no problem on the line. They move quickly and decisively; they want to get back to their table and begin eating. But I'm not talking about the super-fats. Sometimes they can blow a good thing for everybody.

Kenny's Steak Pub used to be the best all-you-can-eat in New York. Really top-grade steaks. One night I sat with Kenny Sheresky, the owner, as he sadly reached the decision to discontinue the buffet.

"I won't cut quality," he said, and then he waved a hand in the direction of a 400-pounder methodically demolishing about a ton of food. "But I'm not in the business of slopping hogs, either."

FINAL RULE: When you're onto a truly great thing, never let go.

The best gluttony in the city goes on in private affairs, elegant things you might get wind of by sheer chance. Thus, on one memorable afternoon, Eunice Fried, the food and wine writer, tipped me off to a caviar-tasting the Iranian embassy was throwing. In carpeted elegance we tasted of the Beluga and the Sevruga, the rare and exotic Golden Caviar, and the Imperial Caviar served only in the royal palace; it was affairs such as these that probably hastened the return of the Ayatollah Khomeini, and we tiptoed softly from table to table, smiling politely and sipping Krug Private Cuvee Champagne and eating enough caviar to finance a revolution.

"I can't go on, I can't eat any more," she said, this food and wine lady who had opened the gates of heaven for me.

"You've got to," I said. "You'll never be able to live with yourself if you quit. You'll never have anything like this again in your life. Sit down for a while. Drink some champagne. Take deep breaths. Then give it one more go."

She did; we lasted till every last grain of caviar was gone, and a few weeks later I ran into Eunice again.

"You were right," she said. "I'm glad you made me go back. I've never wanted a bite of caviar since. If I'd have left when I'd wanted to, I'd have felt unfulfilled forever."

I smiled and nodded. Another convert.

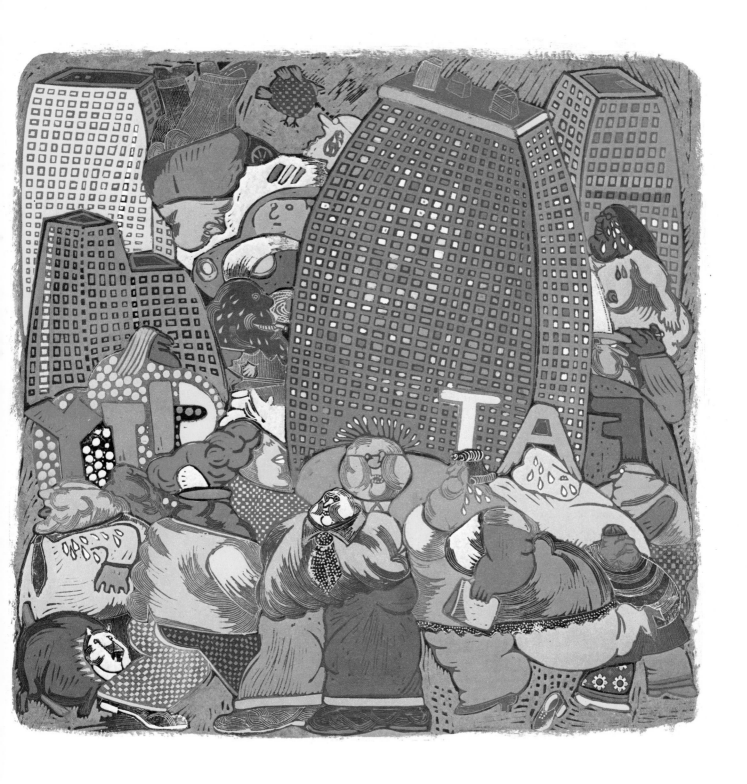

print by Randy Enos

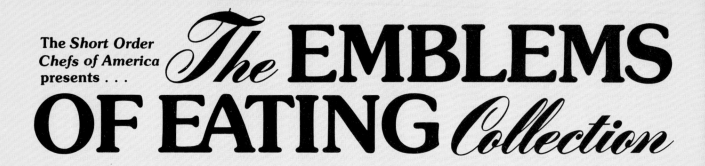
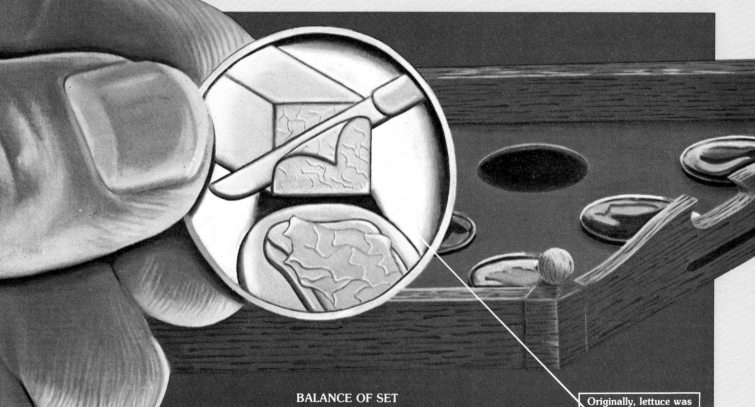

Licking your mother's frosting bowl. . . . Your Dad recalling baked beans in a hobo jungle. . . . Watching the "old ones" eat an ear of corn. . . . That first taste of "extra cheese". . . . Catching the Swedish maid in the liquor cabinet. . . .

Moments like these unite us as a people and link us with our proud heritage. After all, it was a battle over food, the Boston Tea Party, that stirred the Sons of Liberty to cast off the shackles of tyranny and foreign diets. Ever since, food has been a vital part of American life: protecting us from starvation and adapting to our changing life-styles.

Now, as a tribute to the imagination that has kept our food bigger and faster and *more beckoning* than any in the world, The Franklin Kitchen is offering a series of coins commemorating the Great Men, Moments, and Meals in American Food History, "The Official Emblems of Eating Collection."

You will be proud to display this unique collection to friends as they enjoy your summer cookout, and your children will be thrilled to show them off to playmates when they drop by for milk and cookies, or to return anything they may have inadvertently borrowed on a previous visit.

This set of American Culinaria captures 1300 of the people, places, and refreshments that have most influenced our way of eating. Each has been translated into exquisite and *highly detailed* designs by publicity-shunning, meticulous, Old World cake decorators from the Dominican Republic and Mexico, and electro-plated with a bold swirl pattern of *pure* 24-karat gold onto wafers of solid sterling silver.

The wonderful meaning and significance of the moments enshrined forever on these shining discs ("Emblems") is described on the back of each coin in easy-to-understand, everyday language that is both eloquent, educational, and short.

Terrifically beautiful, uncommonly rare

This collection will be treasured for its terrific beauty, its precious metals, as well as for its rarity. Only 443,500 complete sets will be produced, 100 in honor of every American who gave his life in the Revolutionary War. They will be issued 13 at a time, one for each of the original colonies, including Georgia. After the last coin is struck, the molds will be crushed into tiny little pieces, covered with plutonium, and buried somewhere in Canada.

Which means that, except for those collectors, investors, and ordinary people with the vision to subscribe now, absolutely no one will ever have a chance to own a set of these coins. The *only* source for these magnificent medallions ("Emblems") will be those who buy them now, and they are unlikely to part with them no matter how many thousands and thousands of dollars they might be offered. This is truly a once-in-a-lifetime opportunity that is unlikely to recur.

A baker's dozen for just peanuts

The 1300 Series will be released in sets of 13, a baker's dozen, once every four months. Each coin is modestly priced at $34.95, less than what you would expect to pay for a week's supply of fried chicken, onion rings, and a case of Tab.

Years from now, when your collection is complete, it will be prized for its encyclopedic, easy-access information about everything from Apple Jacks® to *zoo food* (those funny 75¢ bags of peanuts? Well, someone *invented* them). Generations yet unfed will share with you the joy of possessing and making regular installments on this priceless heirloom. Long after other bequests have faded from memory, "The Official Emblems of Eating Collection" will frequently remind those who are left behind of their indebtedness to their ancestors.

A source of pride at home—or on the road

Each set will be shipped in a free, distinctive serving tray that may be easily slipped into a drawer or hung on the Family Room wall. It alone is worth $6.79. You will also receive a small circular frame with a magnet base for mounting a favorite coin

text by John Howe, painting by Bob Lambiase

on your car dashboard. Or you may simply want to Scotch Tape several coins to your refrigerator door, as a reminder that it is full of good food which may be quickly thawed and consumed at the first sign of hunger.

A handsome sheet of Cordon Charcuterie—considered the Cadillac of wax paper—protects each serving tray from dust and most spills.

In addition, you will be sent a specially written glossary of terms that will enable you to decipher the secret lingo of restaurateurs, such as "seaboard," "eighty-six," "side of down," "He was a good *man,* he never hurt nobody, who *do* a thing like *this?*" and "Adam and Eve on a raft."

Finally, as an extra bonus, you will get, at no extra cost, an EternaFeast Bronzing Kit, a product of Forever Foods Co., along with instructions for transforming the meal you like best into a lifelike, incorruptible memorial.

Serve yourself—act now

If you set out a bowl of special candies you can only buy in Dallas and your friends come along and wolf them down, perhaps you should think of acquiring some less piggy friends. Then again, you did say they were *special.* And special things tend not to last, like this offering. So please act quickly. All subscriptions postmarked by December 31, 1983, will be entered into our *Calendar '83 Enrollment Charter,* which must close forever at midnight of that day. We are forbidden by law from ever adding to this list.

The Short Order Chefs of America Committee is the official commemorative organization of The Franklin Kitchen. Not associated with any food preparation, nutritional, or menu-planning group, its purpose is to provide a service to patriotic Americans with disposable incomes.

ORDER APPLICATION
The Franklin Kitchen
Century O' Progress, S2-Zone 60609

UNITS	MAJOR CREDIT CARD #	TAX	SALE TOTAL

Name _____

Address _____

City _____

State _____ Zip _____

Signature _____

_____

_____

In accepting this offer I affirm that I am 21 years of age or older and competent to enter into a binding contract. I understand that no prepayment penalties will be levied if I decide to discharge my obligation to The Franklin Kitchen prior to delivery of the complete 1300 Series. Further, I am aware that Franklin Kitchen coins are not legal tender and will not be accepted in payment for monies owed the Company. Should it become necessary to re-finance my commitment, I agree to accept the terms and conditions imposed by The Franklin Credit Corp. YOU REMEMBER WHAT HAPPENED TO COLONEL K. Nine days later the 30-foot steeple broke off a church and impaled him right in the courtyard, like in that movie. Send copies of this letter to people you think need good luck. Do not send money.

- -

RECEIPT		
Date of Order	Amt. Remitted	Amt. Due

Mashed Potatoes

by Cyra McFadden

drawing by Gerry Gersten

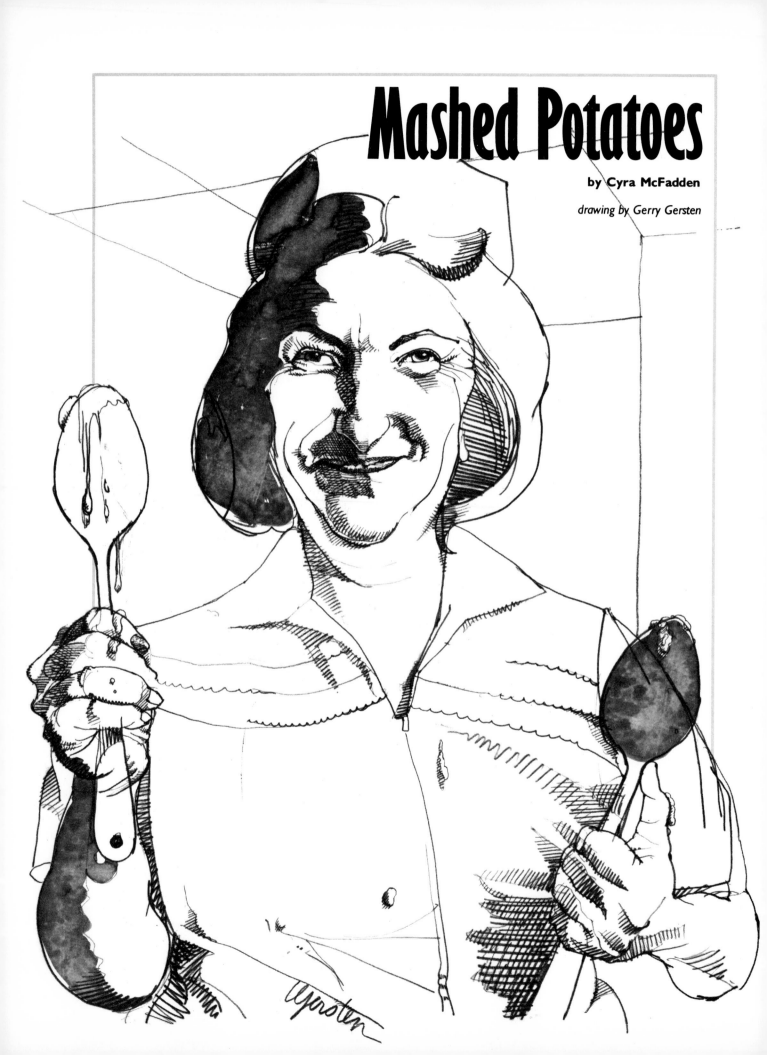

Theme restaurants" abound in California, where people take food consumption for granted in places designed to look like drafty airplane hangars, midget circuses, locker rooms, or gay baths. Still, a new establishment on the Sunset Strip in Los Angeles can only be called unique. Mashed Potatoes serves institutional food in an interior that meticulously recreates a Midwest high-school cafeteria.

"Conceptually, we're an idea whose time has come," explains Ed Ersatz, Mashed Potatoes' tanned, forever blond proprietor. He gazed into the crowd at the restaurant's formal opening with evident satisfaction. "These are all primo people, absolutely primotissimo. They're film and television producers, actors, rockers, roadies ... half the music industry is here, and I mean *names*. And you know why? Because they're basically insecure. They're at the top of their professions. They've got gold records, gofers, groupies, shrinks, and money men, but what they haven't got is a place where they can be themselves ... where they can eat tamale pie and stewed tomatoes, or mess around in a pile of mashed potatoes with a greasy fork and make a lake for the gravy. They've never had a place before where they can eat WASP soul food."

Apparently, Ersatz is onto something, based on a head count of Los Angeles show biz luminaries present, the number of Mercedes sports cars double-parked out front, and the height of platform shoes worn by both male and female guests. "We're going bananas," Ersatz happily told one of the many television interviewers covering the event. "Exactly one half-hour after the doors opened, we ran completely out of Jell-O with fruit cocktail in it."

The restaurant features light-green glossy-painted walls — Ersatz claims the paint has authentically high lead content — asphalt tile floors alternating squares of brown and beige, and illumination from blinking overhead fluorescent lights. No niceties, no menus, and no waiters: Customers push recycled metal Army trays the length of the steam table, with its searing heat lamps and pervasive smell of very old chicken-fried steak. The piped-in Muzak endlessly repeats its single track, "Lara's Theme" from *Dr. Zhivago,* and in keeping with tradition, there are not enough knives.

"Warren Beatty dropped in the other day and called us 'sophomoric,'" Ersatz says. "It blew me away, because that's exactly what we had in mind. I mean, look at these people ... they make maybe a mil, a mil-and-a-half after taxes, but they're only 25 years old, or they have a terrific plastic surgeon and *feel* 25 years old. They know how to fake it with the wine list at the Bistro and Ma Maison — they have to — but what they really crave is the kind of plain, bland all-American cooking they grew up with in Ohio or someplace. Canned corn. White bread with margarine so hard it tears holes in the stuff when you spread it. Corkscrew noodles.... It's the 'Return to Innocence' thing. There's Cher over there on the roller skates, for example; very together, very Big Star, right? Well I have it from an abso-lutely reliable source that what she eats when she's alone is chocolate milk and tuna noodle casserole."

Ersatz's partner in the new venture is "Dr. Dave" Steinmetz, a Los Angeles psychiatrist and personality who treats psychotics who phone in during Channel 7's evening TV news. "He's got the highest image recognition factor in the area," says Ersatz — no small feat when the popular ABC news format also features Disco Dan the Anchor Man and Weatherwoman.

Steinmetz admits he went into the restaurant business looking for a tax shelter. "Right away, though, I flashed that we had something bigger here. As Ed somehow just knew intuitively, institutional food has incredibly powerful associations for most people. They don't know why they feel compelled to come in here, pick up a tray, and get in line, but what we've done is push their buttons. They see those little paper cups with the ice cream in them and the tabs that break so you can't get the top off, and right away, they're back in the hospital having their little tonsils out. They're bundled up all warm in their jammies with their favorite doll, and it's almost visiting hours, and mommie's coming." (Proof: A regular — an ousted Paramount executive — says he goes there because "I happen to like hospital food, but I don't like hospitals.")

Significantly, Steinmetz notes, L.A.'s large population of rebirthers and primal screamers found the restaurant weeks before it opened. "They just stood there on the sidewalk, looking in the windows in the front and eating animal crackers."

Analyzing the success of Mashed Potatoes in what he calls "Jungian/holistic terms," Steinmetz adds, "I think we've hit on something archetypal, something deeply rooted in the American consciousness. I mean, who hasn't eaten government surplus okra off a metal tray at one point in his life or another? The bottom line is, everybody's been to summer camp. Oh sure, we all evolve, call ourselves grownups; but what we really are is the reflection of our culinary culture. Look at McDonald's ... talk about your golden archetypes."

Ersatz puts it all more simply. The 30-year-old former surfer who "finally learned the perfect wave was anywhere I wanted it to be" says he wants the restaurant's customers to "feel real good about themselves here. You look at this crowd at our opening and what *you* see are just a lot of trendies in gold chains and Urdu sheepherders' shirts from Giorgio's and hand-tooled cowboy boots made out of fetal yak. Well what *I* see is a bunch of great big children, perfectly nice kids who grew up in some small town believing in the seven basic food groups."

He pauses, meditatively. "I see the chance to create a space for them where they feel safe to eat the crust off macaroni and cheese. I also see the chance to make a bundle. Because there's a saying in this town: 'Box Office Tells.' And it's telling me we've got ourselves an instant institution."

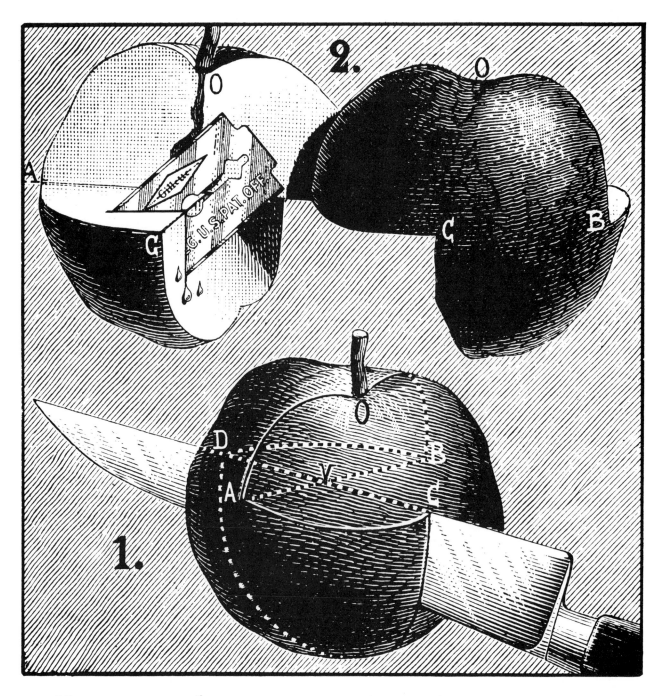

Halloween Sadism

E-Z as giving candy to a baby.

UNICEF BOX into Molotov Cocktail *I. Hack up charcoal into little bits (eensy). 2. Keep the charcoal nice and warm (ovens will do) while you stand your watch. 3. When the goblins arrive, take a dollar bill (with especially young children, you can use Monopoly money, they won't know the difference) and fold the bottom into a small pouch. Fill the pouch with charcoal bits. Then stuff the bill in their Uni Box. A dollar is a lot of money. Watch their faces glow!*
Note: Of course, even under the best of circumstances, in the very best of worlds, your Unicef carton will not always catch fire, as Kerensky was the first to note. Still, the charcoal should heat up the pennies—if not exactly melt them down—which must result in at least 3rd degree burns.

Gag-m-Ade *Just get yourself several tubes (assorted flavors) of Lik-m-Ade—and a standard fire extinguisher recharge kit (H_2O-foam). Pour out the sugary treat and replace it with the powder from the recharge kit...which you may wish to* mix with instant lemonade crystals or lime Kool-Aid, to retain that tangy citric taste. Foam is instantly created on contact with saliva. Average yield: 12 cubic feet. You'll have the neighborhood ghouls going full throttle!

Hydrochloric acid in Nik-L-Nips *I. Buy the H_2Cl at some downtown chemical supply place. They have big vats of it. 2. With a razor blade, remove the top of your Nik-L-Nips and pour off the fluid. (A small pinprick in the bottom may aid this step.) 3. Re-fill with judicious blend of food coloring and H_2Cl. Dilute gently should wax begin to melt. 4. Re-seal the Nips by melting back the tops with an ordinary kitchen match, being careful not to ignite the fumes. Restack in the pack. And wait. Their lives won't be worth a plugged Nik-L.*

Frag-o-Lantern *When a child comes to the door carrying a jack-o-lantern, drop some food in his Halloween bag and some .22 cartridges in his pumpkin.*

Wrathful Grapes *I. Using a syringe, inject bunches of grapes with nitroglycerine. 2. Nitro—which may be manufactured in your kitchen from nitric acid, sulfuric acid, glycerine, and H_2O—is a highly volatile liquid. 3. Quick. Get the grapes into a Fridge. 4. A short time after the little masked pretenders have departed, your "grapes" will warm up, become unstable, and explode. Death stalks again!*

collage by Gary Friedman

Souvenirs of America

MIAMI, FLA. *Brigado de Asalto 2506: the brigade now occupies a small office of the community center in Little Havana, Miami's Cuban enclave. But once the members were holding a beach-head off Cuba's Bay of Pigs. Fiercely anti-Castro and anti-Communist, these veterans of an undeclared war are alleged to be linked to the CIA, political terrorism, and even JFK's assassination. They are nearing middle age now; most are working at jobs, some are professionals, a few own businesses. Ironically, dominoes is the big game on Calle Ocho. Our interviewee insisted only his initials be used. We spoke Spanish.*

JF: *What was your mission?*

DC: *We were supposed to establish a land base on the south shore of Las Villas province in Cuba. With this base in operation, we anticipated that the already disenchanted people under Castro's heel would rise up and we would arm them.*

JF: *Were there any plans if they didn't rise up?*

DC: *Yes. We were convinced that once reminded of what had been lost when Castro seized control, they wouldn't hesitate to revolt. So we brought with us propaganda kits supplied by U.S. intelligence.*

JF: *What was in them?*

DC: *Political leaflets and other things that Cubans would remember.*

JF: *Like what?*

DC: *Well, we have a great passion for sweets—a ''sweet tooth'' you call it—and so the thinking was to bring things like Hershey Bars and Nestlé's Crunch with us. When we arrived in each village, we thought we could win our people back in this way.*

JF: *By giving them chocolates?*

DC: *Yes. We were told that it worked in World War II, especially in Italy when the American GI's were liberating the Italians. The intelligence people thought that what worked there would work in Cuba.*

JF: *What do you think?*

DC: *I don't know. We didn't get a chance to try it, as you know. You have to understand that there was a complete embargo then—there still is—and it was impossible for the people in Cuba to import American chocolates and other things like Coca-Cola. According to some good, hard information we had at the time, the East German substitutes for such items were inferior and not liked by our enslaved countrymen. So the opportunity was there for our Hershey Bars to work.* —**A. Markworthy**

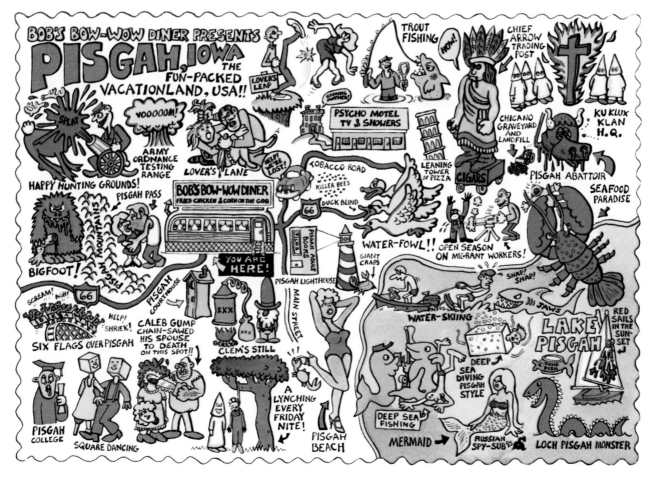

placemat by Ken Weiner

Spaghetti Westerns

by Deborah Young

I. The trouble with Italy. Americans abroad

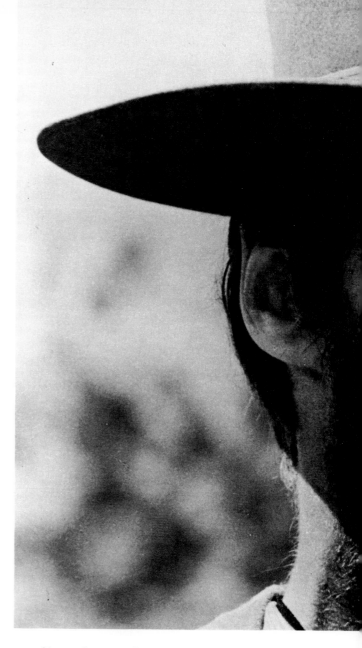

"**F**UCKING GODDAMN SHIT-EATING COUNTRY! With its goddamn unflavored toothpicks!" an enraged young actress from California fumed in the warm after-dinner glow of a cheap trattoria in Campo de' Fiori, where the final sips of espresso were concluding a six-course meal at the English-speaking emigrés table. As though loosened by the thunderous words, a dried red peperoncino fell from its ceiling bouquet into her rippling blonde hair, unnoticed. A group of Roman diners still on the pasta course looked over in mild curiosity. Jill Joy crossed and recrossed her long legs in irritation, as if to articulate an emotion that escaped words. "We have *mint*-flavored toothpicks in the States."

"My dear!" exclaimed the slightly shocked Eleanora MacIntyre, widow of an Italian war hero and, as a result, director of the John M. Synge English Theatre, which the government had given her rent-free for 99 years to ease the pain of bereavement.

"How extraordinarily resourceful of you," piped in Osvaldo MacIntyre, whose father had been an Italian war hero and who was at present the principal actor at the John M. Synge English Theatre. His small black eyes fastened obsessively on Jill's face. "I do appreciate American ingenuity. And yet: the ways of the Old World have their own gracious charm. 'Spurn not the humble shepherd's pie . . .' "

Jill leaned a deeply suntanned arm against the paler one of Patrick De Ville, former tenor of the Metropolitan Opera in the 1940's, and asked him for a Marlboro.

"Darling," Patrick said, as he explored his Gucci men's bag, "you must come over some time and I'll make an absolutely scrumptious southern fried chicken dinner. I just got in a shipment of Crisco and cornstarch from a dear friend at the Vatican black market."

The company murmured in approval. Rob, Jill's incongruously drab escort who had been a New York cab driver before coming to Rome, suggested that Patrick see if bagels and lox could not be obtained from the same source. "If some enterprising young businessman would think to open a franchise in Trastevere," he mused. Milkshakes that don't taste like wash water, dreamed Jill; and real brownies with nuts. Patrick was reminded of reports that the American Army base outside Naples had the only good hot dogs in Italy. Jill demanded a Sunday excursion to see if it was true. None of them had a car, they would have to go by train and rent a car at the Naples train station. Patrick, always capricious, said he would rather roller skate to the base than rent a car from a Neapolitan. The company sighed collectively: Each knew in his or her heart they would never hear more than tales of this Avalon, or meet friends whose friends claimed to have gone. . . . Even Osvaldo and Eleanora appeared moved.

The waiter was serving grilled scampi and fried zucchini flowers at the next table. "I'm going back to the States, I've just decided," Jill announced with resolution ringing through her thin voice. "I'm sick of Italians, I'm sick of making pornographic movies, and I'm sick of these unflavored toothpicks."

"Jill!" cried Rob, who worshipped her.

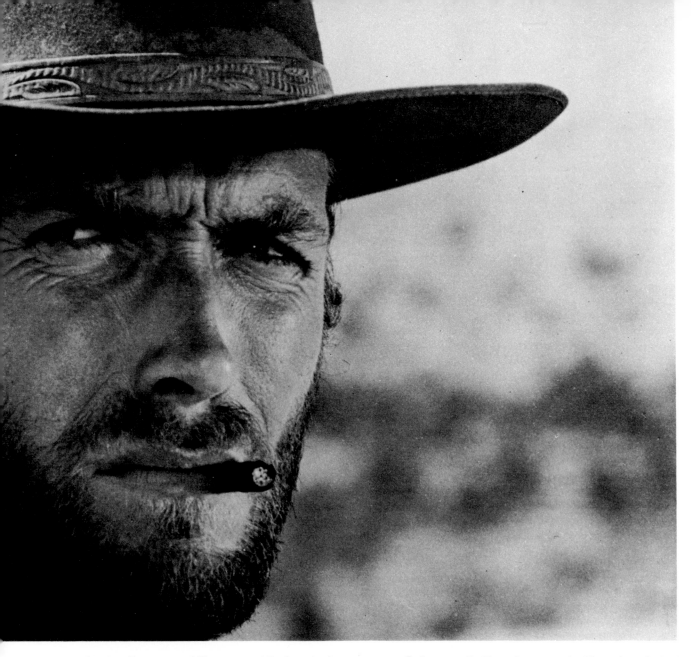

"My dear!" murmured Eleanora, mildly disturbed.

"Can you send me some Product 19 every now and then?" asked Patrick. He adored Product 19. "If you label it 'printed matter' it will go half-price, darling."

They began to discuss the Italian mail service.

2. Nervousness

It was during this conversation that Joe Cecchini, a 28-year-old Italoamerican whose imposing physical presence forestalled criticism of his unpleasant manners, made his appearance. He slung aside the strips of colored plastic dangling at the restaurant's entrance, as if they were saloon doors.

"He-hey!" as he made his way over to the expatriates' table, glimpsed from outside. "Hey, there!" an infectious grin spreading over his bronzed features as he discovered no one he owed much money to. "What'ya say, hey! Finished eatin or startin over here?"

Rob, compelled by politeness, asked him where he had been hiding himself.

"Yeah, I been busy. They been callin me up at Fonoroma for a couple a turns a day, dubbing this Corbucci flick . . ."

Eleanora looked up from her coffee, a half-formed thought on her face. "Joe darling, Osvaldo and I caught you in a ghastly film the other day, what was it Osvaldo dear, it was simply ghastly . . ."

"*Hitchhiking Red Blood,* I believe, Mother," helpfully.

"Yeah, dogshit. But I got ten days work outa it." He straddled a chair comfortably beside Jill. "And got to drive this big Honda around up in the mountains, it was okay. I pretended I was Brando," an indulgence that reminded Joe of the New York premiere of *Last Tango,* which he and his buddy, Mikey, had celebrated in advance by smoking a couple of joints, then packing a couple of bags of beer and sandwiches, and hiding a bottle of Johnnie Walker under their raincoats. A story whose climax was:

"Then I told Mikey to pass me a beer, I was going to open it with this opener, it made a hell of a noise. Well, this guy behind us taps me on the shoulder. I lean over and say to Mikey, 'This guy is really getting on my nerves.' He had no idea who we were. . . ."

"Who were you?" Rob asked politely.

"We were the biggest Brando freaks there are!"

"Quit tearing up the bread," Jill said sharply to Osvaldo.

"So he leaves us alone for a while, we're talking, enjoying the movie, then I open up another bottle of beer and he taps me on the shoulder and says, 'You-two-are-really-getting-on-my-nerves!' I hand Mikey my raincoat and both bags and tell him to turn around at the count of three with his fist out, then make for the exit quick as he can. Without even looking we whip around and wham! hit this guy one." He reached languorously across the length of the table for Patrick De Ville's unfinished glass of rosé. "The whole place broke out in this huge fight, mostly around me, y'know, and I started walking over chairs and people tryin to find Mikey. There were all these people in the aisles after they stopped the movie. But the really crazy thing happened the next day. The next day, Vincent Canby wrote this whole article in the New York *Times* about how 'two young ruffians' (!) 'obviously hoping to see more physical sex than they did, caused a tremendous brawl in the theater where *Last Tango* was premiering.' Can you believe it! He didn't even know that me and Mikey were the *two biggest Brando freaks there are!*"

3. A strange encounter

After these candid revelations, the company shifted back and forth on their unstable wooden chairs, suddenly moved by a common desire to depart. "Eleven o'clock already; too late for the cine, friends!" announced Osvaldo cheerfully. A great burden, that of finishing dinner in time for a second activity, was lifted from everyone's heart. They headed for Piazza Farnese to find more cigarettes.

"What in hell are all these people doing here," Jill commented bad-humoredly, and indeed the square was alive with shouts, music, and human activity.

"Oh dear, it must be another of those noisy little fairs the local Communists put on," apologized Eleanora, who lived nearby above the John M. Synge English Theatre. But they were pulled to the center of the fair like a squadron of magnets.

A brightly lit stage with two enormous amplifiers rose in the middle of the piazza, sheltered by architectural masterpieces of the High Renaissance, and flanked by two fountains of Egyptian granite plundered from the Baths of Caracalla. Lost in the crowd around the outer circle of food stands serving antipasto, fettucine, boiled eggs, and Cokes at popular prices, loaded down with three overflowing paper plates, Michael Winston almost didn't notice his friends. He was a handsome young Ohioan transplanted to

Rome after college an indefinite number of years ago, earning a meager income from English lessons and the occasional translation of books on prestressed concrete. He was highly respected by those who knew him as a frustrated novelist.

"He-hey! How's tricks?" Joe clapped him on the shoulder while carefully examining his meal.

Michael Winston opened his blue eyes in wonder, the arc lights of the *Festa de l'Unita'* adding red streaks to the soft brown hair spilling over his forehead. "I met a wonderful girl last night, I can't stop thinking about her."

The company made its way to an empty row of seats in front of the stage, which was just then being set up, and, between meditatively chewed and swallowed mouthfuls of pasta, Michael recounted his story.

4. A delayed projection

How begin a tale whose ending is still to be discovered in the embrace of a future time? Can a story unfold without an emotional vantage point from which to balance each word, each phrase with its precise counterweight of joy, pain, disappointment, insignificance? Something that cannot yet be assigned to the events of last night . . . as yet but feebly illuminated by a kind of fearful hope, and whose real sense will be revealed only later.

"At the last show of Sergio Leone's *Once Upon a Time in the West*, then: the claustrophobia of the tiny, airless Cine-Club Georges Sadoul with its broken lawn chairs uncomfortably replacing traditional wooden seats. Two spectators in attendance. Myself, a new member to the Cine-Club; and a young woman whose arrival I scarcely took note of, occurring as it did just as a short began. It was a rare print of *Futurist Life* (1916), an early silent whose opening sequence depicted a tableful of Italian Futurists eating risotto in Florence's Piazza Michelangelo and tormenting an old man in a white beard for eating too slowly. Suddenly a protestation; a man who seems to be an American tourist storms over to the table and beats one of the heartless Futurists furiously over the head with his guidebook. Abruptly overcome, I began choking on laughter and a gumdrop, and as I reached into my jacket pocket for a handkerchief posted there for just such emergencies (how often do our physical and emotional selves blend in a single response!), I saw her."

"It sounds ever so romantic so *far*," said Patrick De Ville, who was considering a *gelato*. He was supposed to be on a diet.

"Was it destiny, or just all-too-human mechanical error that the film broke after the first episode? She was sitting nearby, her legs thrown over the chair in front of her, dark glasses in the '50's style covering her undoubtedly soft eyes, as though the brightness of the house lights hurt them. I recognized her as a creature of darkness, like myself . . ."

Come inizia
una storia la
quale fine ve
scoperta
nell'abbracci
un tempo fu
Può una stor
spiegarsi sen
un'impostazio
emozionale c
quale bilancia
ogni parola, e
frase con il se
contrappeso
preciso di gic
dolore, dilusi
insignificanza?
Cosa che ano
non può esse
attaccato agli
avvenimenti
stannotte . . .
ancora non
illuminati che
poveramente
una specie di
speranza deb
ed il vero ser
dei quali si
rivelerà solta
più a lungo.

(Cuanto spes
si combinano
nostri esseri f
ed emozional
una risposta
unica!)

"A bat!" invented Osvaldo freely. "A mole!"

un'uccello bellissimo, nero e notturno.

". . . a beautiful black bird of night," continued Michael, waving a fork to which a few strands of spaghetti still clung, "living, like myself and my own sad nature, in the flickering screen of dreams, desires, and illusions where the image that we see outside of us is only a projection of the hidden things within. I asked her when the Leone film was going to start and she lifted a pale fragile hand, and said:

" 'If it does.'

"And I, enchanted by her deep voice—part English, part American accent—with its sensuous rise and fall and its hidden, no, audible violence, revealed:

ono pazza per Leone.

" 'I love Leone; I think the spaghetti Western is one of the great genres of our time.' And she stared at me through intelligent eyes as though seeing me clearly at last, and replied:

5. Yes?

The destruction of narrative in the American genre we call the Western was proposed, developed, and most brilliantly executed in the work of Italian filmmaker Sergio Leone. Born 1929 of a silent movie actress and a film director, he served an apprenticeship as an actor (we see him at the tender age of 17 in *Bicycle Thieves,* a voluble German seminarian taking shelter from the rain beside the distraught bill-poster at Porta Portese) and as assistant on 58 films by other directors, including Wyler, Zinnemann, Walsh, and Robert Wise before being allowed to direct *The Last Days of Pompeii* (Steve Reeves, Christine Kaufmann, and Fernando Rey). The film, which its director found prudent to sign with a pseudonym, was an immediate and overwhelming success, marking the historic return to the screen of a native Italian genre, the "colossal."

" 'But it was the American West, that is, Hollywood, that was to provide the inspiration for Leone's definitive proposal of a new mass esthetic destined to overturn nationally defined genres and ethnic color—1964 saw the completion of *For a Fistful of Dollars,* the first Italian or "spaghetti" or anti-Western.

" 'Here we should pause to recognize both thematic (ironized violence; the death of human feeling) and formal innovations (narrative deconstruction; expressive humor) so important in gauging the modernity of a contemporary work. But the key question is whether the Italian subversion of the American Western—with Clint Eastwood as its robot hero in Mexican poncho and five-days' growth; its ethical judgments swallowed up in hyperbolized violence, blood, and wholescale death; its unveiling of the American civic sense and respect for law and order as the hypocritical masks of an avaricious capitalism whose only measure of human value is accumulated wealth—whether, in short, such a cynical model should be considered the expression of a country itself no more than a corrupt imitation of the American original, or a critical reproach, in the form of a grotesquely drawn-out metaphor, directed against a civilization which has failed in its mission to renew and regenerate the values of an older, European one? Has Hollywood colonized the Italian cinema, spreading its stereotyped heroes and homogeneous mass culture like butter over the burned bread of neorealism? Or has the innocence of sentiment we perceive in John Ford not been unmasked by the disillusioned irony of a *Once Upon a Time in the West,* which finds the essence of the industrial world—where all pleasure is simple release, all pain mere neurosis—in the death of emotion?' "

"Well I do hope you finally saw the movie, darling," interjected Jill after a long period of patience. "Charles Bronson is fantastic."

They began to discuss their favorite movie stars, leaving Michael Winston alone with his turbulent feelings. He gazed up, up past the electric wires strung around the stage, up to the black night sky over Rome. In half an hour he would be meeting her in Piazza Navona, under the Bernini Triton and seahorse.

With a sense of indulgent well-being he watched Osvaldo wobbling to and fro on the back of a chair that was about to break, and singing to himself.

6. Meanwhile at the Pantheon

A short walk from Piazza Farnese and Campo de' Fiori lies the most fashionable outdoor café in the city, the Pantheon Bar (the café opposite it, though identical in size, price, and refreshments, has no prestige whatsoever and is frequented by tourists). Here a group of internationals was gathered for after-dinner digestives, liqueurs, and conversation: an executive producer both short and bald; an actor called promising several years ago; the well-nourished film director of *Bloody Horses at Dawn* and his attractive young editor; a Yugoslavian movie actress on the crest of popularity; a fashionable intellectual; and an American girl who wore dark glasses despite the late hour. Producer and director had just finished an animated account of the superb meal they had enjoyed together in Fregene last summer, one continually interrupting the other with corrections and refinements.

"The Futurists, of course," extemporized the aging intellectual, who was bored, "detested *pastasciutta* and actively campaigned for its abolition. 'Our *pastasciutta,* like our rhetoric,' said Marinetti, 'suffices only to fill the mouth.' Italians must learn to eat more intelligently, give up heavy lunches *en famille* from 1:00 to 4:00, and adjust to nutritious foods more quickly prepared and consumed," he went on, shaking a finger in thoughtfully mock anger, "in keeping with the exigencies of an industrial society, and the new perceptive schemes of the modern world." A blue-veined hand pushed a dish of marron glacés out of reach.

"*Caramelle più ripugnanti non esistono,*" commented the American girl, a film critic, in agreement. From an

There exists no candy more disgusting.

155

expansive purple sequined bag she extracted, in quick succession, a small Bounty (Italian Mounds), Smarties (M&Ms), Treets (Peanut M&Ms), a Nestlés Gulak, and the large-size Snickers bar that had become so hard to find lately. She kept them handy, she explained, for the cinema.

The soft silk blouse of the Yugoslavian movie star, unbuttoned one too low, was embarrassing the film editor beside her. In the European cuisine—the editor believed—resided the last values of an ancient civilization.

"We discovered this place, you know," the film director whispered conspiratorily to the American girl. "No one came here before we made it fashionable." His watch face suddenly reminded her that it was nearing midnight. The memory of a half-desired encounter mingled with the indolence of the night. Unable for a moment to recall the face of the young man she had met at the Georges Sadoul or, alas! the charming blond streaks in his hair, she allowed a Sambuca to be ordered for her while she hesitated, undecided.

Non potendo ricordare al momento la visa del giovane cui aveva conosciuto alla Georges Sadoul, oppure, Madonna! le affascinanti striscie bionde nei capelli, permise che le venisse chiesto una Sambuca mentre esitò, indecisa.

7. Toward Piazza Navona

At about the same time, a great American writer, descending from the penthouse apartment where he passed various months of the year in reputedly great splendor, set out in search of a bar that sold soy sauce. Tastefully attired in a dark blue suit somewhere between American and continental couture — his handsome face clouded as he tried to recall whether the Café Camerino was closed on Sunday (or Monday?)—he strode from his Renaissance courtyard past the worshipful visage of Michael Winston, who was on his way to Piazza Navona.

"*Volere e potere,*" Michael Winston whispered fiercely to himself. "*Volere e potere!*"

The strange words—the name of a self-help institute housed in the ancient palazzo where the famous writer lived—surged through him with the force of a stiff drink. With the passing. of time they had become inextricably confused with his twin ambitions: first, to meet the great man, and second, to be him. He had entitled his first unfinished novel *Volere e Potere,* the translation of which puzzled him. *To Will and To Can?* Or *To Want To and To Be Able To?* He frowned at the thought of the unfinished Chapter 5 lying sullenly on his desk; then brightened, reminded of the night's pleasures ahead, which far outweighed any desire to give experience permanent form.

8. A girl who knew all Dante once

Stop! Michael Winston! It's your conscience calling!"

There slid into his ears the pitiless mockery of Susan Toober Brontoloni, a college acquaintance (Ohio Wesleyan) whom destiny had coincidentally set down in Rome. Michael, who had deprived himself of her

company since her marriage to an offensively indolent young count, was obliged to inquire about her present condition of life, and whether the nightly parlor games for which their house was famous had continued.

"Oh we've improved them *immensely* now that Mad Mark has replaced boring old Patrick De Ville at the bridge table. His incompetence at the game cost him our friendship."

"I've just left him at Piazza Farnese with the greater part of the Synge Theatre," offered Michael cautiously, never sure how serious his former bio-lab partner was at any moment. Both Susan's ruthlessness and imagination alarmed him.

"Oh not those awful people," she commiserated, offering up a Black Sobranie from a lizard-skin case. "Such dreadful conversationalists (and Osvaldo MacIntyre wanting to break into our nightly circle, can't you just see him trying to memorize the rules to Monopoly and hiding extra hotels in the bathroom?). Though it's just possible I'll do a part in *The Mousetrap* this fall, if Bruno agrees and Eleanora insists; they're both so fond of seeing me on the stage, you know. The last time we did *Earnest,* all the schools wanted to see it; the children were so touching, shouting 'Bravo Gwendolyn!' from their seats and applauding madly. There *was* a rather unfortunate incident at the St. George's performance—" recounted in detail as she lit another Sobranie and blew her nose simultaneously. "How mortifying! Almost as much so as last weekend when Bruno's family aristocracy came down from Milan and found the dried condoms under the bed (we hadn't cleaned the house since the wedding). Actually it hardly mattered, they're perverts anyway; his cousin Tommasso bears a frightening resemblance to James Joyce as a young man and keeps us amused for hours reciting by heart bawdy passages from the letters to Nora in broken Oxford English."

"I'm glad to hear life is enjoyable," Michael, who detested Bruno, got in edge-wise.

"Oh darling!" Susan threw back her unkempt head in an uncontrolled bark of laughter. "I feel so Madame de Guermantes, you can't imagine!"

Michael checked his watch and found it was two minutes of 12.

"Darling far be it from me to halt the progress of a young Romeo to his midnight rendezvous! I was young once too, you know ('*Quant'è bella giovinezza...*'). but just to finish the sentence:

9. A story from the past . . . the upper classes

One day shortly after my summer visit to the heady culture and society of America I received in the post a mysterious invitation from Bruno's savage young cousin, the Milanese Duke, to see at first hand how the then-other-half lived—*cher ami!* you know how curious I am—I could hardly refuse; though Bruno was *senz'altro* furious, poor lamb. . . . He understands intellectual curiosity *pas de tout.* . . . In any case: I was met by a liveried chauffeur at the Milan *stazione* and we proceeded directly to the family manor outside the city, where an impeccably uniformed maid took my knapsack and hurried me into my Watteau-walled chamber. As I attempted to regain full possession of my dizzied senses via a short rest on a duke-sized bed (satin sheets with the family crest), Tommasso having (I thought!) well-educatedly taken his leave, who should pop through the veranda window but a gnomish little person in Valentino-wear and beige gloves who introduced himself as Tommasso's uncle Pippo. A strange gleam in his eye as he asked if I were enjoying my visit should have warned me then and there, yet. . . ."

10. La dolce velveeta/Does all end well?

The moon rose good-naturedly over the great dome of the Pantheon as though to keep the idlers company on their next round of drinks. A church bell, somewhere, chimed 12:45.

All at once, like a hawk alerted to his evening's meal by a timid white flash in the field below, the patrons of the Pantheon Bar turned with one set of hungry eyes to follow the progress of a great American writer across the piazza. He halted abruptly under the obelisk as he heard himself beckoned by an elderly Italian intellectual whose current television program, "Apocalypse and Integration," had made him the *dernier cri* of their very closed circle. Suppressing chagrin, and preparing a few remarks on the servility implied in exploiting the mass media, he gracefully strolled over to the table of his rival.

The latter's thin blue lips curled upward in a malignant victor's smile. "How much water has flowed through the Tiber since we've last caught sight of you, *mio caro!*"

The writer accepted a chair vacated for him. A young American girl, who had been about to leave, sat down again.

"As I was just saying to the *signorina,*" glowed the Italian, "I attribute my own recent overexposure to the perspicacious recognition that the written word has been superseded by the instantaneous expression of sounds and images. By instant gratification of the tactile, olfactory, and taste senses—" popping a potato chip into his mouth "—consonant with the speed, fragmentation, dissonance, noise, and humor of the modern world, which has attracted the lethargic Italians since the days of Futurism. . . ."

"Which perhaps," insinuated the American writer, wondering whether he might not develop this theme in a guest appearance on "Apocalypse and Integration," "is why we have chosen to reside in this underdeveloped country. Sad to say, as the years pass, the blemishes from the ingestion of a foreign culture appear, leveling the charming diversity that originally attracted us to this civilization," and did anyone know if Giolitti's carried soy sauce?

Michael Winston had meanwhile succeeded in convinc-ing Susan to finish her tale of lust, gluttony, and abduction while they walked briskly to Piazza Navona. This forced her too conclude more breathlessly than usual.

At the far end of the piazza, several hundred meters and three fountains away, the middle-aged writer and the American girl appeared from a side street talking animatedly about the role of sentiment in the transformation of values, perception, and art. A paper bag was clutched happily in the writer's sensitive hands. At the edge of the northern fountain he gave a friendly wave to his compatriot, and left her.

As Susan and Michael reached the southern fountain, Susan kissed him wetly on both cheeks and departed for home.

In the silent open space of the long and narrow piazza, eerily deserted at that hour of both tourists and Roman citizens, the iron shutters of the restaurants pulled down and mute, the two Americans slowly turned to face each other.

American expatriates have been consuming the Colosseum since 1946. They are only half done. In this photo, they are washing it down with Fanta Orange. Then they'll take a little riposo.

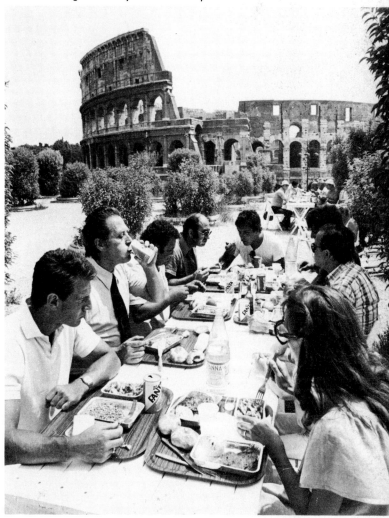

Howard Johnson's, Route 2, William

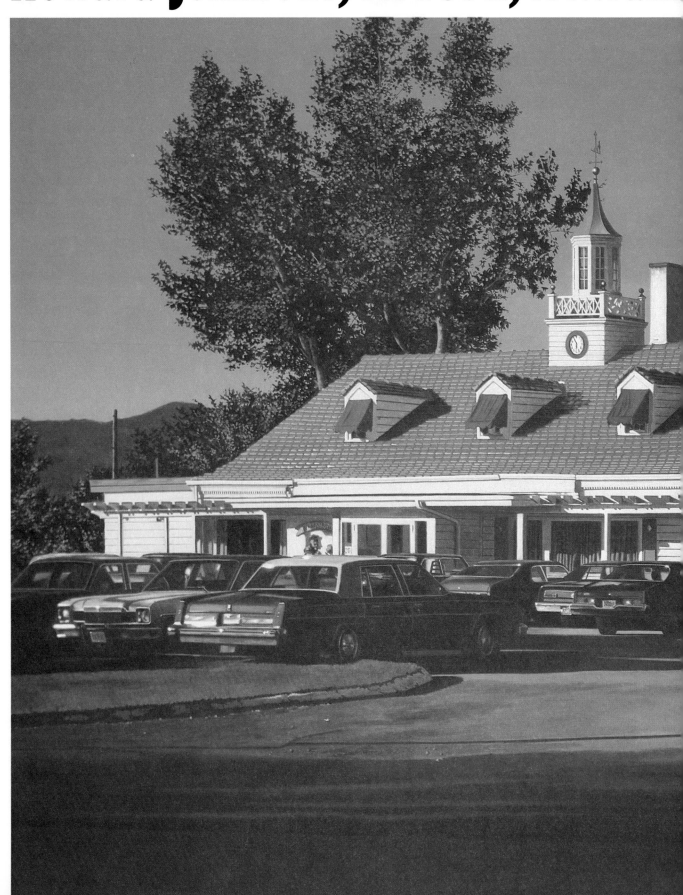

own, Mass.

painting by John Baeder

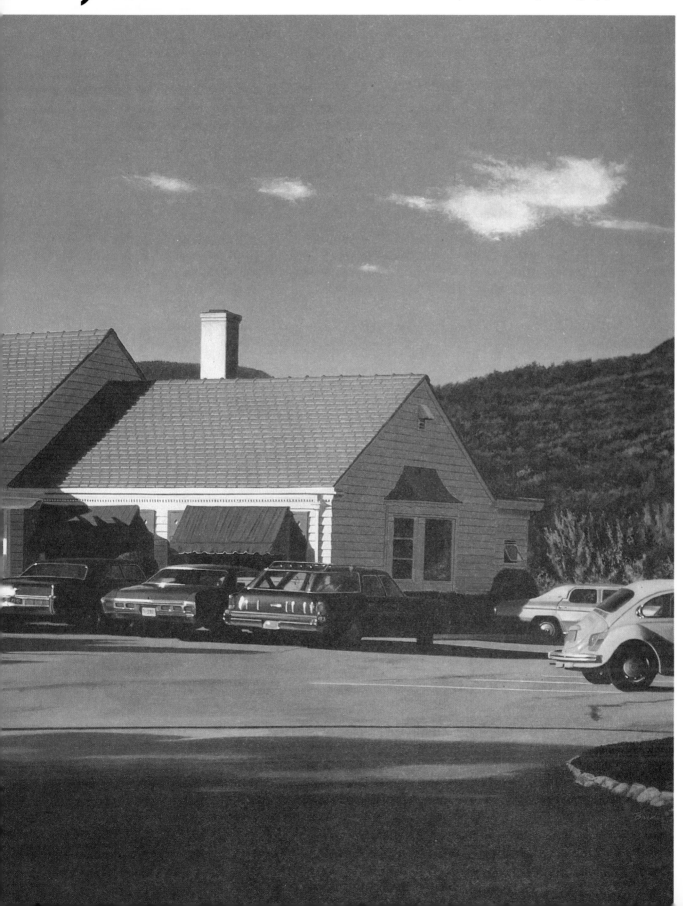

Thomas' English Muffins

It is not necessary to toast an English muffin. Of course it is also not necessary to defrost a frozen waffle or cook a fish stick. All these can be eaten as is with little internal damage. Frozen waffles are just as crunchy frozen as cooked. Sometimes more. An untoasted English muffin is chewy. It does not impose itself upon spreads. Butter makes a clearer statement on the untoasted muffin, staying put, not dripping off, disappearing into illimitable hatches and escarpments. Jam extends, chopped liver gives an even coat, peanut butter and jelly survive each other undiminished. Cream cheese, alas, peels off in hunks. Cream cheese is a good reason to toast.

Thomas' makes the best English muffin. I am told by those who know that Thomas' makes its muffin in the exact same way the English make a crumpet. Indeed, ask for a crumpet in England and you get a muffin à la Thomas'. Which leads one to believe the two are synonymous. The term itself—English muffin—also suggests this (the English being less than likely to lend their name to anything not fundamentally pat). English muffins are essentially pancakes, made with a similar batter, and bubbled with the corresponding holes. Thomas', with its delicate equilibrium of bread and air, comes closest to this flapjack spirit at the heart of the bun, the effervescence of morning.

One summer I occupied a house considerably removed from the local market. Deliveries were made on large orders, but only during the early morning hours. Why spend good money for a house considerably removed from the local market if you have to get up early? Needless to say, food was scarce.

Things you can put on an English muffin in the summer when there is nothing left: chocolate syrup, maple syrup, vanilla flavoring, artificial colors (Red. Yellow. Orange. Brown. Not blue. Purple. Green—trust me), salad dressing, apple sauce, cream of tomato soup, mushroom gravy, butterscotch pudding, banana yogurt, succotash. All of these are edible, some, in fact, pleasant. None fatal. Mustard relish, mayonnaise, sour cream and olive bits, cocktail onions, rhubarb, and candied lemon peel are fatal.

How to make a grilled cheese sandwich in a toaster: Toast an English muffin. Drop a slice of cheese on each half. Press the two halves together. Apply pressure. Apply more pressure. A toasted English muffin will flatten like Coca-Cola in a hot sedan. A toasted English muffin offers little in the way of bulk to impede violence. A toasted English muffin is no charbroiled Beefsteak rye. When flattened to pancake thinness, retoast. The heat of the coils should penetrate through the bread, melting the cheese within. If any cheese protrudes this will explode and spatter pleasingly all over the insides of the toaster. After a while you have to get another toaster. It's about 15 sandwiches per machine.

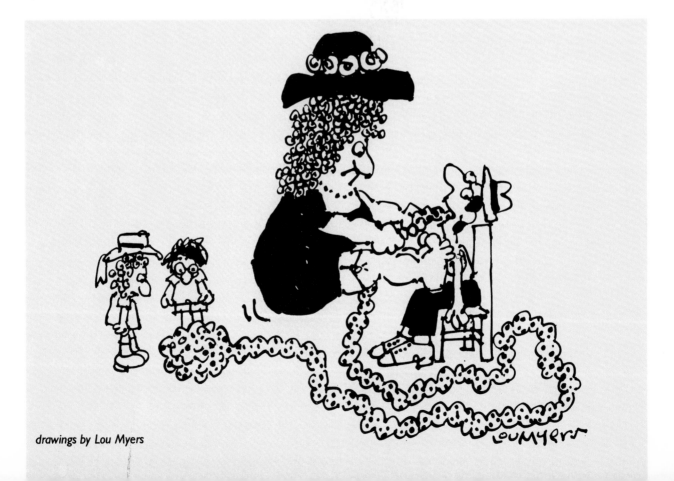

drawings by Lou Myers

I tried to make an English muffin pizza, pouring the tomato paste on the bun, adding cheese, peppers, mushrooms, salami, oil, garlic, oregano, and anchovies, toasting the whole on the grill. Few things disagree with an English muffin. Tuna, egg salad, turkey, butter, jelly, cream cheese, cream cheese and jelly, jelly and peanut butter, tuna and cheese, cheese and mustard, chopped liver, caviar, roast beef, fish sticks, broccoli and hollandaise, hamburgers and onions, hot dogs and sauerkraut, salami and eggs, practically anything fried works. There is, however, one unalterable rule of muffindom: Do not overtax your bun.

English muffins in restaurants are served two ways, burnt with grease, raw with grease. Burnt is better. Raw isn't so bad, but burnt is definitely preferable and an art if properly essayed. The secret of burnt English muffins is to keep the burnt on the outside. Burnt insides are depressing and remind one of Gus Grissom. As for burnt through and through: Remember Pompeii.

Always order burnt English muffins with something on the side, even if it is only cottage cheese and a lump of slaw. The contrast is essential. An acquaintance of some years who lived on nothing more than burnt muffins and narcotics always surrounded himself with garniture, salads, vegetables, appetizers, aspics in abundance. "It cheers me up," he said. "The eyes must also eat." Anorexia notwithstanding, he finished law school and works now for a large midtown firm. There is such a thing as hope.

English muffins may be eaten alone. They are one of the finest lonely foods in the universe. Their simplicity and elegance make them simultaneously easy to prepare yet uplifting to consume. One is never pathetic with an English muffin as, let us say, with a scone. One is often hungry (famished may be a better word), unfulfilled, disappointed, but never lost. The English muffin has very great karma. I attribute this to butterability.

Beware of English muffins with things already in them: blueberries, raisins, cinnamon, bran. Beware of corn muffins masquerading as English muffins, and be especially alert to the cadaverous allure of those Gallic pretenders, croissant and brioche. Weak, crumbly, and flavorless, they aspire to muffindom but cannot hold the spread.

No, one needs the original itself, unencumbered by distraction, unadulterated, pure, a moon without footsteps, sex without hot tubs, a salad without cheese. Do what you will to it, put what you will on it, make what you will of it, but underneath let it be as it was in the beginning, simple and serene, the Ivory Soap of baking.

When you run out of English muffins there is no more hope. I have been to the bottom many times, sometimes for short, other times almost the count. I have learned over the years always to take along a good supply of air, change of socks, and to pack lunch. Lunch is the tough part. It can't be hot because the temperature fluctuates. It can't be complicated because eating is on the run and baggage a liability. It can't be too plain because, after all, one does need reassurance in a hostile place. Normally I take along a piece of fruit, a candy bar, Fresca, a cheese danish, and an egg salad tuna fish English muffin sandwich. I have always come back.

—Jonathan Etra

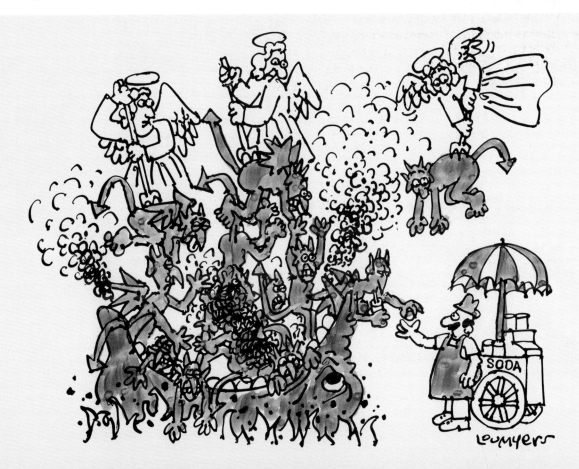

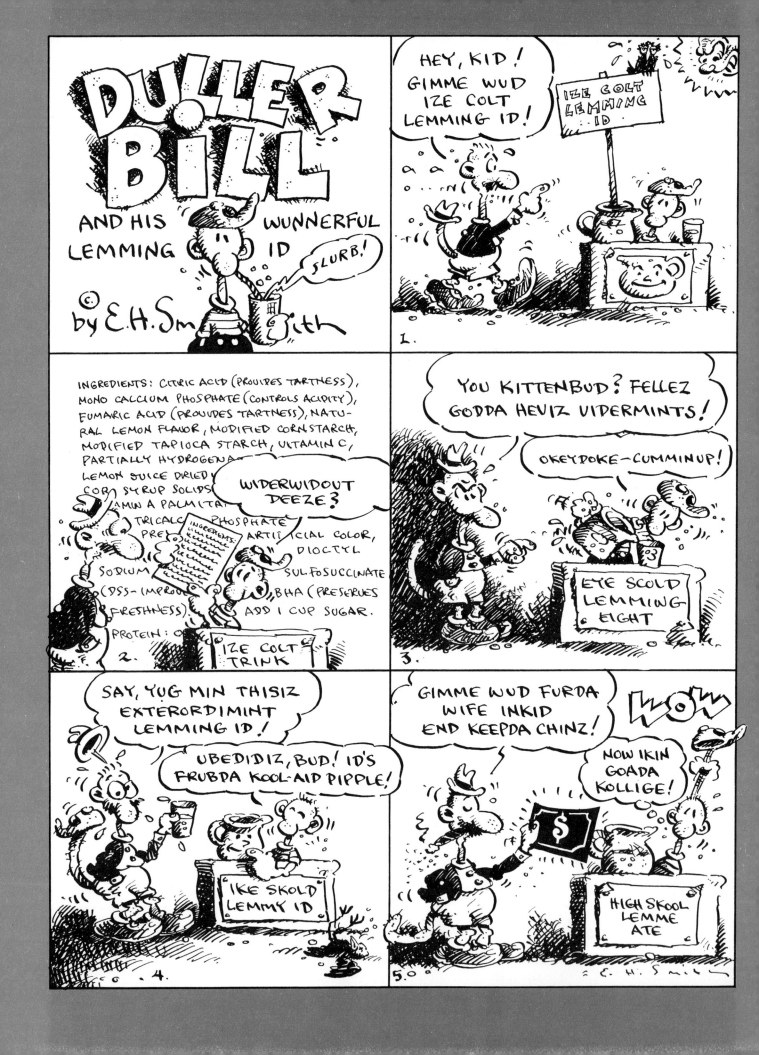

The Junk Food 69

by Paul J. Isaac

Company[1]	Junk food businesses	Approx. 1978 junk food business sales (in millions)[2]	Major brand names	Total sales in millions 1978[3] (1968[4])	Earned after-tax 1978 (1968)		Profit/ dividend per share 1978 (1968)	Stock price range 1978[6] (1968)	Notes
					millions	% earned on equity[5]			

Behemoths

Company	Junk food businesses	Approx. sales	Major brand names	Total sales	millions	% earned on equity	Profit/dividend	Stock price range	Notes
Beatrice Foods	a) candy	390.0	Now 'n' Later, Clark Bar, Milk Duds, Switzer's Licorice, Jolly Rancher, Fisher's Nuts	6314.0 fye 2/28/78 (1433.00)	≈240.0 (50.1)	≈16.0% (16.1%)	2.60/1.05 (.96/44½)	28¼ – 22 (21⅛ – 14)	One of the nation's largest, least-known companies, Beatrice buys up firms with strong brand-name ID and good records at marketing a consumer product, and then runs them superbly, viz. Tropicana, La Choy, Hotel Bar Butter. Not bad for an ex-dairy.
	b) grocery products	700.0	La Choy, Mario's, Krispy Kreme, Rosarita, Little Browny						
Borden	a) bottles Pepsi	NA		3800.0 (1683.0)	136.0 (47.0)	13.3% (9.0%)	4.19/1.68 (1.65/1.20)	31⅜ – 25¼ (37¾ – 28⅛)	If you ever out-grow your need for milk, Borden will still be in business.
	b) serves a buffet	1190.0	Campfire Marshmallows, Drake's Cakes, Bama jams and jellies, Flavor House Old London snacks, Wyler's drinks, Wise Potato Chips, Cracker Jack, Cremora						
Consolidated Foods	a) processed foods	1100.0	Sara Lee, Russette, Kahn's, Bryan, B+G	3536.0 fye 6/30/78 (1445.0)	100.6 (51.5)	16.9% (19.0%)	3.21/1.60 (2.08/.97½)	27 – 21 (48½-37)	Another tribute to the joys of acquisition.
	b) beverages & confections	653.0	Shasta drinks, Popsicle, Fudgsicle, Dreamsicle, Butternut, Zero, Payday & Milk Shake candy bars, Delson, Merrimint						
General Foods	a) beverages and breakfast foods	2473.0	Kool-Aid, Country Time, Awake, Orange Plus, Tang, Start, Postum, Log Cabin & Country Time syrups, Post cereals	5376.0 fye 3/31/78 (1894.0)	169.5 (103.4)	14.5% (16.2%)	3.40/1.64 (2.08/1.22½)	35¼ – 26½ (46⅞-37½)	Lives at the mercy of El Exigente. 40% of last year's sales came from coffee, but only 4% of profits, which is why Burger Chef pushes so hard. Packaged foods and "Other" contributed 60% of sales but almost all the profit.
	b) food products		Birds Eye, Minute Rice, Stove Top, Shake'n Bake, Jell-O, Open Pit, Cool Whip, Dream Whip, Minute Tapioca, Pop Rocks						
	c) restaurants	752.0	Burger Chef						
General Mills	a) cereals	1860.0	Cheerios, Wheaties, Total, Trix, Lucky Charms, Cocoa Puffs, Franken-Berry, Count Chocula, Kix, Frosty-O's, Corn Total, Country Corn Flakes, Boo•Berry, Fruit Brute, Crazy Cow, Nature Valley Granola and Granola Bars, Breakfast Squares	3243.0 fye 5/31/78 (885.0)	129.0 (36.0)	16.7% (20.4%)	2.58/1.04 (.88/.40)	34⅛ – 26⅝ (21¾-17)	A company that keeps a fairly high profile. Maybe it's necessary for morale: Would you rather be an assistant vice-president of General Mills, or the managing director of Fruit Brute? Also a very big toy & game manufacturer. It bought Parker Bros.
	b) snacks		Tom's Snacks, Slim Jims, Andy Capp's Potato Snack						
	c) other foods		Hamburger Helper, Tuna Helper, Gorton's						
	d) restaurants	350.0	Delimatic Vending, Red Lobster, Betty Crocker Pie Shops						

NA = not available
NM = not meaningful
fye = fiscal year ending

[1]Company. The list does not include foreign firms, e.g., Nestlé (Swiss), Keebler (part of United Biscuit—U.K.), Peter Paul (part of Cadbury-Schweppes—U.K.), Crush International (Canada), and Baskin-Robbins (J.Lyon & Co.—U.K.). Also not included are companies primarily involved in merchandising rather than production and licensing of production (e.g., franchise holders rather than franchise grantors).

[2]Approximate 1978 sales. Calculated by multiplying total sales X the percentage of sales represented by the narrowest product line containing the junk food product(s) whose sales the company will disclose. Where 1977 product mix was known, but not 1978, and where there were no major 1978 acquisitions, the 1977 mix was used.

[3]1978 total sales and 1978 after-tax earnings. 1977 figures, where used, are marked. Source: applicable annual report or Standard & Poor's.

[4]1968 figures are derived from same sources as 1978 figures, 1968 calendar year or the closest fiscal year to it.

[5]Percent earned on stockholder's capital, 1978. 1978 profit divided by the net shareholder's investment at the start of the year.

[6]Stock price range, 1978. For listed companies: the range of actual prices at which trades took place. For unlisted companies: the high and low bid prices in the over-the-counter market.

Company	Junk food businesses	Approx. 1978 junk food business sales (in millions)	Major brand names	Total sales in millions 1978 (1968)	Earned after-tax 1978 (1968) millions	% earned on equity	Profit/ dividend per share 1978 (1968)	Stock price range 1978 (1968)	Notes
Heublein	a) wines	238.0	Italian Swiss Colony, Ingelnook, Annie Green Springs, T.J. Swann	1190.0 fye 6/30/78 (304.0)	56.5 (16.6)	14.1% (44.6%)	2.66/1.40 (1.27/0.74)	31⅜ – 23¾ (43⅞ – 32)	An old distiller (Smirnoff, Don Q), Heublein acquired Kentucky Fried Chicken, July 8, 1971, for about $200 million in Heublein stock. They have had problems with KFC. Including: competition from other fast-food chicken outlets such as Church's Fried Chicken; failure to penetrate luncheon trade because of emphasis on take-out food; sloppy store management; & embarrassing criticisms of KFC products by KFC founder Col. Harlan Sanders.
	b) grocery products	87.0	A-1 sauce, Escoffier sauces, Ortega Mexican Foods, Grey Poupon mustard						
	c) restaurants	320.0	Owns (747) and franchises (4414) Kentucky Fried Chicken units, also 83 H. Salt Seafood restaurants, 84 Zantigo's Mexican restaurants						
H.J. Heinz	prepared & frozen foods	NA	Mrs. Goodcookie, Star-Kist, Heinz, La Pizzeria, Weight Watcher's Dinners	2150.0 fye 4/30/78 (790.0)	99.2 (28.4)	14.5% (11.1%)	4.13/1.61 (1.52/0.53)	44¼ – 33¾ (23⅜ – 13½)	A 19th-century pioneer in brand-naming foods and in food canning, Heinz has stayed pretty close to what it knows best: processed foods and vegetables, condiments, etc.
Kellogg	a) breakfast cereals	1100.0	Corn Flakes, Rice Krispies, Special K, Sugar Frosted Flakes, All-Bran, Raisin Bran, Sugar Pops, Sugar Smacks, 40% Bran Flakes, Froot Loops, Cocoa Krispies, Pop-Tarts, Danish-go-Rounds	1691.0 (467.0)	145.0 (42.3)	25.6% (22.3%)	1.90/1.20 (.59/375)	25 – 17 (11¾ – 9⅜)	Founded by W.K. Kellogg, a leading 19th-century nutritional faddist who derived breakfast cereals from the diet he served at his Battle Creek, Mich., spa. The products were promoted as health food. As of 1978 the W.K. Kellogg Foundation Trust owned over 43% of the company's stock, worth some $600 million.
	b) desserts	NA	Mrs. Smith's pies and pastries						
Kraft	a) cheese	2211.0	Kraft, Velveeta, Cracker-Barrel, Philadelphia Cream Cheese	5670.0 (2428.0)	184.0 (76.2)	17.0% (12.9%)	6.57/2.65 (2.67/1.57½)	49⅞ – 41⅞ (46½ – 33¾)	Another big old-line dairy products outfit. Still the titan of Wisconsin cheese.
	b) vegetable oil-based processed food	2155.0	Parkay, Miracle Whip						
	c) ice cream & frozen desserts	317.0	Breyer's, Breakstone						
Norton Simon	a) food products	NA	Snack Pack pudding, Reddi Whip, Orville Redenbacher's Popping Corn	2429.0 fye 6/30/78 (967.0)	115.8 (31.6)	14.1% (12.7%)	2.37/0.69½ (0.94/zero)	20⅞ – 16⅜ (20¼ – 15⅝)	Named for the man who combined Hunt-Wesson, Canada Dry, and various smaller companies.
	b) beverages	340.0	Canada Dry, Barrelhead, Orange Spot, Wink, some liquor						
Pepsico	a) beverages	1700.0	Pepsi-Cola, Teem, Mountain Dew, Patio	4300.0 (848.0)	225.8 (46.5)	25.4% (19.4%)	2.43/0.82½ (0.70/0.30)	33⅞ – 24½ (19 – 12⅛)	Leads a charmed life. Who else could cozy up to the Russians, hire ex-Nixon aides, join the Arab boycott of Israel, and unleash oceans of Pepsi and a billion-dollars-plus of pizza and chips on the national complexion, yet still be considered a down-home piece of corporate Americana? (cf., Coca-Cola.) In Nov., 1977, it bought Pizza Hut for over 13 million shares of Pepsico stock (approximate market value: $325 million).
	b) snacks	1300.0	Frito-Lay, Fritos, Lay's Chips, Ruffles, Cheetos, Doritos, Rold Gold Pretzels						
	c) restaurants	470.0	Pizza Hut, Taco Bell						
Pillsbury	restaurants	650.0	Burger King, Steak & Ale, Poppin' Fresh Pie Shops	1704.0 fye 5/31/78 (569.0)	72.5 (14.4)	15.9% (10.7%)	4.14/1.34 (1.48/0.62½)	47¾ – 33½ (28⅜ – 19¾)	As with a lot of food processing companies, Pillsbury is trying to escape the perils of being in a fluctuating commodity business like flour or grain. So far, battling Ronald McD has proven just about as tough as trying to out-speculate the rest of the Chicago Board of Trade.
Procter & Gamble	convenience foods	1863.0	Crisco Oil, Jif Peanut Butter, Pringle's Chips, Duncan Hines mixes	8099.0 fye 6/30/78 (2708.0)	512.0 (187.0)	19.9% (16.9%)	6.19/2.70 (2.25/1.25)	93 – 73⅜ (55⅞ – 41)	Famous for its marketing and persistence. You haven't seen the end of Pringle's yet.

Company	Junk food businesses	Approx. 1978 junk food business sales (in millions)	Major brand names	Total sales in millions 1978 (1968)	Earned after-tax 1978 (1968): millions	Earned after-tax 1978 (1968): % earned on equity	Profit/dividend per share 1978 (1968)	Stock price range 1978 (1968)	Notes
Quaker Oats	a) cereals and breakfast foods b) other processed foods c) restaurants d) cookies	747.0 152.0	Cap'n Crunch, Life, Puffed Wheat, Puffed Rice, Quaker Cereals, Aunt Jemima products Celeste Frozen Pizza, Wolf Brand Chili 72 Magic Pan restaurants Burry's	1686.0 fye 6/30/78 (554.0)	73.6 (25.7)	15.6% (14.9%)	3.34/1.01 (1.36/0.56⅔)	27⅝ – 20⅛ (32⅜–21⅛)	A major manufacturer of Girl Scout Cookies.
Standard Brands	a) desserts b) nuts c) consumer foods d) confectionary	1839.0	Royal Planters Piñata Mexican foods, Egg Beaters Baby Ruth, Butterfinger, Reggie, Curtiss, Sun Maid	2358.0 (1346.0)	75.8 (33.0)	18.2% (29.4%)	2.68/1.34 (1.24/0.71¼)	29⅝ – 22½ (27½ – 16½)	Silver anniversary recently celebrated. Chocolate bars make up 75% of candy sales. Case in point is Baby Ruth's fudge center surrounded by caramel and peanuts. Case not in point is the Reggie bar, which is not chocolate but "chocolaty."

Cookies

Company	Junk food businesses	Approx. 1978 junk food business sales (in millions)	Major brand names	Total sales in millions 1978 (1968)	Earned after-tax 1978 (1968): millions	Earned after-tax 1978 (1968): % earned on equity	Profit/dividend per share 1978 (1968)	Stock price range 1978 (1968)	Notes
American Brands	cookies	less than 500.0	Sunshine, Krispy, Hydrox, Cheese-it, Hi-Ho	5180.0 (1898.0)	211.6 (92.9)	17.1% (15.1%)	7.93/3.63 (3.38/1.87½)	53 – 39⅜ (41⅝ – 30⅛)	Ex-American Tobacco. Like most tobacco companies, it entered other businesses to diversify out of cigarettes. Ironically, when the government restricted cigarette advertising, American Brands saved a pile of money while smoking continued to grow anyway, only less rapidly. The result was a flood of tobacco earnings which AB could put to less harmful uses, such as buying Sunshine, or Franklin Life Insurance.
Big Drum	baked goods	9.0	None	32.6 (9.6)	2.3 (0.6)	17.0% (NA)	1.86/0.42 (0.42/0.18)	19¾ – 8⅞ (6½ – 4⅛)	The biggest manufacturer of sugar cones in the country.
General Host	a) meats b) baked & frozen goods c) pretzel stands	460.0	Cudahy, Bar-S Van de Kamp, Eddie "Hot Sam"	660.0 (202.0)	– 2.6 (3.3)	deficit (8.7%)	– 1.50/0.60 (1.30/zero)	12 – 8⅝ (45⅜ – 21¾)	Struggling conglomerate, but very happy with its 130+ "Hot Sam" pretzel stands.
International Telephone & Telegraph	a) baked goods b) other foods	NA NA	Wonder Breads, Hostess Cakes Genuine Smithfield Ham, Gwaltney	15,300.0 (4067.0)	661.8 (180.0)	(15.0%)	4.49/2.00 (2.58/0.87½)	34⅜ – 26⅜ (62½ – 44⅞)	Wonder and Hostess are so insignificant within IT&T that they're just lumped in with Sheraton Hotels and Scott Seed.
Nabisco	a) cookies & crackers b) cereals c) candy d) frozen foods	1380.0	Fig Newton, Lorna Doone, Oreo Creme, Ritz, Premium, Triscuit, Graham Crackers, Mister Salty, Uneeda, Biscos Shredded Wheat, Cream of Wheat, Team Sugar Daddy, Junior Mints, Chuckles Freezer Queen frozen entrees	2197.0 (770.0)	101.5 (42.0)	20.8% (15.9%)	3.16/1.35 (1.13/1.10)	28½ – 23 (27½ – 23½)	Born as the National Biscuit Company, it has paid a dividend every 3 months since 1899. Compare the 1968 and 1978 statistics to see the decreased esteem in which stocks are held.
Tasty Baking Co.	a) baked goods b) packaged Mexican Food	121.0	Tasty Kake, Juniors, Krimpets, Kandy Kakes Ole South, Dixie Frost	166.4 (75.0)	3.0 (2.3)	9.6% NA	1.15/1.18 (1.07/0.72)	16½ – 11⅛ (20¼ – 16⅛)	May 1979 — Tasty begins phasing out Ole South.

Candy

Company	Junk food businesses	Approx. 1978 junk food business sales (in millions)	Major brand names	Total sales in millions 1978 (1968)	Earned after-tax 1978 (1968): millions	Earned after-tax 1978 (1968): % earned on equity	Profit/dividend per share 1978 (1968)	Stock price range 1978 (1968)	Notes
American Home Products	a) candy b) snacks c) home food	675.0	E.J. Brach Jiffy Pop Chef Boy-Ar-Dee, Gulden's	3277.0 (1086.0)	348.4 (111.9)	33.5% (29.5%)	2.21/1.32½ (0.70/0.40)	32¾ – 26⅛ (22½ – 16⅞)	One of the classic, consistently profitable consumer goods companies. A doted-on darling of institutional portfolio managers.
American Maize Products	candy	12.0	Mallo Cup, Smoothies, Jamboree	319.0 (101.0)	6.8 (4.6)	8.5% (NA)	1.43/0.42 (0.95/0.267)	10⅞ – 6½ (16¼ – 10½)	As of June 1979, the candy business was taking a backseat to AM's hot new field, gasohol.
Blue Chip Stamps	candy	49.0	See's Candies	144.0	14.3	16.0%	2.62/0.24	22¼ – 15½	(No 1968 figures, Blue Chip was not then in the candy business.)

Company	Junk food businesses	Approx. 1978 junk food business sales (in millions)	Major brand names	Total sales in millions 1978 (1968)	Earned after-tax 1978 (1968)		Profit/dividend per share 1978 (1968)	Stock price range 1978 (1968)	Notes
					millions	% earned on equity			
Culbro Bros.	snacks & proprietary products	54.0	Bachman, Ex Lax	443.0 (235.0)	− 5.1 (3.2)	deficit (21.3%)	− 1.52/1.32 (2.11/1.20)	23⅝ − 19½ (37¼ − 28⅛)	Ex Lax (not *really* a candy) is phenomenally profitable. About 50% of the sales price is gross profit.
Hershey Foods	a) confectionary	668.0	Hershey bars, Reese's Peanut Butter Cups, Mr. Goodbar, Kit-Kat, Y&S, Nibs, Hershey Cocoa, Hershey Kisses San Giorgio Macaroni	768.0 (296.0)	41.5 (19.9)	17.1% (13.6%)	3.02/1.22½ (1.67/1.10)	23½ − 18½ (33⅝ − 24⅞)	Hershey is a company with a stodgy reputation: 60.4% owned by a school for orphans. It finally took the plunge in late 1978, paying something over $158 million for 97.6% of Friendly's Ice Cream, and enriching the Blake family (who founded Friendly's) by some $44 million in the process. At the time of the acquisition, Friendly's was running along at a clip of about $200 million in sales and $9 million in earnings.
	b) food services	100.0							
	c) restaurants	200.0	Friendly's						
Mars, Inc.	candy	≈800.0	Snickers, Mars, M&M's, Milky Way, 3 Musketeers	1500.0	90.0	NA			Mars is entirely owned by the Mars family and foundations. It releases no information it doesn't absolutely have to. It will not even confirm whether Forrest Mars, its founder, is still alive (as of late 1978, he was). With 30 − 32% of the U.S. candy market vs. 20% or so for runner-up, Hershey, it is the biggest U.S. candy company and a major factor in Europe as well. It is paternalistic, secretive, obsessively devoted to quality control and efficiency, iconoclastic, and determinedly antiunion.
E.R. Squibb	a) candy, gum, baked goods	364.0	Life Savers, Fruit Stripe, Carefree, Beech-nut, Pine Bros. Breath Savers, Table Talk pies	1516.0 (615.0)	117.3 (38.3)	15.1% (21.6%)	2.60/1.03½ (1.03/0.75)	37⅜ − 21⅜ (26½ − 17⅝)	Squibb's largest business is pharmaceuticals; but as long as you're in the drugstore, anyway…
	b) restaurants	227.0	Dobbs House airport food, Le Snac, Steak 'n Egg restaurants						
Tootsie Roll Industries	candy	61.3	Tootsie, Tootsie Roll & variations, Mason, Bonomo	61.3 (30.6)	3.6 (2.0)	17.0% (14.0%)	1.53/0.394 (0.80/0.29¼)	14⅜ − 7⅜ (22⅛ − 13½)	One of the last major independent candy manufacturers.
Topps Chewing Gum	candy, gum, baseball cards	61.5	Bazooka, Smooth 'n' Juicy, Ring Pop, Pop Bottles, Big Buddy, Gold Rush, Blockbusters	61.5 fye 2/78 (22.5)	1.8 (0.1)	14.0% (NA)	1.01/0.28 (0.06/zero)	14¼ − 5¾ (initial sale) 6/72 @ $17½	The dominant baseball card company. In fiscal 77 − 78 Topps paid $1,035,119 in royalties for use of sports players' pictures under agreements with athletes' players' associations and team owners' associations. Topps also received $1,426,000 in royalties from overseas on its products. About half came from Canada, Argentina, and Nigeria. Fleer Corp. has been trying to break Topps' hold on the sports card market since 1975. In April 1978 the U.S. Supreme Court let stand a ruling that Fleer may pursue a private antitrust suit, charging Topps with monopolizing the baseball picture card market.
Warner-Lambert	a) Chewing gum, mints, proprietories	865.0	Dentyne, Chiclets, Clorets, Adams Sour Gums, Freshen-up, Bubbilicious, Trident, Rol-Aids, Dynamints, Certs	2878.0 (718.0)	208.0 (60.5)	18.6% (20.9%)	2.61/1.17½ (1.01/0.51)	32½ − 22⅞ (30¾ − 19⅝)	If your major business is giving people pills to pop, you might as well cover the more innocuous side of the market. Warner-Lambert bought American Chicle some years ago. In August 1978 this manufacturer of pharmaceuticals and Listerine shelled out $231 million for 99% of Entenmann's, Inc., a big northeastern regional bakery. Entenmann's earned $11.2 million in 1977 on $142 million in sales: meaning Warner-Lambert shelled out about 50% more per dollar of Entenmann's earnings than the then-current market valuation of IBM.
	b) baked goods		Entenmann's						
Wm. Wrigley, Jr., Co.	chewing gum	401.0	Wrigley's Spearmint, Doublemint, Juicy Fruit, Freedent, Big Red, Orbit, P.K.	446.0 (160.0)	31.8 (15.5)	17.3% (15.6%)	8.08/3.90 (3.93/2.75)	77½ − 56¾ (58¾ − 51⅜)	Biggest domestic chewing gum manufacturer. Has 40 − 45% of the market.

Company	Junk food businesses	Approx. 1978 junk food business sales (in millions)	Major brand names	Total sales in millions 1978 (1968)	Earned after-tax 1978 (1968)		Profit/dividend per share 1978 (1968)	Stock price range 1978 (1968)	Notes
					millions	% earned on equity			

Behind the Scenes

Company	Junk food businesses	Approx. 1978 sales	Major brand names	Total sales 1978 (1968)	millions	% earned on equity	Profit/dividend per share 1978 (1968)	Stock price range 1978 (1968)	Notes
Golden State Foods	meat supplier	272.3	None	272.3 fye 7/31/78 (20.3)	2.1 (0.1)	17.6% (NA)	1.96/0.20 (0.16/zero)	15¾ – 9½ (first sold 1972 @ $13 share)	One of several independent companies that do McDonald's beef shopping and processing in large regions.
Idle Wild Foods	food supplier	19.0	Idle Wild Farms	458.0 fye 8/78 (created by merger 1973)	7.2 (NA)	25.6% (NA)	4.18/0.57 (NA)	18½ – 15 (NA)	Idle Wild Farms was the pioneer in flash-frozen, portion-controlled gourmet food entrees for "better" restaurants. Now Le Bistro de Syosset doesn't even need a chef.
International Flavors and Fragrances	a) synthetic flavors b) and fragrances	113.0 253.0	None None	366.0 (82.5)	56.2 (11.6)	25.7% (20.8%)	1.53/0.59 (0.32/0.11)	27⅝ – 19⅝ (19⅝ – 14⅝)	The minds behind all those artificial flavors. For fun, the research labs at IFF will whip up something unusual, like "cave-smell" or the lion house at the zoo.
UMC	vending and food dispensing equipment	112.0	NA	288.0 (134.0)	12.1 (6.0)	14.0% (11.1%)	2.35/1.20 (1.16/0.72)	22⅜ – 14 (27⅜ – 17⅜)	Also an important manufacturer of advertising matchbooks.
Vendo	vending equipment	97.1	NA	111.0 (99.9)	– 2.8 (4.6)	deficit (NA)	– 1.06/zero (1.72/0.60)	9⅝ – 4 (34 – 23¼)	

Guzzlers

Company	Junk food businesses	Approx. 1978 sales	Major brand names	Total sales 1978 (1968)	millions	% earned on equity	Profit/dividend per share 1978 (1968)	Stock price range 1978 (1968)	Notes
Coca-Cola Bottling Co. of New York	a) bottles soft drinks b) produces wines	325.0	Bottles Coca-Cola, Dr Pepper, Welch's, 7-Up, Country Time, Lipton's Iced Tea Mogen David, Franzia Bros., Tribune	425.0 (74.0)	4.2 (4.9)	13.5% (21%)	0.74/0.40 (0.53/0.30)	9¼ – 5½ (9⅛ – 5⅞)	One of the biggest, but just one of a legion of soft drink bottlers across the country.
Coca-Cola Co.	a) soft drinks b) wines	2900.0	Coca-Cola, Tab, Fresca, Fanta, Sprite, Simba, Mr. Pibb, Minute Maid, Snow Crop, Hi-C, Real Gold Taylor, Monterey, Sterling	4337.0 (1186.0)	375.0 (110.0)	25.4% (27%)	3.03/1.54 (0.97/0.58)	47¼ – 35⅛ (40¾ – 31)	America's largest soft drink manufacturer. Despite some stiff competition, still quite profitable and thriving. There is a coca leaf extract in the confidential Coca-Cola formula. The top-secret extract probably isn't drugs, though it is manufactured in a closely supervised plant in New Jersey by the Stepan Chemical Co.— ironically, one of a handful of plants in the U.S. licensed to manufacture pharmaceutical cocaine.
Moxie Industries	a) soft drinks b) chocolate drinks c) bubblegum		Moxie, Monarch, Nu-Grape Brownie, Chocolate Soldier	36.8 (2.9)	0.8 (0.1)	NM (NM)	.24/0.10 (0.06/zero)	5½ – 2¾ (10 – 5⅜)	Moxie, Inc., made a big mistake back in the late '60's. It changed the formula of its stern-tasting Moxie (a northern soft drink that once outsold Coca-Cola) and lost its old New England customers while gaining few new ones. The company has made a comeback recently with chocolate drinks, grape soda, health food supplements, and "Old Fashion" Moxie.
Royal Crown	a) soft drinks b) restaurants	203.0 38.5	RC, Diet-Rite, Nehi, Kick Owns (75) and franchises (672) Arby's roast beef sandwich shops	390.7 (83.8)	10.0 (before extraordinary charge) (5.3)	11.1% (24.1%)	2.28/0.85 (0.93/0.48)	20⅛ – 13 (31½ – 17⅜)	According to The Wall Street Journal, per capita consumption of soft drinks in the United States in 1978 exceeded that of any other type of beverage except water, and, at present rates, soft drinks would surpass water within the next decade. RC proves you can be a cola also-ran and still do OK.
United Brands	soda, fast food	245.0	Makes A&W root beer and franchises A&W stands	2725.0 fye 6/30/78 (555.0)	11.5 (30.9)	7.7% (8.8%)	1.05/zero (3.73/1.40)	15½ – 6¾ (55¼ – 21⅛)	A&W root beer is one of the healthier limbs on this sick pup. UB is the once-mighty United Fruit Co., titan of Central America, whose Chiquita brand is still the signal factor in the banana business. It just isn't very profitable.

Fast Food Out

Company	Junk food businesses	Approx. 1978 junk food business sales (in millions)	Major brand names	Total sales in millions 1978 (1968)	Earned after-tax 1978 (1968)		Profit/ dividend per share 1978 (1968)	Stock price range 1978 (1968)	Notes
					millions	% earned on equity			
Bonanza International	restaurants	≈52.0	Bonanza Steak Houses	≈52.0 (7.7)	2.1 (0.9)	9.0% (NA)	0.42/zero (0.33/zero)	9 – 3⅜ (47½ – 6½)	Fast food has been to the '60's and '70's what gold and silver mines were to the late 19th century: a golconda where any venturesome investor or entrepreneur with luck or pluck might discover the fabled mother lode. Only after some years did people realize that skill and technical expertise might make a difference in an operation's success. As in mines, it wasn't necessary for the venture to be profitable for the promoter to do well just from organizing and running it. And there were some Comstock Lodes.... McDonald's in 1968 earned 56% on its stockholders' investment (the average of all American manufacturing companies usually runs 12–15%), and in 1978 it was still earning 27%, although the company was about 20 times larger than it had been 10 years earlier.
Investors' high hopes were reflected in the prices paid for the stocks. Compare their 1968 prices with the companies' profits that year. In 1968 the average stock sold for 15–20 times earnings.
Although fast food continues to grow as more and more meals are eaten out of the home, a glance around the nearest shopping mall will show how competitive and, in the words of securities analysts, "mature" an industry it has become. Hard-rock mining and engineers have replaced the prospector and his pan.
Chart House	restaurants	237.0	Owns (70+) Cork 'n' Cleaver and Chart House Steak Houses, operates (270) Burger Kings	237.0 (5.9)	10.9 (0.4)	24.7% (NA)	2.75/0.80 (0.26/zero)	26⅛ – 15⅞ (not traded)	
Chock Full O'Nuts	restaurants	16.0	Owns Chock Full O'Nuts, Beef Corral	131.0 fye7/31/78 (43.0)	3.7 (2.2)	NM (14.1%)	0.77/zero (0.47/0.45)	7⅞ – 3⅜ (16⅜ – 7)	
Church's Fried Chicken	restaurants	302.0	Owns and operates 900 fried chicken and 18 hamburger outlets under the names Church's and G.W. Jr.'s	302.0 (7.2)	28.0 (0.6)	38.0% NA	2.22/0.395 (0.06/zero)	30⅝ – 14½ (not traded)	
Denny's	restaurants	429.0	Owns and operates 735 Denny's and 877 Winchell's Donut Shops	546.0 (138.0)	24.3 (6.4)	15.4% (13.1%)	2.82/0.65 (1.68/0.45)	35 – 21⅞ (60 – 33⅝)	
	donut shops	117.0							
Dunkin' Donuts		57.1	Owns (100) and licenses (800) Dunkin' Donuts, also owns 11 Howdy Beefburger restaurants	57.1 (14.3)	3.8 (1.1)	19.0% (NA)	1.75/0.20 (0.58/zero)	17¾ – 7⅞ (55½ – 20)	
Frisch's Restaurants	restaurants	82.0	Owns (107) and franchises (114) Big Boy restaurants, also owns (21) and franchises (1) Roy Rogers Family Restaurants	88.8 (34.7)	1.9 (1.3)	11.2% (16.9%)	1.09/0.29 (0.73/0.21)	9⅛ – 5¾ 15⅛ – 8¼	
Furr's Cafeterias	restaurants	84.5	Furr's	84.5 (14.7)	3.8 (0.5)	16.3% (NA)	1.63/0.44 (0.34/zero)	15¾ – 7⅞ (first offered 1969 @ $12.25/share)	
Gino's, Inc.	restaurants	311.4	Owns (359) Gino's [which also sell Kentucky Fried Chicken along much of the eastern seaboard], and operates (147) Rustler Steak Houses plus a few Chubb's Pier restaurants	311.4 (43.3)	6.8 (2.6)	8.8% (28.9%)	1.38/zero (0.55/zero)	12¼ – 6¼ (48¼ – 28¼)	
Hardee's	a) restaurants	138.0	Owns (419) and franchises (714) Hardee's restaurants and supplies them	214.0 fye 10/78 (41.0)	9.0 (1.4)	26.2% (19.0%)	2.20/0.20 (0.68/0.15½)	18⅞ – 8¼ (not traded)	
	b) restaurant supplies	75.3							
Horn & Hardart	restaurants	35.0	Owns 5 restaurants, 3 cafeterias, and operates 15 Burger King franchises	77.6 (50.3)	0.6 (0.2)	NM (0.2%)	0.61/zero (0.07/zero)	7¼ – 3⅞ (46⅝ – 22)	H & H is trying to overcome its poor image and financially recover through New York City Burger King franchises. As long as the flashers steer clear of the burger palaces, the strategy may succeed.
Host International	a) airport and inflight food	180.0	None	316.6 (75.0)	14.0 (3.7)	23.0% (23.3%)	2.55/0.48 (0.98/0.31½)	27 – 12 (45 – 32¼)	
	b) specialty restaurants	38.0	13 Charley Brown's, 13 Red Onion, and 10 Casa Maria Mexican restaurants						
	c) fast food restaurants	42.0	Owns 185 Jim Dandy fried chicken units and operates 81 Church's Fried Chicken franchises in Houston						

Company	Junk food businesses	Approx. 1978 junk food business sales (in millions)	Major brand names	Total sales in millions 1978 (1968)	Earned after-tax 1978 (1968)		Profit/ dividend per share 1978 (1968)	Stock price range 1978 (1968)	Notes
					millions	% earned on equity			
Howard Johnson	restaurants	435.0	Owns 891 Howard Johnson's; another 254 are licensed; also owns 100 Ground Rounds	555.0 (237.0)	33.5 (9.6)	13.3% (NA)	1.53/0.39 (0.48/0.09)	17−9 (15¼−8⅜)	10 years ago this was bigger than McDonald's. Look at 'em now.
IHOP Corp.	restaurants	60.0	Owns (21) and franchises (449) International House of Pancakes; owns (20) and franchises (33) Love's Family Restaurants; owns (8) and franchises (1) Copper Penny coffee shops	61.2	2.5	≈50%	0.47/zero	6¼−1⅜	This company was formed as a result of the bankruptcy of International Industries, its previous incarnation, which had managed to lose $80 million between 1973 and 1976. In the reorganization of International Industries, each old common share (closing price, 9/30/70, 16⅞) was exchanged for 1/15th of a new IHOP corporation share. In March 1979, the balance of International fast food power shifted. Control of IHOP was purchased by the Wienerwald Group, a large German chain of fast-food operations.
International Dairy Queen	drive-ins	71.2	Licenses 4778 Brazier and Dairy Queen units	71.2 (27.7)	3.3 (0.8)	NM (NA)	0.71/zero (0.11/zero)	6⅜−2⅝ (not traded)	
JB's Big Boy Family Restaurants	restaurants	34.9	Operates 75+ JB's Big Boy, Bob's, Scoreboard, VIP restaurants	34.9 (4.7)	1.3 (0.3)	33.0% (NA)	0.70/zero (0.16/zero)	5⅛−2⅞ (Stock first sold 1970 @ $5/share)	
McDonald's	restaurants	1672.0	Owns (1500+) and franchises (3600+) McDonald's fast food restaurants in U.S. and 12 foreign countries, principally Japan, Australia, & West Germany	1672.0 [4600.0 including franchises] (97.8)	162.7 (9.4)	27.0% (56.0%)	4.00/0.32 (0.29/zero)	60½−43⅞ (11⅛−5⅝)	The GM of fast food operations. Rumors abound: but USA earthworms go for at least $5/lb. Whatever McDonald's culinary sins, earthworms in the beef isn't one of them.
Mr. Steak	restaurants	55.9	Owns (57) and franchises (225) Mr. Steak restaurants	55.9 fye 9/28	1.6	36.9%	1.00/zero	12½−3¼	Company went public in 1975.
Nathan's Famous	restaurants	31.9	Owns (38) and franchises (17) Nathan's Famous	31.9 fye 3/78 (10.4)	−0.6 (0.3)	deficit (NA)	−0.35/zero (0.18/zero)	4½−1½ (43½−8)	Nathan's got started as a hot dog concession at Coney Island in 1916. For a variety of reasons, it never really prospered in the fast food boom. It is still controlled by the descendants of founder Nathan Handwerker.
Orange-Co	restaurants	57.3	Owns (182) and franchises (570) Arthur Treacher's Fish & Chips	117.0 fye 8/78 (0.7)	2.2 (0.3)	7.0% (NA)	0.47/0.20 (0.11/zero)	10⅞−4⅝ (Stock first sold 1972 @ 11⅜/share)	
Pizza Inn	restaurants	83.0	Owns (305) and franchises (348) Pizza Inns in U.S., Mexico, South Africa, and Japan	98.0 (4.0)	2.5 (0.2)	11.5% (NA)	0.61/zero (0.15/zero)	10⅝−5⅞ (Stock first sold 1969 @ $9/share)	Pizza is now the favorite fast food of adolescents by a wide margin, according to food-industry surveys. Also, according to Forbes magazine, pizza has the lowest ingredient cost relative to price of any fast food. (Hence, Pepsico's paying a fancy price for Pizza Hut.)
Ponderosa System	restaurants	197.0	Owns (417) and franchises (200) Ponderosa Steak Houses; also owns 5 Scotty Sandwich Shops	197.0 fye 2/78 (3.5)	9.7 (0.3)	19.9% (51.5%)	2.17/0.22½ (0.09/zero)	30½−13½ (7½−6½)	
Sambo's	restaurants	531.0	Operates 905 Sambo's Restaurants	572.0 (3.3)	7.6 (0.9)	6.3% (41.3%)	0.59/0.60 (0.12/zero)	21¾−9¾ (Stock first sold 5/69 @ $19/share)	What's in a name? Sambo's has always maintained that its name combines those of its co-chairmen: Sam Batistone and F.N. Bohnett. Its promotional material, however, played up the story of "little black sambo," though sambo was changed to a brown Indian with a turban. Some communities have passed legislation to try forcing Sambo's to adopt a less racially offensive name. As of June 1979, Sambo's was still successfully defending its present name in the courts. But Sambo's has other problems. It used to sell interests in its restaurants to supervisors, but a change in that program had prompted about 600 defections by May 1979.

Company	Junk food businesses	Approx. 1978 junk food business sales (in millions)	Major brand names	Total sales in millions 1978 (1968)	Earned after-tax 1978 (1968)		Profit/ dividend per share 1978 (1968)	Stock price range 1978 (1968)	Notes
					millions	% earned on equity			
Shoney's, Inc.	restaurants	144.0	Owns (89) and franchises (171) Shoney's Big Boy restaurants; also operates 19 Kentucky Fried Chicken outlets and owns (82) and licenses (90) Captain D's self-service restaurants	144.0 fye 10/78 (8.2)	8.2 (0.5)	17.3% (NA)	1.03/0.05 (0.19/zero)	16 – 8⅞ (Stock first sold 4/69 @ $12/share)	
Steak 'n' Shake	restaurants	85.6	Owns (143) and franchises (5) Steak 'n' Shake restaurants	85.6 fye 9/78 (17.8)	1.7 (0.9)	9.6% (NA)	0.34/0.22 (0.18/0.10)	9⅜ – 3¾ (5¼ – 1¾)	
Victoria Station	restaurants	101.1	Operates 77 restaurants, 72 under the name Victoria Station	101.1 fye 3/78 (started 1970)	4.9	16.1%	1.74/0.10	19¼ – 9	In 1972, this company had sales of $5.5 million and earnings of $340,000, or 24ᶜ a share. That same year, the stock was first sold to the public at $15/share.
Wendy's International		195.7	Owns (250) and franchises (1100) Wendy's Old Fashioned Hamburger restaurants	195.7 (started 1970)	23.2	41.5%	1.66/0.14	39 – 16¾	First sold to the public 8/76 @ $10/share. Wendy's has been the hot item in fast food in recent years. A top Wendy's executive had been with Kentucky Fried Chicken in its pre-Heublein era.

Hold Onto Those Bonds, the South Will Rise Again!

Company	How many shares sold to the public	When?	By what firm?	At what price?	Amount raised	Subsequent History	Date of last quoted market	Last quoted market
Emersons, Ltd.	200,000	6/72	Filor, Bullard & Smyth	12½	$2,500,000	Filed for bankruptcy 2/77, formerly known as General Restaurants and before that as Franchised Food Systems.	No quote	
Franchise Management Corp.	250,000	10/69	Company	6	$1,500,000	9/71 changed name to P.K. Management Corp. Still alive and operating Italian restaurants. For fiscal year ended 4/30/78 lost $187,000 and had a negative net worth of half a million dollars. 3,600,000 shares outstanding.	1978	25 cents bid
Franchise Management Systems	300,000	10/69	First Devonshire	5	$1,500,000	8/72 name changed to FMS Management Systems, Inc. Profitable IHOP franchise in Florida.	1979	4 bid (up from ½ bid in 1975)
Frank n' Stein Systems	150,000	10/69	Amswiss Int'l.	5	$750,000	3/71 name changed to Gene Browne Systems.	1975	1/16 bid – ¼ offer
Hamburger Dens	120,000	6/69	Granite Securities	6½	$780,000	Name changed to Burlingame Foods and then Burlingame Western.	1975	no bid – 25ᶜ offer
Performance Systems	392,000	5/68	Kleiner, Bell & Co.	20	$7,840,000	Originally Minnie Pearl's Chicken Systems. Name changed again 9/78 to DSI Corp. and 5 old shares were exchanged for 1 new share.	1979	6½ – 7¼ equal to 1.30 bid – 1.45 offer on old stock
Plain n' Fancy Donuts of America	100,000	6/68	Roth & Co.	5	$500,000		1975	8 cent offering
Steak and Brew	300,000	4/72	Faulkner, Dawkins & Sullivan	20	$6,000,000	4/76 name changed to Beefsteak Charlie's. Still operating.	1979	1½ bid – 2½ offering
Der Wienerschnitzel International	500,000	6/69	Slerman, Gowell & Co.	5	$2,500,000		1975	no quote
Wetson's Corporation	220,000	5/69	White, Weld & Co.	11	$2,420,000	5/74 filed for bankruptcy	1977	¼ bid

painting by Les Cabarga

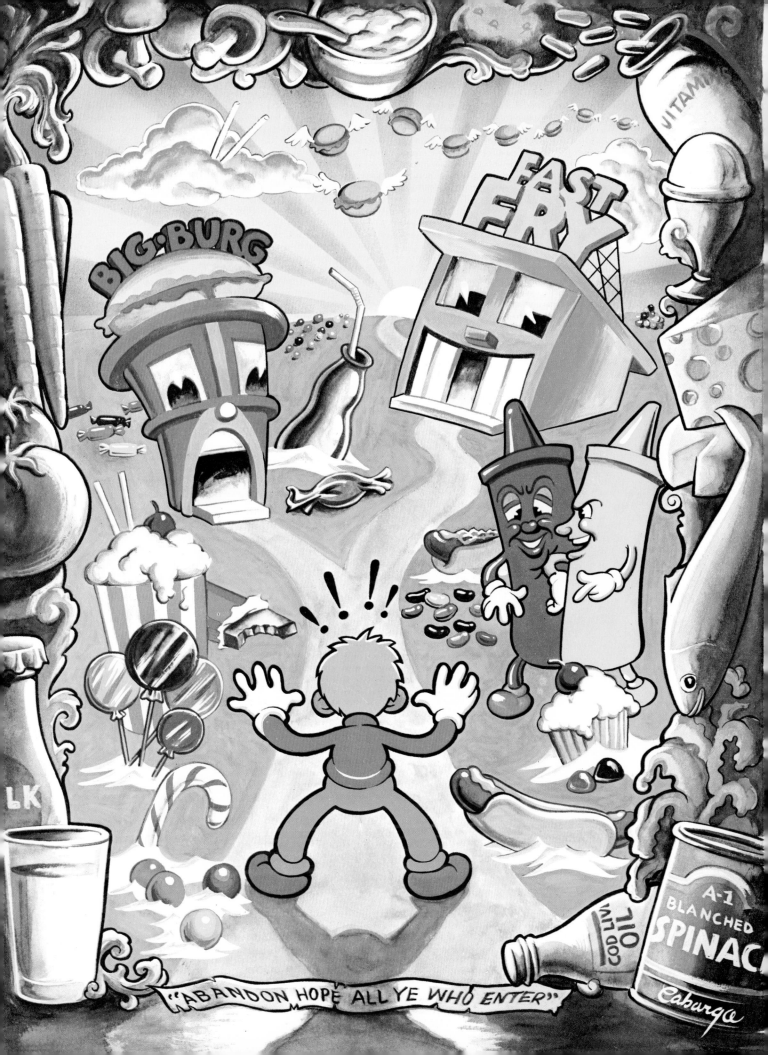

About Falafel: Some Dreams & Broken Dreams along Queens Boulevard, & Slightly West, in the Village

Definition: It's a deep-fried little ball (or two) of mashed-up chick peas stuffed into a small slit-open loaf of flat (pita) bread, along with vegetables and a tart white (tahina) sauce. You had to ask?

by Richard Rothenstein

This area was *dead* previously," Jack Zubli assures me, posing near his Cafe Baba of Israel, a nightclub drenched in the sort of pink and silver sequins my Aunt Ida from Florida would call "psychedelic." Zubli displays the mandatory requirements for running an Israeli place in Queens: rings around every body part but the collar, Qiana shirt unbuttoned to panoramic chest hair, an imported tan, and, please, a spiel.

"People come from all the boroughs to the Baba," he says. "We're like Studio 54—the biggest disco in New York—we give the people what they want." He pads into the club. "I wanted to give it the Las Vegas look, but still be Oriental," Zubli says of the interior. "It's always sparkling. It's an illusion." On the tables are prime ribs au jus and menus that promise "To add the Israeli flavor to your party, Houmus—Tahina—Falafel will be on your table at slight extra charge."

Zubli is 51 and overweight, but expensive tailoring and the fact that he is, apparently, always in motion tend to disguise this. Now he bounds onto the zebra-striped stage and announces, "This is a 35th anniversary for Evelyn and Sal and a 40th for Roslyn and Harry!" 250 mouths shape "Mazel tov!" Evelyn and Sal and Roslyn and Harry are persuaded to join Zubli onstage and *naches* pours like sweat on this humid summer night.

Checking a list, Zubli wishes a happy 80th birthday to Poppy—the Baba Band vamps into "Hooray for the Red, White, and Blue"—as waitresses in maroon mini-skirts and pink tops revolve from the kitchen with a stream of cakes and candles.

"Finally," Zubli says, palms upraised, fingers wiggling, "let's have a big hand for the newlyweds. . . ." Steve and Rima encircle a cake and Zubli winks, "Steve, see if you could kiss your wife for the longest time possible." Rima blushes, looks up in protest. Zubli smiles mischievously. And counts: "One." The couple's lips meet. "Two. Three. Four. Five. . . ."

The audience joins in the crescendoing chorus, many standing, until the couple break at "Twenty-six!" to waves of applause. The in-laws hora around them. Then Zubli introduces headliners Daniel & Dimitri, "the Captivating Continentals," who belt out Catskillized versions of "Ba Sha Na" and other Israeli finger-snappers.

Zubli ushers me into his office. It has mirrored walls and a pink whipped-cream rug. He books an affair for next month on the phone, agreeing to include champagne in the price. "I'm not really worried about competition," he begins quietly, whistling as he talks, a nervous tic that appears to relax him. "I really don't care. We're the oldest Israeli club in existence. You open a place because there is a taste for everybody. I know the other Israeli places in New York because we use same entertainment, compare same food prices. There are a lot of Jewish people around, and if you cannot have several places for them to come in and patronize, there's something wrong."

He must excuse himself to work the stage lights for Daniel & Dimitri's big finale. Next, he hits a spot to bring on Zarefah, an energetic, if not endowed, Lebanese belly-dancer who clacks onstage, tambourine keeping time, shaking her veiled tuchis into cocktails at ringside.

Moshe the sax player grabs the mike. "Don't worry, Rabbi. She's strictly kosher."

Two elderly women squeal coquettishly. Then one clucks, "Enough already! Today, there are no ifs, ands, or buts!"

photographs by Carol Jayne Rubin

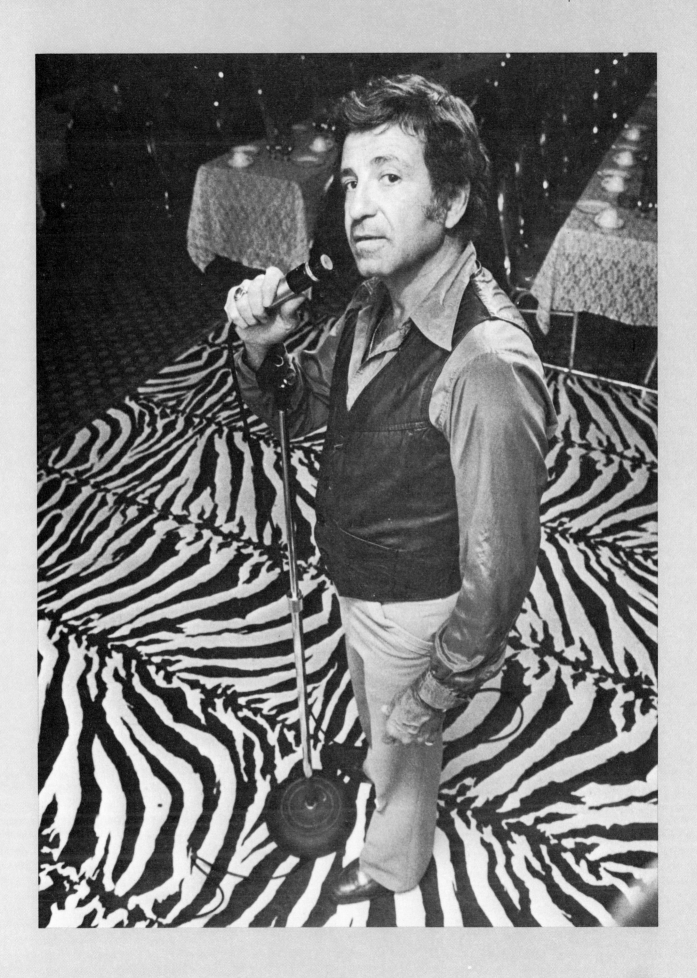

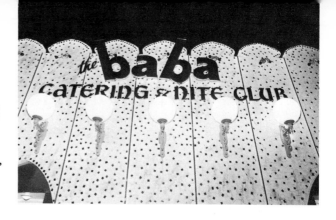

"Or buttocks," her husband says. "Eeefs. Ands. Or—"

One of the wedding party confides to a waitress that, on vacation next week, she's going to see Isaac Bashevis' singers.

In the back of the room, Jack Zubli gleefully surveys the noise, his guests, his Baba. "The only problem with falafel," he cautions, "is that it still has too much of that mid-Eastern taste. It's too ethnic. The secret is for somebody to come in, play around with the mix, and Americanize it." His voice is rising. He dreams. "And change the shape: Instead of round and open, you have to make it either flat or long."

The Baba was built in August, 1968. Zubli designed it, having studied architecture at the University of California at Berkeley in 1949, a year after immigrating from Iraq. Later, he worked on the First National City Bank and Ford Motor Company pavilions at the 1964-65 World's Fair in Flushing Meadow Park, and he consulted on the American-Israel Pavilion, which had boulders "hewn" (said the official Fair guidebook) from King Solomon's mines scattered at the entrance, and snack bars serving falafel: then hyped as Israel's "cousin" to the hot dog.

The Baba, which Zubli owns in a three-way partnership with his brothers, Albert and Avi, did an estimated $250,000 business last year. Recently, Zubli negotiated to buy the Kosheria, a thriving falafel booth in Queens College's student union. The deal fell through. He is anxious to expand beyond his present location in Rego Park, where the Baba's pink glow looms on a landscape most often visited for the Alexander's department store a few blocks away. He'd like to franchise Babas in Los Angeles and Long Island "for the availability of parking, but it's only at the dream stage."

Actually—quitting Zubli for a moment—the highest concentration of falafel in Queens is 10 minutes east of Baba on Main Street, Flushing, where the residential west side is interrupted by a one-mile strip of kosher cuisine crammed between chiropractors' offices; an Angelo's Pizzeria; a Wing Luck; and a 5&10 featuring Yom Tov Bingo, Barton's Nut Clusters, and the "Shlomo Carlebach Live" album in the window. Emanuel Dahari, the manager of the prosperous

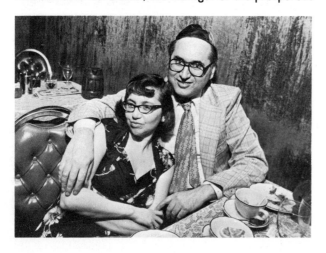

Levy's Kosher Pizza & Israel Falafel, claims that his aunt opened New York's first falafel restaurant on Pitkin Avenue in Brooklyn more than 20 years ago. (Whatever, on this night a long line had formed outside Levy's, waiting for the Sabbath to break. Two teenagers wore I AM A ZIONIST HOODLUM T-shirts.) Dahari adjusts his A&P OUR PLEASURE TO SERVE YOU whites and observes, "A lot of people didn't know what falafel was 10 years ago." Levy's has three other branches.

Eight blocks away, the Magic Pita has a fancy new brown awning. The awning obscures a weather-beaten 3-D falafel—glossy lettuce, the works—that used to be the restaurant's come-on. In fact, Magic Pita used to be called Steak & Pita. Its owner, Ronnie Shelley, says, "I tried to give people the McDonald's but substituted pita instead of a bun." He tugs at an orange yarmulka knitted by his wife, who's a waitress there, and keeps emphasizing that falafel contains no preservatives and is *very* popular among vegetarians. He's added a Thursday and Saturday night all-you-can eat "Special Israeli Salad Bar" (falafel, babaganouj, fried eggplant at $2.95 per person). He's put parve cheesecake on the menu. Cappucino. "When I come from Israel three years ago," Shelley explains, "my friend bought me vanilla sundae. I don't know what the hell it is. Now I know. I love it. It's same with falafel. *Sunday* is our big day. The religious people come out on Sunday. You go into an Italian neighborhood—you see pizza slices." Right now one customer is up at the counter ordering Coke, otherwise the place is empty. "Maybe," shrugs Shelley, "we should take the Hebrew lettering off the sign and paint one saying 'Health Food'?"

Several weeks later, Jack Zubli models his black sequined sports jacket at the Baba and introduces Intamar as "one of Israel's great names." Intamar sings Elvis with an Israeli accent and in black bellbottoms so tight he doesn't need a circumcision certificate. When the crowds are herded out—not before being reminded by their M.C. that Intamar's records are available in the lobby—Zubli doubles wooden seats on the tables, so the floor can be mopped.

Plopping into a lone chair, he mutters, "My problem is . . . Saturday night, Sunday morning all day, I slept three hours, and I could see now, for me to concentrate, and get my mind, you know, to uh, *you know,* I don't think that I could do anymore. I'm in competition with nobody. I don't wish to have these other places in Queens be closed and stay all by myself. That's no good. I'll be lonely. Anyway, I've discussed it with my partners, my brother, Avi. They won't allow me to do anymore. Most people love publicity. I don't want it. I gave you all there is the first time. I shy away from publicity, because my life is so boring. I have accomplished nothing. It's private, right? But I have a great person for you to talk to."

Oh?

"His name is Avram. Avram Grobard. Has a big Israeli place in the Village. And he *loves* to talk, loves publicity, very colorful. We're both Israeli clubs. El Avram is a Village type of nightclub, here I try to impose a little bit of Vegas in it. . . ."

You spend much time in Vegas?

"Yeah. Yeah, I been there a couple of times."

Ever worked down there?

(Quick) "No, no, I try to show that again, that Vegas impression. I don't mean gambling, I mean, the glamour, if it's possible. You know, the front and the inside. I'm not trying to bring gambling into the club. But Israel should be glamorous, why not?"

T his isn't what you'd call a swinging bar," observes the bartender at El Avram. "They won't ask you for a Sidecar or a Green Lizard." A silver Torah clings to his neck, an unsteady toupee to his scalp. "The people who come here are of the Zionist persuasion." He serves up some seltzer—"the Jewish aphrodisiac"—and describes his boss: "He's Jewish, short, and middle-aged. A Jewish Burt Reynolds. And he plays the accordion."

Downstairs, in the dimly-lit dining room decorated in Spanish murals, the chef says he sells 3,000 falafel a week: "a more refined, native New York brand" on a combination platter. The chef says his last job was "head administrator" for Horn & Hardart.

Avram Grobard finally arrives from his home in New Jersey, hurrying down the spiral staircase of "New York's only kosher Israeli/Mediterranean restaurant and nightclub." He wears tailored dungarees, a matching vest that dramatizes a slight paunch, and white vinyl shoes. Smiling steadily, he orders drinks and remembers when there were, maybe, 35 Israeli places in all the boroughs combined, and when Jack Zubli used to visit his club after it opened in 1967, two weeks before the Six Day War.

"He used to come here often, looking around, see what I'm doing and try to imitate me," he begins tensely. "Gabe Kaplan used to come here, too, always doing his imitation of Ed Sullivan. On the big shows, he always said he used to take bellydancer home after work. He was talking about *this* place, my bellydancer. He worked here a year almost. So did David Brenner. He drops in once in a while. The other guy's too big, I think, too snobbish, Kaplan. He should drop in, 'cause this place used to be a home for him. But okay." Sighs. "We'll meet in the graveyard, maybe in the same area."

Drinks come, Avram raises his glass. "L'Chaim. See," he continues, "Jack tried to do his own thing, which he eventually did quite well. I've never been to the Baba, but it's not a nightclub, it's a catering hall. He used to come here and see my operations, ask me questions. Every time I had an entertainer, he used to ask me how is he, you know, good or bad? When I first started, El Avram was *the* in-place for Jewish people." Then, Avram retained a press agent who nicknamed him "Playboychik of the Western World," and booked him on shows like *Eyewitness News,* to share falafel recipes. "Unfortunately, I must say, the war in Israel brings people together. Business improves whenever there's a war. Now it's dropping."

Avram failed at franchising El Avrams in Florida. As he watches his evening's band, The Five Russkys, set up, he seems to see his failure clearly, and says, "If I could have gotten one condominium coming once a week, every condominium once a year, they have now about 400 condominiums, just *one* condo working with a social director, coming down to have some falafel, that would have been all we needed." Now he's not sure if he's getting out of falafel altogether, or just New York. "Maybe New Jersey," he reflects. "A lot of Israeli live there. A lot of rich people." He's tired of the clientele: "It's a very rough business working with Jews, they want to pay and get something extra. They want an extra dollar, just to come in. They want to get something for free." He leaves to confer momentarily with

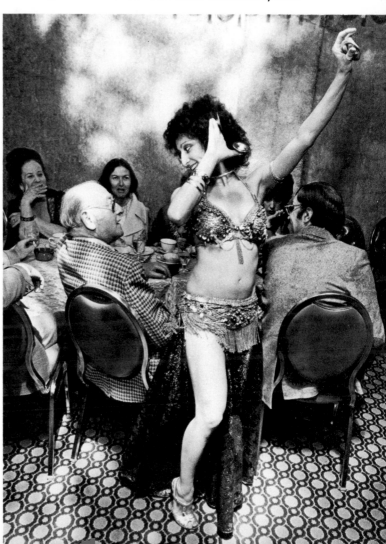

a man who booked a bachelor party, and had Avram make up a cream cake inscribed MAZEL TOV, SHMUCK! When he returns, a friend who has been at Avram's side all night says he's got the name for the first drive-in falafel chain . . . JAP-In-The-Box. Avram smiles, but it wasn't his joke. His eyes burn with the potential of falafel.

"See, it's a fantastic thing for appetizers," he says. "For bar mitzvah instead of playing with the meatball." He thinks waiters and advertising should talk up the ingredients. "You should want to try it, like you come to a Chinese restaurant, and be daring with a pu pu platter. People stop here for falafel after the movie, before the movie. In Israel, that's what they call Ben Gurion's Revenge!" He laughs, as if on cue. "—Because after you eat it, it doesn't forget you!" That's *your* cue. "The problem," continues Avram, satisfied, "is that when falafel isn't done fresh, it becomes soggy. It has to be crisp. Many years ago, I had a friend who tried to find a system how to freeze falafel and sell 'em in the supermarkets. He thought he had a big thing in his hands. He tried it for a long time, but couldn't find the right recipe. I mean, frozen falafels, gevalt!" Avram Grobard leans intently across the table. "I think it can be done," almost whispering, *secrets,* "but as a powder."

If Jack Zubli manages to bring Baba to Long Island, a conspicuous competitor will be Tsachi Liron, who owns the Gates of Lion cabaret in Oceanside. Liron and his wife worked the Baba years ago as a singing duo.

"Jack's doing totally different thing than we are doing," says Liron. "*We're* the only Israeli place. You can use Jewish place, or Israeli imitation. Baba, if I compare, is Middle Eastern, more like Turkey place, all those bright colors. In Israel, you don't find so much the bright and very different, strong colors. It's too European. I can tell you between us . . . Baba, you need a band, so he has the people who make noise onstage. Sometimes luckily, they're good. He picks one from there, one from there, he's busy taking other one. We do dis with the dishwasher."

I mention that Zubli may have his eye on the territory, and Liron strokes his neatly trimmed beard. "I think I heard about dis," he replies. "I don't know. He relate to different Glatt Kosher people. They concern mainly about food. If the rabbi stand there and say it's Glatt Kosher for them, it can be worst food in the world. They eat it."

Although Gates of Lion is only four years old, it is already popular with the Sisterhood/Men's Club set, the kind of "package deal" audience for which the Baba is normally a magnet. Simultaneously, Liron—himself, in his early 30's—is trying to attract younger customers. During summer he sets up a special falafel stand for the beach crowd. He reasons, "After visiting the Baba, I say, 'If I have the opportunity, I do it better, I do it my way.' I didn't like nothing about the place. Jack, I like very much. But he's doing his way. Which has his Arabic background. I want to do something that relate to Israel. You cannot say that

Arabic nightclub is Israeli nightclub." His cheeks flush. "As far as I know, he's architect. I don't like his tastes. What you see in Israel is what we bring you. The music has to be perfect. Like Las Vegas show."

Liron has escorted me outside the Gates of Lion: Miniature plaster lions guard the door. "My wife and I sing mixed," continues Liron. "We sing songs from films, like 'Feedler on the Roof.' We sing 'All I Ever Need Ees You,' Sonny and Cher have big hit with dis song, 'Little Green Apples,' and do new American song 'Raindrops Fallin' on my Head.' We feed the people with teaspoon, the Israeli thing. We cannot sing all the time Hebrew, 'Jerusalem of Gold' and 'Ba Sha Na.' We have a stage act with slides. People say about us when they leave, 'You move me something. . . . I feel something toward Israel.' "

Jack Zubli answers the phone the next day with his customary exuberance: *"Baba!"* He is very busy—and tells someone in his office, "You look faaaaaaaantastic!"—puts me on hold, and returns five minutes later, shuffling through his appointment book. I tell him about Tsachi Liron's comparisons between Gates of Lion and the Baba and he cries, "I don't know what he means by Arabic. If you go, for example, to Vegas and you see all of these glamorous-looking hotels, either Mexican, Arabic, or Spanish, they give it that motif. So what does it matter? Let's face it. If you want to go to Israel, you see all of those things he calls Arabic there, in Tel Aviv, in Jerusalem, all the arches. . . . If he wants to call this Arabic and give credit to the Arabs, then I think he's wrong. Like outside I have the stucco entrance to give it that Oriental/Middle-Eastern flavor."

Zubli has spent his afternoon paying bills, buying food, booking entertainment, and disposing of a Russian comedian who brought nervous titters the night before. "He's very good, but not good enough," Zubli explains. "The public here are businessmen, doctors, lawyers, professional people who have been around and seen professional shows—you can't fool them." He has also spoken with the Cafe Baba in Tel Aviv, "just a side cafe near the Yarkon River" that has no live entertainers.

Zubli begins to whistle: "Baba means two things: either grandma or father. I think it mostly means grandmother and we picked it up because a lot of people, when they heard of the Ali Baba & the Forty Thieves, they would remember the name real quick." He whistles. "And I believe I've told you everything. One day, maybe I can tell you. Deeper into that, nobody would be interested. Falafel will grow and there'll be problems—you hear of MacDavid's in Israel being sued? They serve roast beef, fries, cheeseburger, American franchise claims they're misleading people. That's the best publicity this MacDavid's could have gotten!" Zubli says he must go to a meeting and then get ready for tonight's Baba bash, a bar mitzvah. He hangs up the phone decisively, suffering from an apparent case of Chai Anxiety.

drawing by Gerry Gersten

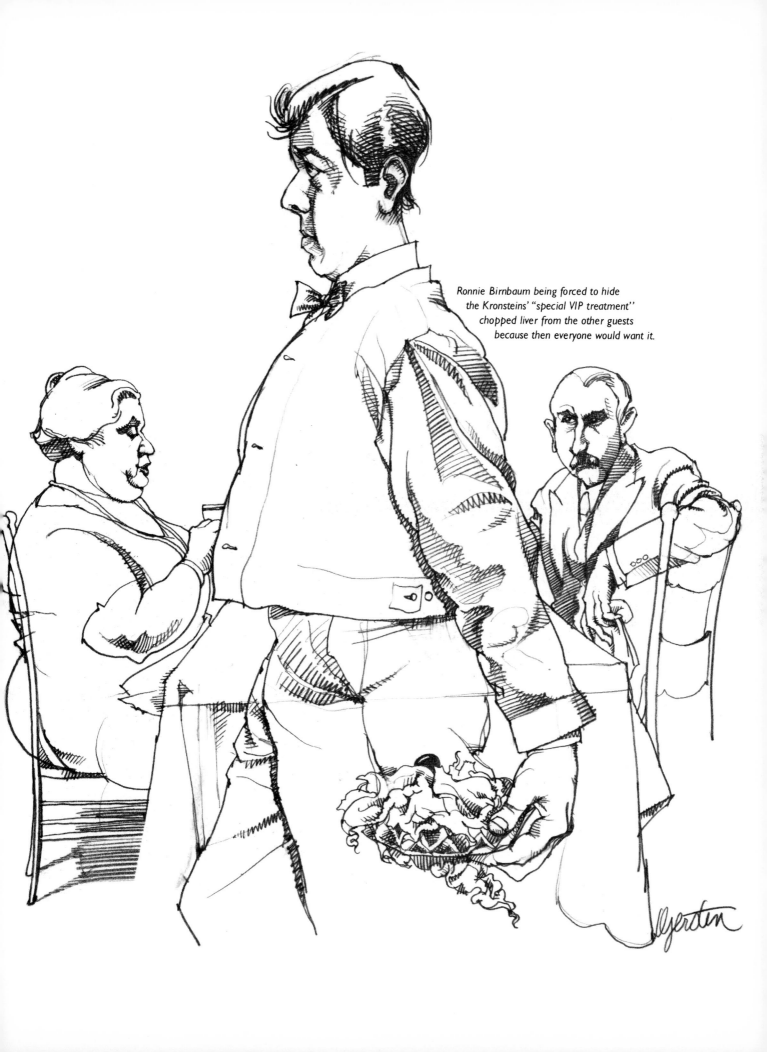

Ronnie Birnbaum being forced to hide
the Kronsteins' "special VIP treatment"
chopped liver from the other guests
because then everyone would want it.

Phyletic Size Decrease in Hershey Bars

by Stephen Jay Gould

The solace of my youth was a miserable concoction of something sweet and gooey, liberally studded with peanuts and surrounded by chocolate—real chocolate, at least. It cost a nickel and was called Whizz; its motto proudly rhymed on the wrapper, "the best nickel candy there izz." Sometime after the war, chocolate bars went up to 6¢ for a while, and the motto changed without fanfare — "the best candy bar there izz."

Little did I suspect that an evolutionary process, persistent in direction and constantly accelerating, had commenced.

I am a paleontologist—one of those oddities who parlayed his childhood enthusiasm for dinosaurs into a career. We search the history of life for repeated patterns, mostly without success: But a generality that works more often than it fails answers to "Cope's rule of phyletic size increase," which states that, for reasons yet poorly specified, body size tends to increase fairly steadily within evolutionary lineages. Some have cited the ordinary advantages of larger bodies—greater foraging range, higher reproductive output, more smarts with larger brains. Others claim that founders of long lineages tend to be small, and that increasing size is more a drift away from diminutive stature than a positive achievement of greater bulk.

Whatever, the opposite phenomenon of gradual size decrease is surpassingly rare. There is a famous foram (a single-celled marine creature) that got smaller and smaller before disappearing entirely. An extinct, but once major group, the graptolites (floating, colonial marine organisms, perhaps related to vertebrates) began life with a large number of stipes, or branches bearing a row of individuals. The number of stipes then declined progressively in several lineages, to eight, four, and two, until finally all surviving graptolites possessed but a single stipe. Then they disappeared. Did they, like the Incredible Shrinking Man, who must now be down to the size of a muon, simply decline to invisibility? Or did they snuff it entirely, like the legendary Foo-Bird who coursed in ever smaller circles until he flew up his own you-know-what and disappeared. What would a zero-stiped graptolite look like?

But the rarities of nature are often commonplaces of culture; phyletic size decrease surrounds us in products of human manufacture. There was the come-on once brandished on the covers of comic books—"52 Pages, All Comics." They only cost a dime.

And consider the Hershey Bar. To my mind, the unadvertised symbol of American quality. It shares with Band-Aids, Kleenex, Jell-O, and the Fridge that rare distinction of attaching its brand name to the generic product. It has also been shrinking fast. I have been monitoring this process informally, and with distress, for more than a decade. I have not been alone. The subject has become sufficiently sensitive that an official memo emanated last December from corporate headquarters at 19 Chocolate Avenue, Hershey, Pa. This three-page document is entitled "Remember The Nickel Bar?"

I do indeed, and ever so fondly, for I started to chomp them avidly in an age of youthful innocence, ever so long before I first heard of the nickel bag.

Hershey defends its shrinking bars and rising prices as a strictly average (even a slightly better than average) response to general inflation, an assertion I do not challenge. I use the bar as a synecdoche for general malaise—as a typical, not an egregious, example.

The accompanying graph has been constructed from tabular data in the Hershey memo, including all information from mid-1965 to now. As a paleontologist used to interpreting evolutionary sequences, I spy two prevalent phenomena: gradual phyletic size decrease within each price lineage; and occasional sudden mutation to larger size (and price) following previous decline to dangerous levels. I am mostly innocent of economics, the dismal science. But I think I finally understand what an evolutionist would call the "adaptive significance" of inflation. Inflation is a necessary spin-off, or by-product, of a lineage's successful struggle for existence. For this radical explanation of inflation, you need grant me only one premise—that the manufactured products of culture, as fundamentally unnatural, tend to follow life's course in reverse. If organic lineages obey Cope's rule and increase in size, then manufactured lineages have an equally strong propensity for a decrease. Therefore, they either follow the fate of the Foo-Bird and we know them no longer, or they periodically restore themselves by sudden mutation to larger size—and, incidentally, fancier prices.

We may defend this thesis by extrapolating the tendencies of each price lineage on the graph. The nickel bar weighed an ounce in 1949.

And it still weighed an ounce (ignoring some temporary dips to 7/8 oz.) when our story began in September, 1965. But it could stall its natural inclination no longer and decline began, to a steady 7/8 oz. in September, 1966, and finally to 3/4 oz. in May, 1968, until its discontinuation on November 24, 1969, a day that will live in infamy. But just as well, perhaps, for if you extrapolate its average rate of decline (1/4 oz. in 32 months), it would have become extinct naturally in May, 1976. The dime bar pursued a similar course, but beginning larger, it held on longer. It went steadily down from 2 oz. in August, 1965, to 1.26 oz. in January, 1973. It was officially discontinued on January 1, 1974, though I calculate that it would have become extinct precisely on August 17, 1986. The 15¢ bar started hopefully at 1.4 oz. in January, 1974, but then declined at an alarming rate far in excess of any predecessor. Unexpectedly, it then rallied, displaying the only (though minor) reverse toward larger size within a price lineage since 1965. Nonetheless, it died on December 31, 1976—and why not, for it could only have lasted until December 31, 1988, and who would have paid 15¢ for a crumb during its dotage? The 20¢ bar (I do hope I'm not boring you) arose at 1.35 oz. in December, 1976, and immediately experienced the most rapid and unreversed decline of any price lineage. It will surely die on July 15, 1979, before this volume goes to press. The 25¢ bar, now but a few months old, began at 1.2 oz. in December, 1978. Ave atque vale.

The graph shows another alarming trend. Each time the Hershey Bar mutates to a new price lineage, it gets larger, but never as large as the founding member of the previous price lineage. The law of phyletic

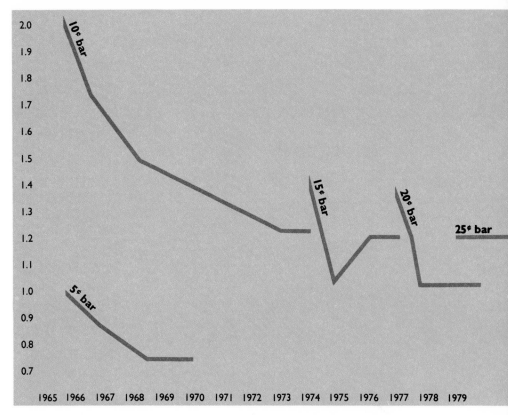

size decrease for manufactured goods must operate across related lineages as well as within them—thus ultimately frustrating the strategy of restoration by mutational jump. The 10¢ bar began at 2 oz. and stood there still when our story began in late 1965. The 15¢ bar arose at 1.4 oz., the 20¢ bar at 1.35 oz., and the quarter bar at 1.2 oz. We can extrapolate this rate of decrease across lineages to its final solution. We have seen a decrease of 0.8 oz. in three steps over 13 years and 4 months. At this rate, the remaining 4½ steps will take another 20 years. And that ultimate wonder of wonders, the weightless bar, will be introduced in December, 1998. It will cost 47½¢.

The publicity people at Hershey's

mentioned something about a 10-pound free sample. But I guess I've blown it. I would remind everyone of Mark Twain's warning that there are "lies, damned lies, and statistics." And I will say this for the good folks in Hershey, Pa.: It's still the same damned good chocolate, what's left of it. A replacement of whole by broken almonds is the only compromise with quality I've noticed, while I shudder to think what the "creme" inside a Devil Dog is made of these days.

Too bad, still. A 10-pound bar titillates my wildest fancy, though even at that weight it should disappear into the void by . . .[1]

[1]Ed. note: August, 3685.

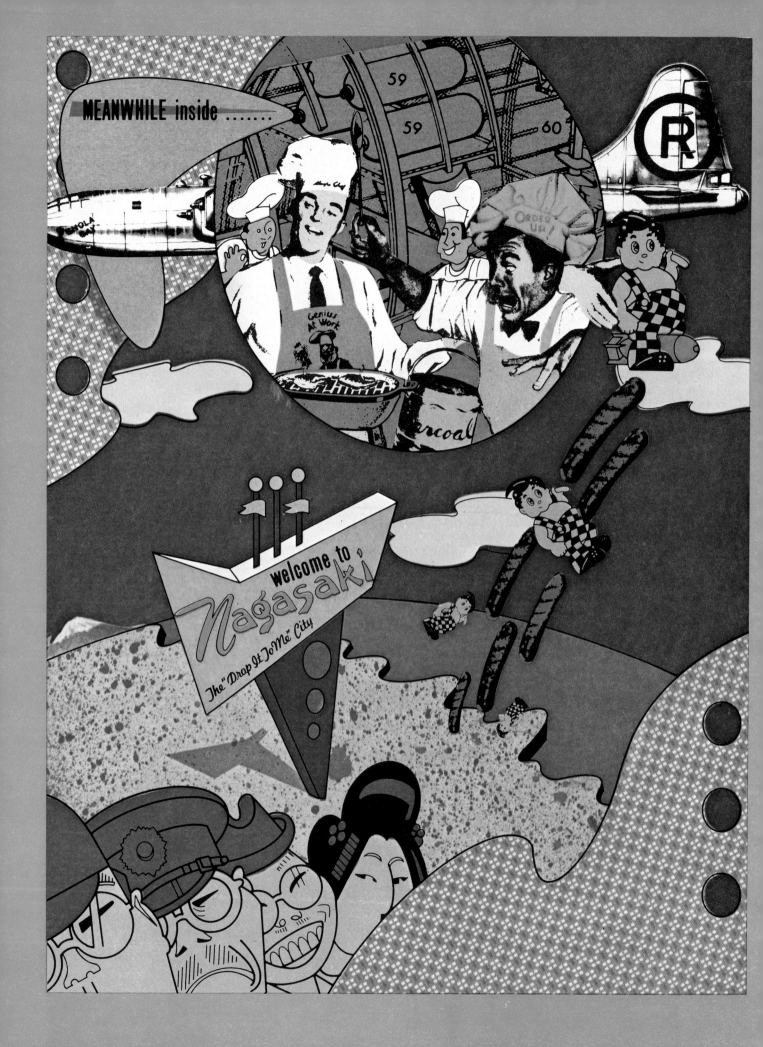

Black Smoke

An interview with John Paul III

by R. Bruce McColm and Doug Payne

G. C.—George Clinton—the Cosmic Father of Funk and referee of a large, nomadic subculture known as P-Funk, a conglomerate of bands and groups with interchangeable tags like Parliament, the Brides of Funkenstein, the Horny Horns, Parlet, Funkadelic, and Bootsy's Rubber Band, reclines on his hotel Barcalounge musing about the ubiquitous Placebo Syndrome.

"Fast food is Muzak for your stomach. It's been programmed to hit those tiny places. It won't kill you but it ain't going to do nothing for you either. It just satisfies. They've got all the colorations, all the things that just hit certain spots of your stomach. Click! — tastes good. After a few years, you'll get sick of McDonald's Big Mac. But they can change to the modern tempo of where you've gone and give you the same thing with a twist. Call it another name, wrap it in another package. They can regulate how long you can stand something."

The Syndrome is everywhere. In Nairobi on a street named after Jomo Kenyatta's ivory-smuggling wife; around the corner from the Thorntree, Hemingway's hangout named after a stump afflicted with jungle rot, now redone in early Ramada Inn; and one block from the Catholic bookstore specializing in cardboard-covered editions of Tanzanian political philosophy, stands the Colonel Sanders Fried Chicken emporium on the former location of the Tom "Shot from Guns" Mboya Shoe Shine Parlor. The marquee has junked *Kentucky* because it's too exotic, and *Southern* to avoid reference to minority tribes who drink cow's blood and gnaw on the raw, pulsating livers of antelopes. *Colonel* will soon be stencilled over to eliminate all allusions to the military.

"I was looking at B. F. Skinner. He's bad, really bad. The motherfucker really learned his lessons good. But what do you do after you make a rat walk a figure eight a hundred thousand times? You can do like advertisers: Can you make this man walk to the Safeway and back to the food lever? Nobody cares but advertisers."

And hidden in the noontime crowd are two KGB agents on recess from snorkeling around the UNCTAD conference held at Nairobi's only skyscraper, the Kenyatta Center, a futuristic spire of prefab elegance and dysfunctional toilets. In their zoot suits and Yuri Gagarin neckties, the two Pillsbury Doughboys wobble with alcoholic bilge in front of the life-sized, 3-D plastic holographic representation of the Colonel beckoning like Ahab to the passers-by. Would they be reported to Lusaka headquarters for nibbling an Extra-Crispy drumstick? (Or would they opt for the Gus Grissom Barbecue Pit across the street? *Have Him Your Way/French Fried or in the Ashtray*.) Inside, assorted Ugandan backcountrymen with Halloween teeth filed during circumcision rites man the counter and ring up orders beneath a sign reading MORE YUKS FOR YOUR BUCKS. Behind the Colonel a band of Hindus in alligator shorts and green polyester leisure suits snort at the agents' indecision. Well, as Ed Filene of bargain basement fame used to spout, "Advertising is America's answer to Bolshevism" — the Soviets eventually capitulate to a Family Bucket.

"People want to be sedated. So make the tempo quick, comfortable, and fast. I don't eat the stuff myself. It tastes suspicious. And all the colors. I'm suspicious of all the pretty colors. I deprogram it out of me. The program they're giving us should carry messages, like on cigarette packs. The side of a hamburger should say: 'This Will Make You Lazy, Passive, and Give You Nothing to Do.' They're taking everything away from us so people are trying to find something to do. They're ad-libbing like crazy now. A bunch of people are fucking watermelons and carting out the whips and chains. They hit you with all those catchy little primal phrases like 'The System Is the Solution' and that shit works deep. That's why I do prune juice all the time. So nothing stays in me. I'm a real believer in the hassles of being full of shit."

What were Gus Grissom's last words? Snap, Crackle, Pop.

Meanwhile, back at the UN's Dag Hammarskjöld Plaza, the orange flowers and Babylonian ziggurats spray-painted on the jungle gyms are rusting. The diminutive Jack Ling, Worldwide Director of Information for UNICEF, grappled with the buttons on his Ozzie Nelson suit and blanched Caucasian as he grasped the black pole of a ONE NATION UNDER A GROOVE flag handed him by Warners' PR wags. From a silver celebrity-mobile leaped G. C., decked out in Americana shades, silver-yellow satin jacket with script Dr. Funk over the arrow-shaped pocket, and red leather, thigh-high, 17-inch platform boots. The funkateers in sheriff-badge sunglasses, Jim Bowie jackets, black leather gaucho pants, and assorted helmets joined him from the Mothership, in its present incarnation as a hulking white charter bus. Mr. Ling accepted G. C.'s petition to the UN General Assembly calling for the recognition of One Nation

collage by Jim Heimann

Under A Groove as a viable global force based on the proposition, "Think, It Ain't Illegal Yet."

Funkentelechy, the musical mindset Clinton promotes and plays with, is the quest for self-actuality as distinguished from the long dormant potential of robots. ("We're just an ugly commercial.") *The comic/cosmic war is waged between Dr. Funkenstein and Sir Nose D'Voidofunk, who zaps people with his Snooze Gun making them yawn, consume, and not dance. With the aid of clones from the intergalactic UFO—the Mothership— the Doc has discovered that visitors from another galaxy stashed the secrets of funk in the pyramids where they've festered for aeons. The messianic Star Child has entrusted the Doc with mankind's secret weapon, the Bop Gun, which counters the Placebo Syndrome, the conspiratorial web of Mad Ave, carry-out disco, fast food, Melvin Laird, and other technological voodoo used to —*

"Every time we come to New York we have some kind of media event," said some bag-flanked slime soldier from the platter company to no one in particular. A passing tape deck broadcast "Lunchmeataphobia," and an American dip-

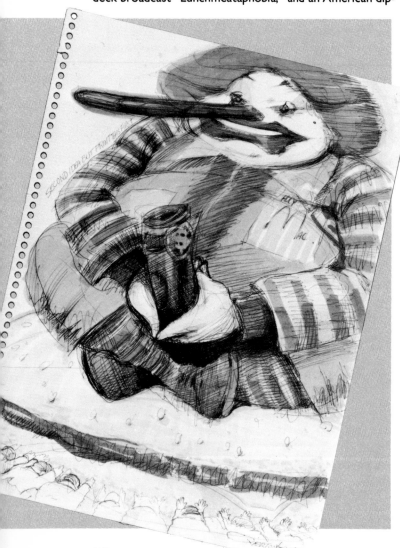

lomat said to a roadie in rasta do, "You're doing your own thing in your own place and time," with the tone of some-one who regularly converses with walls.

"They're still dabbling with your head and you can't contest *that* in court. The Placebo Syndrome just wants us to stick to the brand names."

After one too many glances at G. C.'s funky figure, Jack Ling bolts out of the crowd and sprints four blocks past the rubber displays of Sushi and Jun fading in the windows of local eateries. The Warners crowd rounds up three children with banana bellies and Love T-shirts for a photog session with P-Funk to help in the International Year of the Child hype. The grinning American attaché takes the royalty check for the UNICEF slush fund and slithers away to a cabbie who makes book. The chocolate dome of the UN's souvenir wing glows in the sunset as the flag of Equatorial Guinea is folded into triangles, and the entourage, finally, gets to rest up from the previous night's extravaganza at Madison Square Garden.

"I see it all as they just divide us up — 'You take a piece of the head, I take a piece of the head, and we all get his ass.' Remember when you were kids? — 'Psyche your mind! Psyche your mind!' I mean that's what they're doing and the rat ain't got no notion."

Inside, everything was dark. Except for the concession stands where toothless archons in frayed Knick caps doled out chocolate-covered smegma balls and cat salad sandwiches, and Beagle wafers, and cellophaned Beagle Jerky sticks. In the mezzanine, upwardly mobile black couples stepped gingerly over prostrate dope hounds hoping not to find relatives. If Sonny Werblin was up in his box counting Gulf & Western stock certificates, he wasn't turning on his lamp.

The curtain opens and life as you know it stalls out, replaced by a 30-foot, albino Kong skull peering ahead with orange eyes and air hammer bass lines bottoming out the ax chops of Gary "Dowop" Shider, Throbbasonic Funk-geetarist, who leaps from the giant ape mouth and revs up the chanting — "Shit, Goddam, get off your ass and jam." As he is joined by the rest of the Funkadelic Main Invasion Force, the heaving throng lunges forward. Then, gliding through gyrating Brides and Parlets and sporting strobo-scopic aqua-suit, waist-length blond wig, and headlight sunglasses, comes Doctor F., the phoenix rising from Atlantis. The pulsating flesh down front spills over onto the stage, nearly getting char-broiled by giant torches simulating waterfalls. Blue-uniformed phalanxes of NY's finest at-tempt to peel the funkers back as the Doctor declares — "A mind's a terrible thing to waste or give away. A mind's a terrible thing to waste or give away . . ."

"The head is such a vast thing. It's like a giant CB, and they're always wiggling into it. With the stuff they got, they can override it, put that voice in there saying 'Do this, go ahead, you'll like it, you really will,' and eventually you *will* like it. You know how the FCC claims the rights to the airwaves? Well, when we're able to mental telep, they're going to claim the rights to your head."

For anybody who came with shit for brains, it was time to get their Doo Doo chased by the Doctor: "The world is a toll-free toilet . . . our mouths neurological assholes . . . in a state of constipated notions." But P-Funk wields the "neurological enema . . . prune juice of the mind . . . designed to rid you of moral diarrhea, social bullshit, crazy do-loops, mental poots.'"[1] Then a giant yellow pterodactyl soared back and forth over the stage screaming — "Fried Ice Cream is a reality! Fried Ice Cream is a reality!"[2] Those few who didn't get it were too afraid to tell anybody.

We whizzed over to the Juan Pizarro Motor Lodge on Central Park South. The flags at the Plaza alerted the Trinidadian steel drum player that the U.S. was in, the West Germans were in, the UN was in, Atlantis had sunk, Carmine Galante was out, and Georgie Jessel was in bed. The lounge lizards, embalmed women of the ethnic persuasion, waltzed with their cotton candy boyfriends à la Paul Henreid past the 20-mule team manure factory parked along the curb waiting for romance to rear its ugly head.

After a momentary logjam near the Blimpie Base complete with High Tech logo, our chuck wagon pulled up alongside the Sanitation Department's meat grinder. Juan's lobby was full up with Odd Fellows donning Aztec plumage and dreaming of duck hunts and the big skeet shoots held on foggy mornings spent wallowing in a swampy blind. As they piled into the Mamie Eisenhower Bar & Grille for pâté à la squat, furburgers, and bearded clams, we skated past the last of the Golden Horde only to find Roy White and Joe Franklin holding down the knish booths outside the chromium elevator banks camouflaged by Beaux Arts grape leaves. On the 10th floor, a mammoth steak or facsimile thereof was hung between the mirrors at the end of the hallway, subliminally flashing the big Eat Me. We headed on down to the room marked 00.

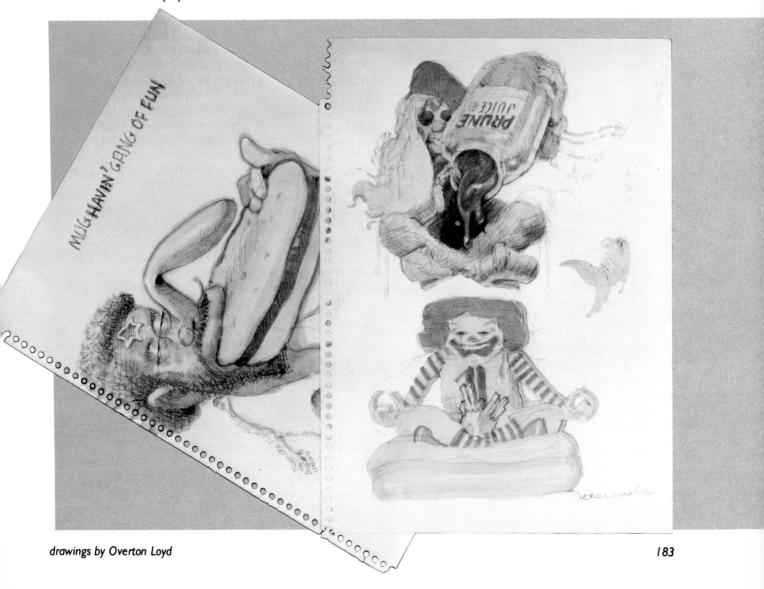

drawings by Overton Loyd

As he talked, the Captain of Funk stared out over Freddy Olmsted's playground and watched as Elks and Rotarians grazed the Sheep Meadow looking for the eschaton. In the background, we could hear the muted jabber of a peg-legged PR man explaining the R & B origins of P-Funk to an eager Richie Cunningham.

"But you know when you get right down to it, it takes a lot of energy to fight the Syndrome. Maybe it ain't worth all that energy. I'll dabble every now and then, buy a bag of chips or something and have a few, but I throw the rest *away*. And if I go home to my mother's house, just the memory of eating chicken and those pork chops will make me dabble a little bit. But if I do too much, I'll get real bad migraines and it makes me want to shit. So I try and deal with it, treat it as a joke, play with it. Because, you know, the Syndrome is funny, When you look at it, the shit is funny. If it ain't funny then you got to jump out the window because it's *that* serious. We'll probably evolve to the point where we'll have to get off the planet and begin some hellified basic training. But for right now I'm wondering if this place has any room service 'cause I want to get me a lobster."

[1], [2] From the song "PROMENTALSHITBACKWASHPSYCHOSISENEMASQUAD (The Doo Doo Chasers)," by George Clinton, Gary Shider, and L. Brown © 1978 Malbiz Music, Inc.

Chewing the Fat with Uncle Harry at Lewis' Cafe in the Heart of Town

ST. CLAIR, MO. *Uncle Harry, Packy Wheeler and Joe Spradling are passing the pleasant morning hour of 8-9 in a high-backed wooden booth in the only place to eat in St. Clair, Missouri (besides Coach's), Lewis' Cafe. The coffee is 20¢ the first cup and 10¢ for refills, served by a waitress who's leaving the week after next to teach at the Lutheran school, but they don't pay nothin. Joe asks her rhetorically if there's a charge for loafin. All six adjoining booths are filled with St. Clair's over-80 crowd, 8-9 in the morning and 2:30-3:30 in the afternoon. They eat before they come, to save money. Harry says he has raisin bran for breakfast and supper and one meal a day at lunch. Packy sometimes picks up the special at Lewis': Mon., hamburger; Tues., chicken; Wed., beef pie; Thurs., can't remember; Fri., fish and barbequed hamburger. Joe says the barbequed hamburger is just awful. Once in a while they surprise us, Packy continues — the other week we got liver and onions that just melted in your mouth. Uncle Harry remembers the time they had beans and ham hocks.*

The conversation turns to food. The other day, Harry says, he fixed him some cornmeal mush. Joe, who eats liver because it's healthy, prefers whole-wheat mush. You go out and grind some fresh whole-wheat, fry it up in a little butter or oleo, and eat it with honey on top. Harry likes to put gravy on it too.

Packy had grits once when his cousin from North Carolina was up. Lewis' does not include them on a modest standard menu. Joe says they've had the same menu since they opened in '37—that's what happens when you don't have no competition, except Coach's. The other day he tried this I-talian place the other side of Washington, $8 and all you got was a salad, this thin little piece of meat, hardly nothin at all, bread and butter, and a dessert. You could get more than that at Lewis' for $2. Harry used to eat the Senior Citizens lunch at the high school cafeteria till his eyes went bad and he had to give up driving his Ford. Other day Homer Girady sold him a jar of honey this big, wax and all, for $3.65. Joe tells a funny story about a doctor he had once who had a Bible saying on the wall of his office: "Eateth thou honey for it maketh thee well." Harry says he doesn't put it on bread, he just eats a spoonful when he feels like it.

They order a refill on the coffee. A large pile of donuts in a tempting array of colored glazes does not interest them. Good thing there's no charge for loafin. A raw-boned farmer in a straw cowboy hat comes in and Joe complains that they hardly know half the people who come in here nowadays. Harry says he sure can't remember names. In fact he has forgotten Joe's last name, although he's known him well nigh 60 years. Packy is thinking of a huckleberry cobbler he used to eat quite a bit. Huckleberry is another name for blueberry but it sounds better. They used to pick 'em. Joe imagines he'll have the roast beef plate for lunch: roast beef with gravy, bread and butter, dessert extry. People eat too much these days.

"Yeah, Joe's a nice guy," Uncle Harry comments on the way out, "but he's awful p'ticular 'bout what he eats."

—Deborah Young

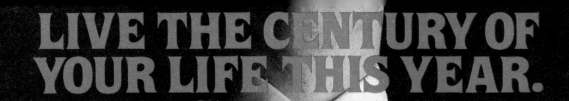

LIVE THE CENTURY OF YOUR LIFE THIS YEAR.

BURDY

Join the People Who've Joined the Fair.

"When I first signed up with the Ranger Chefs, I was sure they'd wash me out in a week. That was three months ago and I've learned a lot since then. It used to take me near half an hour just to make my own breakfast, but now I can turn out 200 meals in nearly half that time. Hell, I can even field-strip a 20-lb. turkey, drumstick, dressing and all — and put it back together in 30 seconds."

RANGER

Feast on Life. Join the Century O' Progress Ranger Chefs.

Proudly We Serve It — Motto of the Combi-Nations, the Ranger Chefs of Tomorrow.
Are you a boy with a talent for taking orders? Then get in touch today.

Food Fight

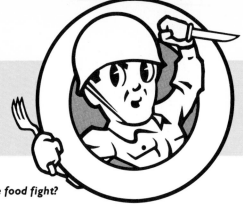

Q: What was your most memorable food fight?

JULIA CHILD, legend: "I remember flipping butter onto the ceiling with one's napkin at children's birthday parties. That was in the old days when you had linen napkins and you'd just put it in the napkin and then go pull your two hands, far far apart, you go flip, and it just flips up onto the ceiling. It just stays up there and then gradually comes down."

RON GALELLA, paparazzo: "As a child, I would go in gardens. North Bronx Italians . . . had a lot of gardens, a lot of farmland. My brothers and a whole gang of kids used to grab tomatoes and have tomato fights, smashing tomatoes in each other's faces. I had them up until sixteen, I'd say, and the fights did have a release—it was self-expressive."

AARON LATHAM, author: "I was sitting in bed one day, and my girl friend came in and started throwing raw eggs at me. I was in graduate school, working on my dissertation—F. Scott Fitzgerald's movie career. I was going with a girl who was studying acting, named Sigourney Weaver, now an up-and-coming actress. She used to have dreams about her father: the recurrent dream was that the father would take her over his knee and take down her underwear and crack eggs on her behind and then spank her, thereby scrambling the eggs. So she had some special psychological interest in eggs. So one day we were not getting along too well, and I was sitting in bed working, and she thought I shouldn't be. And this was in a borrowed house, I was house-sitting in New York on East 93d Street, practically total stranger's home, and I look up and there she's standing in the doorway, with a carton of eggs. And she just started throwing and I kept thinking, 'What if there'd been a gun in the refrigerator instead of a carton of eggs?' And the eggs kept hitting lamps and splattering on the wall behind me, really exploding, and then one hit me right in the head. And I just knew if it had been a gun, I'd be dead. The bed and walls were covered. I was furious. Kind of frightened. What I did immediately was grab her and twist her arm behind her back and force her out in the backyard and turned the garden hose on her, and drenched her. It was an incredibly phallic fight, with her throwing eggs and me getting out the garden hose and spraying her up. Then we finally made up and then we had another fight about who was going to clean it up. The eggs were on walls, the beds, and the lamps for a couple of days before we settled who would clean it up— which turned out to be me, since I'd borrowed the house."

RUDY MAXA, gossip columnist, Washington Post: "The Kennedy kids' food fight was in the summer of '75, it happened at Clyde's in Georgetown. Ethel Kennedy's daughter, Courtney, was there at a table with Jean Kennedy Smith's son, Steve, and they were sitting with Dustin Hoffman, who was in town filming **All the President's Men**. They had been drinking that night and Hoffman suggested that he and the Kennedy kids have a food fight. The rules were that you had to sit still while your opponent dumped all manner of goo over your head. And the first guy to flinch lost. So Hoffman went first, of course, he emptied a can of whipping cream on Steve Smith's head. Then Smith poured an entire bottle of catsup over Dustin Hoffman. Hoffman went into the kitchen and began mixing vegetables and chili and any food he could find into a very large mixing bowl. At that point, Clyde's manager kicked the Kennedy kids out. You have to understand, in Washington, the only people who get any respect are movie stars."

FRAN LEBOWITZ, author: "My food fights are largely contained to arguing about which restaurant to go to."

VIDAL SASSOON, barber: "During the early, frustrating years, trying to create a niche out of hair, I organized a birthday party for Georgia Brown. It was attended by friends from all runs of life—this was a very fast crowd. Somehow I became involved in a heated argument. I have no recollection about what. The birthday cake was sitting benignly on the table. The wildest urge came over me. Could I really activate a

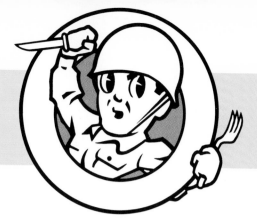

fantasy? Yes, I hurled the cake straight at a wall. I have never seen a party end with such alacrity. I have never wanted to throw another cake. Once you have done it, there is no point, is there?''

NANCY FRIDAY, author, **My Mother, My Self:** "When I'm invited to somebody's house for dinner, and I'm not fed enough or well—which I think is a terrible thing to do to people, because it's very easy to give them enough food—I become withdrawn and very grumpy. So while I don't actually pick up food and hurl it, I'm, I'm . . . angry. I can't understand some people who have all the money to provide food and even maybe help to prepare it, and <u>still</u> insufficient or bad food comes to the table. I find it very hard to contribute to the rest of the evening. It brings out a kind of childish belligerence in me.''

LEONARD MELFI, playwright: "Hot chocolate. H. M. Katoukas would get very emotional sometimes. And he happened to have a play on at La Mama, in 1967. My play had opened up the Festival. I was working there, also, as a waiter, serving the hot chocolate and the coffee and the tea. The second play of the Festival was his play, and he directed it, too. One night he was just upset by things in general—like the audience—and what happened was the pay phone had rung the night before, the first night of the show, it should have been off the hook but it

rang right in the middle of the play. So he went over there and he pulled it, and when he pulled it, he pulled it out of the wall. Then it wasn't fixed right away, so people couldn't make reservations to come see his show. And he was very disappointed. So he just got up, and he threw hot chocolate and we had whipped cream on it, he just took it off the counter and started throwing it at the audience while going into this dramatic thing about theater . . . something like 'I will kill for my play!' Then he went out in the hallway.''

GAEL GREENE, food critic: "I am told by my brother that my sister and I once hid some green grapes in his pudding and that he was traumatized for life by that. He didn't eat fresh fruit, and he considered it one of the great betrayals of his childhood. That's my only violence with food.''

SOUPY SALES, comedian: "The only food I've ever thrown would be what is called a pie. My first time was in 1950, I was working at a station in Cleveland, and at the time there was a movie out called **Broken Arrow,** Jeff Chandler, it was the story of Cochise. They got me a loincloth, horse and a feather, and I got them to get a cavalry outfit and we put it on a guy and shot the scene completely over his shoulder, with just a hat and an epaulet and they played the music and it was **Son of Cochise.** I came riding over the hill, on this horse, bareback, scared to

death, and I got up and said to the guy who is right there in front of the camera, 'White man come and take away happy hunting grounds, kill all of red man's deer and buffalo and antelope and what is there left for the Injun?' And with that, he hit me in the face with a pie, which was done with egg whites, because the shave bomb, which we used later, didn't come about till 1954, so up to that time, you had to use whipping cream or egg whites. We'd put it in a piecrust, not in a tin pan. And so he threw it at me and I said, 'That's not-um what I had in mind.' The most famous, of course, was in 1965, in California, when Frank Sinatra came on. I ran into his daughter one night and she told me he was a big fan of the show. And he called me when I was gonna go network, and he wanted to go on the first show, but he would only do it on one condition: and that is, he wanted to come on and get hit in the face with a pie. Which was just fantastic because up to that time, I had no idea of hitting a celebrity in the face with a pie. The last time Frank did the show, in '65, he brought on Sammy Davis and Trini Lopez and we did the waiter bit where we threw about 300 pies, and of course, people were always complaining that it was a terrible thing to waste food while people were starving . . . you remember your mother used to say . . . but I always said, 'Listen, if people want to eat shaving cream, that's all right with me.' ''

DON RICKLES, comedian: "My greatest food fight was when I went into the kitchen and boiled an egg while my mother was watching.''

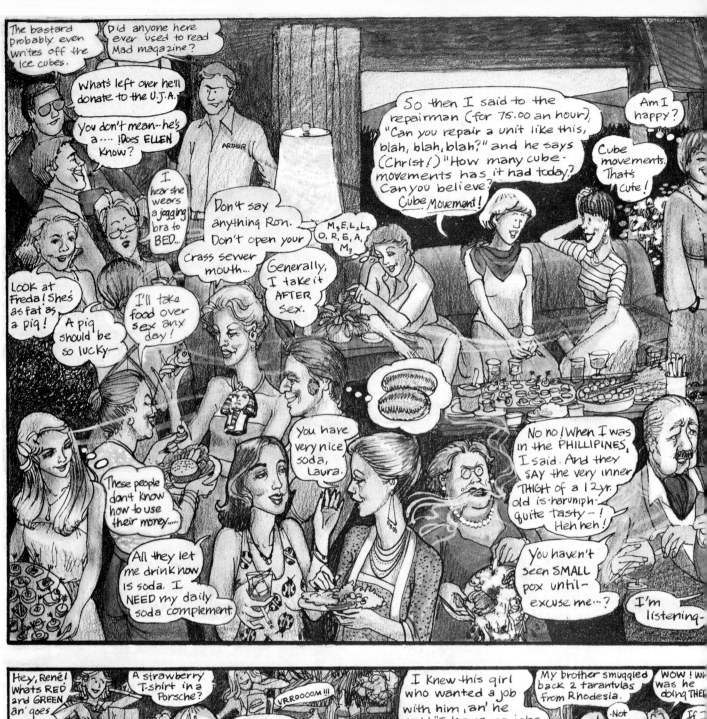

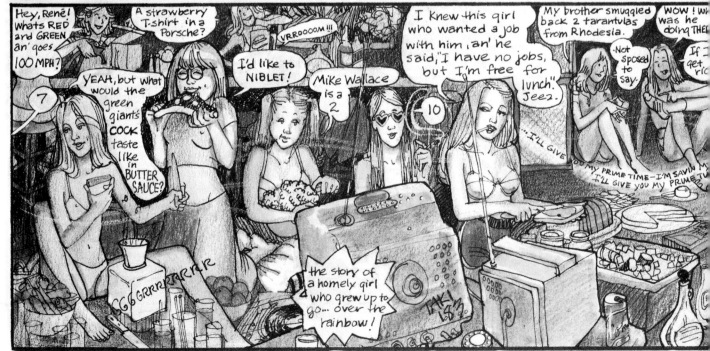

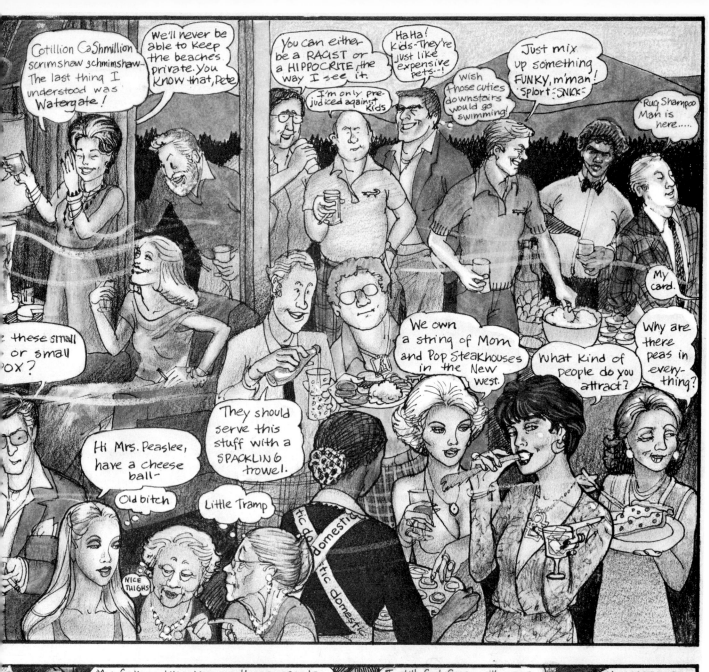

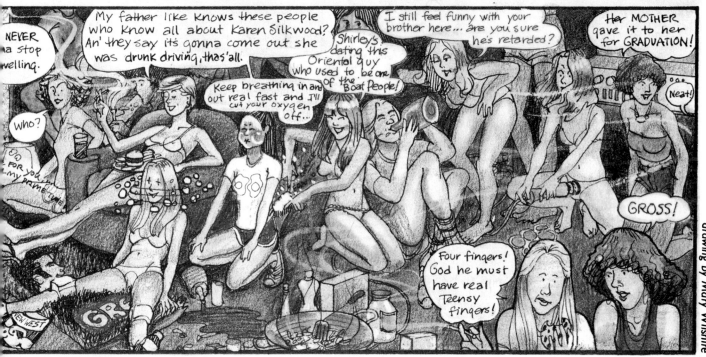

drawing by Mary Wilshire

The Potable Oxford Book of Literary Wining

by Andrew Zimmerman, Esq.

"I have a Vision, but I keep it to myself."

The eminent John Henry Newman, later to turn Papist and Cardinal, had invited Quern, Jervis, me, and a few other pious scholars over to his room for a religious supper. For His Flesh and His Blood we were to have sherry biscuits and claret. The biscuits proved to be dry, rock hard, and slightly sour — in short, exquisite. But my first sip of claret was attended by a shock that could not have been greater had there been an electrical eel coiled in the dregs. Newman had adulterated the claret with sherry!

I called on Newman to confess and he coolly owned up to the deed in these words: "As you know, it has long been my desire to reconcile, insofar as is possible, science and religion. Therefore when Huxley informed me that blood is composed of a ratio of fifty-five per cent of the white element to forty-five per cent of the red, I resolved to formulate a corresponding mixture of white sherry and claret."

A few days after the event, poor Jervis and Quern openly professed Atheism. My own faith was severely tried for some time afterwards.

It was the yearly custom of the Port-and-Claret Society to host a combined luncheon and scholarly debate. That year the subject was to be the nature of ancient Athenian civilization. Championing a case for the essentially juridical-patriarchal nature of Athenian society in the 6th century B.C. was Cambridge's Humphrey Chadwick. His opponent, our own Sir Arthur Edward Sherry.

After the claret bottles were cleared away and the port brought out (the good, glutinous **stuff), the** debate commenced. Surrounded by stacks of journals and buttressed by his own immense monograph, Chadwick brilliantly presented his argument.

We were, to say the least, apprehensive of Sir Arthur's and Oxford's chances. Apprehension gave way to despair when we saw that Sherry was crawling towards the stage without a single note. Chadwick was positively smirking. Bravely grappling with the lectern, Sherry held forth. "To my way of thinking, all society may be divided into two types. On the one hand, the primitive and repellent" — here he stared pointedly at Humphrey Chadwick — "juridical-patriarchal society. And on the other hand the refined and congenial port-and-claret society. I should say that Athens of the 6th century B.C. was undoubtedly a port-and-claret society."

Spontaneously and to a man we rose and acclaimed Sir Arthur the victor. Once again, Oxford had carried the day!

It was said of the undergraduate Wilde that he never took port except with petits fours. Asked by Beardsley to verify this report, Oscar replied in his inimitable way, "Actually what I said was 'I never drink port except on all pretty fours.' Care to play horsie and see?"

The eminent scientist Huxley, on leave from Cambridge, dined with me at Commons. Over our third sherry trifle and fourth bottle of port I mused aloud, "I can drink as much sherry and as much claret as I please with no untoward effect; but after my second bottle of port, I invariably see double. I wonder why?"

From under the table Huxley's kindly and reflective voice explained, "As Newton tells us, light is composed of corpuscles. I should say port is composed of paired <u>identical</u> corpuscles, and that one of each pair migrates to the left eye and the other to the right, resulting in double presentation of the image. You laymen name this double vision. To correct for such phenomenon, you must place an opaque body over one eye. Whether said body be a patch of stout cloth, a stone, or the rosy bottom of a freshman is of little consequence."

I have since tried all three remedies and have met, in every instance, with complete success. Another testimonial to that great man's easy genius!

At the table, Jowett had fallen into a bitter and voluble funk occasioned by what he believed to be the Lower House's declining powers of expression. The sherry suggested to me a tack which might divert his thoughts and conversation from that melancholy subject.

"It's a funny thing," I said. "My old nurse Grey, rest her soul, used to dose me with sack whenever I suffered from a fit of the colic."

No sooner were the words out than I regretted their impertinence. With his eyes dripping thunderbolts Jowett commented, "Then, sir, your Grey was nothing more nor less than a quack and mountebank. Commons have been guzzling the spirit for nigh a century — which practice has done nothing to arrest the deterioration of that body's vocal organs."

A PUBLICATION OF CONSUMO UNION • NO ADVERTISING • APRIL 1983 • FOUR DOLLARS

Consumo Reports

Brand name ratings

- ☐ cattle prods
- ☐ microwave blankets
- ☐ aerosol burger makers
- ☐ hovercraft
- ☐ ivy league schools
- ☐ gasohol bar-b-q's

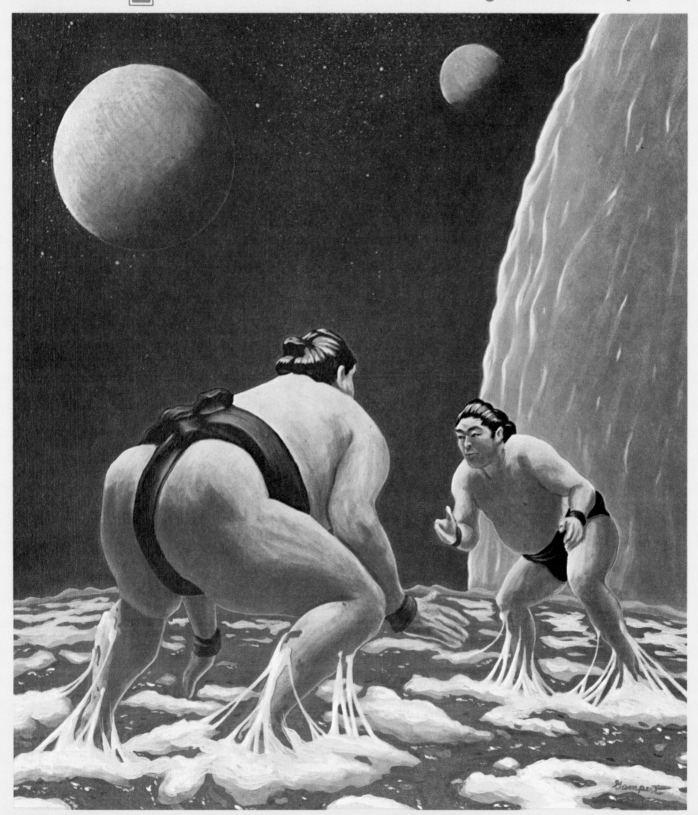

Vacu-Mac Burger Maker

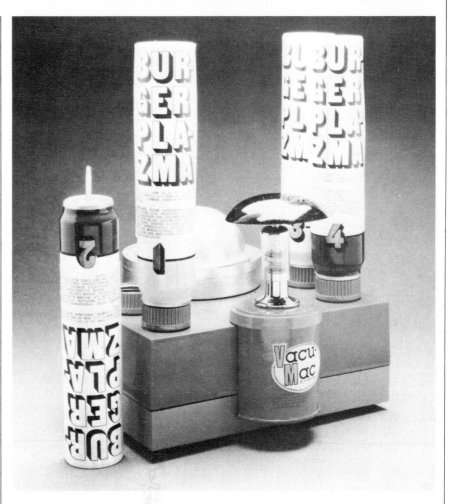

During the last several years, CU has evaluated a number of so-called "educational" toys from the Hun Co. that, in our judgement, taught children little of value and often exposed them to serious bodily harm. For example, the company's *Acupuncture for Pets* and its *Fingernail Removal Kits* offered little in the way of useful instruction. We rejected its entire health series, including the *Chemotherapy for Dolls* and its *Enema Sets* (1 and 6) on the same grounds, and didn't recommend the manufacturer's collection of magic tricks due to its faulty Crib Death Illusion.

It's small wonder we were pleased when Hun announced a new product that we can endorse, the *Vacu-Mac Burger Maker (CLR 2576)*. We rate it highly because of the valuable lessons it provides youngsters about high-pressure, low-density, polyethylene diets.

How It Works

Attached to the side of the *Vacu-Mac* are six pressurized metal canisters containing an organic blend of nutrients known as Burger Plazma, the basic building block of hot sandwiches. What makes this device unique among foodstuffing machines is that different formulations of this plazma are used to make the bun, pickle, and cheese.

When Plazma 1 is exposed to 225F, it undergoes a chemical change giving it the appearance and texture of broiled hamburger. When Plazma 2 is heated it becomes a lightly toasted bun. These thermally-initiated transformations are made possible by chromosomological/microencapsulization: a technology that impregnates the plazma with the genetic coding necessary for it to develop into a mature sandwich component during a 20-second gestation period. All together, Hun makes four different plazmas and has plans for 700 more.

The machine we tested was simpler to operate than a *Slinky*. After installing the canisters and selecting a mold, we pushed the appropriate plazma selector button. Next, we pumped the air out of the molding cavity, forcing in the plazma where it was heated.

Our initial efforts were not all that successful. The pressure gauge was not precisely calibrated, causing our hamburgers to expand to more than 5 feet in diameter. We judged that result much too large for luncheon purposes.

Another problem involved cleaning up afterwards. Unlike ordinary foods, the remains of *Vacu-Mac* burgers tend to drift around the room, soiling walls and ceilings. If you plan to dine inside, first be sure there is sufficient cross-ventilation.

Durability. Prototype *Vacu-Mac* burgers would often turn stale after 5 or 10 minutes, but improvements in the plazma formula have overcome that problem; our tests indicate an average half-life of 70 months before the sandwich decays into a canapé. Care should be taken not to expose them to high humidity, however, as that tends to promote condiment corrosion.

Noise. During its start-up cycle, the *Vacu-Mac* emits harmonic frequencies of 500,000 cycles per second that may cause tooth enamel to darken temporarily.

Options. Four optional attachments may be purchased at extra cost, but we didn't think any of them worth the money:

Running Lights: Unnecessary. A 25-watt bulb or any ordinary flashlight provide more than enough illumination.

Rangefinder: Judged of marginal use. Could not be calibrated for snacks. Plastic lens.

Read Only Memory (ROM): Capacity limited to 16K bytes. Slow access time (350 nS).

Stamen and Pistel: Cross-pollinator prone to jamming.

From an operational standpoint, we think, despite some shortcomings, this device provides an effective way for children to learn how to make meals that are high in polyunsaturated vapors.

How They Taste

Taste tests are difficult to conduct because they are so subjective; what is delicious to one person may taste like flounder marinated in an unflushed toilet to someone else.

Nonetheless, we have attempted to describe as precisely as possible the flavor of a fully-operational *Vacu-Mac* burger.

All the patties we made had a nicely corrugated texture and the fresh aroma of delicately-spiced nitrogen, which mixed delectably with the light perfumy odor of the hydrogen. The buns, however, had a somewhat vapid taste. Despite the crisp, nutty flavor of the ionized argon there was no mistaking the odor of day-old oxygen, probably accounting for the lack of body characteristic of these sandwiches. This deficiency may be corrected if the cooking pressure is held at 5 pounds per square inch *below* what the manufacturer recommends.

Overall, we rate the burger's taste as Good. We would have judged it Excellent except for its tart undersmell of carbon dioxide and its rather bland garnish of particulate matter.

Recommendations

Because the *Vacu-Mac* is such a unique toy, we could not find a similar appliance with which to compare it. So we did the next best thing and tested its performance against other equipment that seemed capable of making a credible facsimile of an aerated sandwich.

As can be seen from our Ratings, the *Vacu-Mac* proved superior to all other machines evaluated. The cyclotron was able to turn out a convincing burger in only 1/1000 second, but at a quarter million dollars each. The Hun sandwiches, although they took two minutes to cook and assemble, were a much better bargain.

Our experiments with a carburetor met with no success. We were unable to arrive at a suitable air:plazma ratio.

The sewing machine gave somewhat better results except when we used plaid buns, which produced a slight case of nausea when they clashed with the tweed patties. Also, the double-breasted sandwiches tended to lose their buttons.

As expected, the iron lung turned out a well-formed product, but—as feared—it tasted like something that had come out of a can. The hoe did little better. Although it could make an inexpensive burger, it took us months to gather enough material for a meal.

Jovian's Interrositer, a marvelous machine that turns mental images ("thoughts") into three-dimensional objects, created sandwiches at great cost. In addition, our tester found it difficult to concentrate on nothing but plasti-form food for 72 consecutive hours, as required.

The Hun Co. is now constructing an improved version of this unit, to be displayed at the CENTURY O' PROGRESS, using heavy hydrogen (deuterium and tritium) and converging laser beams to produce a high-yield (100,000 giga-calorie) sandwich. Although the meal it generates measures barely 1 micron in diameter, it should be able to feed the entire population of Illinois, and transients, for an entire year. We'll report on it soon.

At press time, the Hun Co. announced that it had shortened its name to HunCo to reflect changes in the character and scope of its operations.

Ratings

Aerosol Burger-Making Machines

	Unit Cost ($)	Cost per Serving ($)	Prep. Time	Predicted Repair Incidence	Words per Min.	Toasts	Power (watts)	Product Nutrition	Advantages	Disadvantages
V-M Burger Maker (Hun, CLR 2576)	13.95	0.75	20 min.	○	NA	Yes	40	Does Not Apply	E,F,H,L,S	B,E,H,R
Cyclotron (Brookhaven Labs)	2.5×10^7	2.5×10^5	1 millisec.	○	NA	Yes	3×10^9	0	D,F,O,Q,W	B,C,I,O
Carburetor (Holley Mfg., Model 4160)	110	NA	NA	○	NA	Yes	NA	NA	E,F,J,X	A,B,F,Q
Sewing Machine (Singer, L1209)	230	10	6 hr.	○	NA	No	25	No	B,D,F,R,U	B,F,J
Iron Lung (Climax Medical Products, L22A3)	2500	27	20 hr.	○	NA	No	100	Zero	C,E,H,M,V	B,E,L,P,T
Hoe (Koch Garden Equipment, 1009TM)	10.95	1	Summer	○	NA	No	NA	—	A,E,F,I,P.	C,K,M,S
Interrositer (Jovian Engineering, 471FP6)	150,000	10,000	72 hr.	○	NA	Yes	1000	None	F,G,K,N,T	C,G,N,U

KEY TO ADVANTAGES
A — Comes with chopping blade.
B — Available in 57 colors.
C — Doubles as an ice chest.
D — Operates on batteries.
E — Tapered.
F — Responds to gravity waves.
G — Has child-proof containment vessel.
H — Dealers welcomed.
I — Beautifies as it protects.
J — Teflon lining.
K — Lifts and separates.
L — UL approved.
M — Sizes AAA to EEE.
N — Uncirculated, mint condition.
O — Landau roof.
P — Compounded daily.

Q — E-Z gradient separation.
R — Free storage bag.
S — Inflatable.
T — For eggs only.
U — Dolby.
V — Mounted on casters.
W — Jeweled satin finish.
X — Nihil Obstat.

KEY TO DISADVANTAGES
A — Light bulb replacement somewhat difficult.
B — Has moving parts.
C — Non-kosher.
D — Non-kosher.
E — Whir, whir, whir!
F — 30 ft. turning radius.
G — Lacks space age styling.

H — When opened, butter compartment door hits 1 lb. block of butter.
I — Egg tray can be dislodged if accidentally jostled.
J — Subjunctive mood.
K — Manual pause control.
L — (R.-Neb.)
M — Contains no owner serviceable parts.
N — Has back-mounted condenser coil with floral pattern.
O — Arm rests not detachable.
P — Single ratchet system.
Q — AMORC.
R — Seams glued, not sewn.
S — Decals do not adhere.
T — Affected by parallax.
U — Not self-sealing.

text by John Howe, model by Jim Wilson, photo by Carl Waltzer

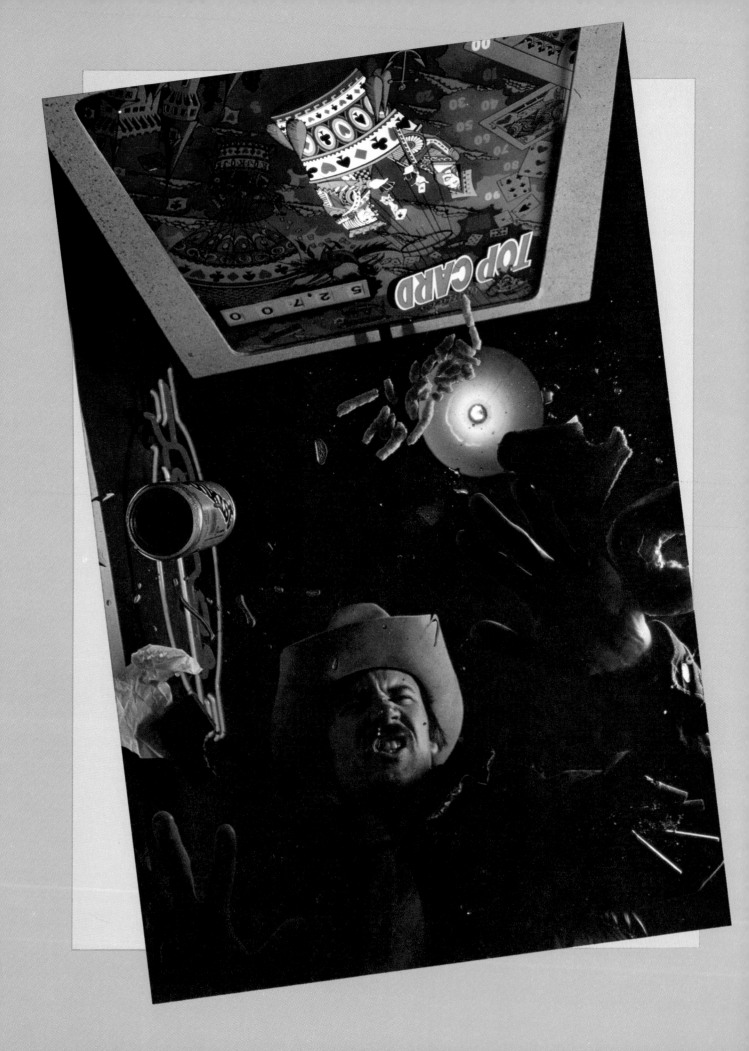

THWOCK!
Your Score Matches Your Food, & Other Contradictions

Playing with your food.
Play fast ... it's being O'Progressed.

by John Walker

I used to spend six hours a day playing pinball and now I don't. Just like Chum Fergason used to kill ten Dr Peppers in an afternoon and now, don't.

"This ain't Dr Pepper," said Chum, much later in life in reference to the aluminum can he was nursing through an entire evening. "They just *call* it Dr Pepper."

And, apart from a pious handful who tout the joys of "Flipper Skill Games," they still call it "pinball."

But I just can't get hot for some machine that trills "The Mexican Hat Dance" every time a ball drops. Meanwhile ... none of the Big Three execs are talking about a certain designer who was canned for sinking $3000 of company bucks into "No Exit," a machine intended to exploit pinball as the ultimate existentialist activity: That's five minutes of scoreless pinball—lots of lights and bells, and drop targets—no holes.

You can go out and *buy* an old machine. You can also build a soda fountain in your basement and wear a cap with "Jerk" written on it. I don't have to tell you it ain't the same. You can't buy your way back into the Golden Era. I quote Floyd, from Floyd's Drive-In:

"Who's gonna bust their butt to win a free game when all they gotta do is push a button? It's like those dogs in Russia. Soon's they found out they could get a seven-course dinner just by ringing a bell, they stopped runnin those mazes even though maybe they secretly enjoyed it." Smartest thing Floyd said ever.

You should have seen Texas in 1965. Pinball machines like weeds. An entire chapel of pinball in the Dallas airport. Pinball machines in supermarkets.

"The dumbest place for a pinball machine I ever saw was on a boat."—Floyd, of Floyd's Drive-In.

There you have it. Pinball on *boats*.

In the summer of 1965 I was darting around every point of the star in a '64 Impala a drunk had given me the day Kennedy got shot. Pulling into our Texaco, he announced that the car was tainted by "unholy Dallas," jammed the pink slip into the pouch of my coveralls, and lurched off. It set in our garage for a year and a half before I managed to latch onto a doctored driver's license saying I was 14 (legal minimum, then), and I got a mustache from Chum's Gags to enforce it. In those days, as in these days, the worst offense was in not looking your part.

I would get up at 5:30 and drive a case of empties to the Coca-Cola plant on the outskirts of Paris. There, I'd buy a case of Coke for our cooler at the Texaco and a six-pack of Tab for my mother. While the guy was getting the Tab, I'd steal the case of empties back off the pile and stick them in the trunk. Then I'd burn it back to town, stock up the cooler, and wait for the Piggly Wiggly to open. Then I'd sell the empties to the Piggly Wiggly. Then I had money. Then I'd go to Chum's.

From the outside, Chum's looked fairly tasteful, for a gag shop: no catchy display of latex excrement or razz cushions, the only window being a small porthole through which Chum shoved slices of frozen pizza.

Directly inside was Chum's little gag emporium, a shrine to the back cover of a comic book. No matter what a man's pleasure was, Chum had something to ruin it. But Paris was not exactly a knee-slapper's town, and the legitimate attraction of Chum's was the game room out back, a purist's delight: six pinball machines, period. All tuned for maximum volume.

What drew me to Chum's was the fact that it opened at 8:00 a.m. (Chum labored under the delusion that if there was an early-morning clientele who needed a stink bomb to take to work, it was his duty to make it handy to them.) Other regulars began filtering in around 10:30, heading straight for the back without so much as a glance at the novelties. This disdain just served to twist the rubber dagger in Chum's gut. He took real pride in his "hobby merchandise"; hell, everybody had pinball, but Chum had four varieties of itching powder. He made no effort to hide his resentment, forcing us to weather a daily impersonal hail of rubber fingers and exploding matches, and the sight of a lit Special often reminded Chum to "test" his main power switch.

Chum had a machine which never failed to match on 8. If you were into your last ball in what was clearly a losing game, you got somebody to tell you when the score was 6,308 or 22,468 (or whatever) and then tried letting the ball drop without racking up another point. The 8 would match its twin on the backglass and the machine would make that noise like one of the Three Stooges getting clopped by a two-by-four—the sound of winning—and you had yourself a free game. It was a cheap way to win, often necessary. But I once saw Chum reduce Teddy Lorton to a staggering mass of tears after a three-hour binge that had cost Teddy deep in the purse. Lorton was showing all the danger signs of last-dime desperation, yelling "Is it on eight? Is it on eight?"

Chum, who disapproved of this method, strolled by and casually eyed the score. "It's on eight," said Chum.

Lorton recoiled from the machine. The ball drifted slowly, bounced off a dead flipper, and rolled out of sight. Lorton whooped for joy.

Do I have to tell you that his score read 7,602? Sweating, Chum retreated to the gag counter.

There followed a three-day mope that had everybody on guard. Finally Chum stormed into the back room with his little edict: that the machines were a "special service" for *customers,* that he, Chum, was not a change machine; and that, starting tomorrow, you had to buy a gag first if you expected to play pinball. So every day the same, sorry lot would drift in one by one to purchase the cheapest item available, which was "pucker" chewing gum. Most of them actually chewed it. I got lucky when a Mexican mechanic at the Texaco wanted a case of rubber vomit for his trip home (apparently hard to come by in Mexico, and highly coveted). I arranged to pick it up for him and wangled a two-month credit for the big buy. I was no fool; I was brilliant.

With the '64 Impala, I could skip off to Dallas for a bit of variety. Chum's was hardly the end-all in selection, and the only other place in town with a comparable assemblage was the "fancy" bowling alley which had countered riff-raff with an enforced rule that you had to rent bowling shoes to play pinball.

I should've caught on. From the jump, pinball was always pushed as the great enhancer of on-premise consumption, and neither Chum's nor the "fancy" bowling alley fit neatly into that scheme. Bowling is bowling, serious stuff for those who do. Pinball isn't going to perk up bowling or pucker gum any more than good gravy improves a bad slice of pie; the basic quality of bowling, or pucker gum, doesn't change much. Food—on the other hand—trots across a whole spectrum of quality; in a Place Of Food, pinball is the ultimate bluff. When a player's mind is on knocking out the 3

and the 7, the subtle taste of whatever slithers off the grill can't be his main concern; so if your food stinks, get yourself a pinball machine.

Floyd's Drive-In was a cheap meat/deep fry place nestled in what we used to call "Ruby Territory." Next door was a "Near-Topless" lounge I liked frequenting, until the air-conditioning in the Impala conked out and my mustache sweated off. I squeezed by for one more day with the story that I'd had to shave for a funeral, but when I showed up the next afternoon with a new mustache they gave me a one-way shove toward Floyd's.

Floyd, a South Philadelphian, had wound up in Dallas through some branch of the military and married a Mexican girl who spoke only in the loving tongue. They had three kids who weren't too long in the English department, either. The kids wandered around chawing on frozen corndogs, sometimes playing the machines, sometimes just sort of clinging to them. "Just kick 'em out of the way," was Floyd's advice.

"Papa! Papa! Lo tengo 'Free Game'!" I remember his oldest kid howling when the BIG DEAL matched his pitiful score during peak hours on a July 3.

"Good goin," noted Floyd. "How'd you like to bite Jayne Mansfield on the ass?" The kid grinned. "That," said Floyd, "is the *dumbest* kid I've ever seen."

Floyd's specialty was pinpointing the *dumbest* example of any genre. Some winners: Push-button transmissions, poodles, artificial wood, and squid in tins. Dumbness and Floyd were no strangers, to be sure. Floyd's Drive-In wasn't even a drive-in. Sometimes you had to park three blocks away.

For a while Floyd sponsored a contest called "Win A Cheeseburger," a real nice idea marred considerably by Floyd's overzealousness in awarding the cheeseburgers. The gimmick had nothing to do with pinball skill, you just had to be playing a particular machine at a particular time. Once an hour Floyd would shout, "We got a winner!" and charge up to some player and shove a cheeseburger at him. Who in hell wants to *accept* a cheeseburger in the middle of a game? Ultimately, some chronic winner threatened to make Floyd eat a cheeseburger backwards if he ever came near him again and Floyd dropped the whole idea.

Floyd's credo was "Pinball and hamburgers go together like pretzels and beer," a line he'd gotten out of a catalogue. Floyd just never understood that you don't put the pretzels into the beer and *stir.*

Now I don't want to make too much of this next story, but I don't want to make too little of it, either. I made a few calls to Chicago, the Bethlehem of pinball, trying to scrounge up some great anecdotes to put the delicate balance of food and pinball into some sort of historical perspective. Like: After a tense round of negotiations, do the Amalgamated

Meat Cutters cut loose with a sausage sandwich and a fistful of dimes? Well, I got nothing so romantic, but I did get what amounts to a first-rate argument for maintaining a token separation of ingestion and competition:

"There was this great marathon pinball craze in the summer of '77," recounts Tom Nieman, who does P.R. for the Bally Corp. "Someone discovered that the Guinness *Book of Records* didn't have an official time for longest continuous pinball play, so everybody ran out and was gonna play pinball for a little longer than anybody else. Finally Guinness and the Steel Pier in Atlantic City decided to co-sponsor an attempt to set a world's record. They had four kids, and one of them was huge, a *blob,* with this pushy mother who must've forced him into the damn thing. It was a hot, humid time but they got through 24 hours. The Blimp's mom spent the first night next to him on a cot. They hit the 48-hour mark and the kids looked pretty ragged. They were only allowed a five-minute break every hour, and they had security guards who'd take these kids and stick their heads under water to keep them going. Then, after the second night, a Gino's connected with the Steel Pier saw the publicity and offered, gratis, all the food the participants could eat, for as long as they could go. There's two kids left at this point—a real thin kid, and this heavy-set young lad and his mother still sitting there, prodding him on. But the mother's getting real tired, and finally says she's going home, she'll check back first thing in the morning. Right off her kid starts ordering and goes on a food binge in the middle of the night. Pizzas, chicken, burgers . . . he made up for a long dry-spell and it caught up to him instantly. The kid goes into a retching routine, pukes his brains out and . . . fades from the competition. They take him home and send him to bed. Now I guess the scene next morning is the mother doesn't know the kid's home, and she wakes up, finds him, starts screaming at him, and drags his ass back to the Steel Pier, insisting he be allowed back in the competition: That it must have been the *food.* That he is still ready to *go.* But the kid looked green. The other kid continued—I think he went 93 hours and 30 minutes before he literally collapsed. But his trick was that *he didn't eat much.*"

Dilettante players can't fathom the effect of residuus crud on the serious game. You don't want to gunk up what ought to be a precision machine: That's just good sense. Mainly, though, you don't want to deal with anything that's going to foul your concentration. (Of course, if pinball didn't take two hands, there wouldn't be such a problem; or if each machine came equipped with a slop-trough, there wouldn't be such a problem.) The only alternative to cramming everything into your mouth is to let a friend hold it while you play, and then, odds are, he's going to start eating it for you. You can't worry about keeping him honest and play decent pinball simultaneously.

Drinks in paper cups are poison to the game. Not only does a large Slushee cut deep into your field of vision just *sitting* on the glass, but its precariousness amounts to a second tilt mechanism. I once saw a businessman in Floyd's knock a whole Jumbo cola down the front of his white suit. He had another six games racked up and played off 30 balls with an expression of pure misery on his face. After he left, Floyd doused the machine with a pail of sudsy water. The next day Floyd *oiled* the machine. It was a destructive cycle.

You couldn't really fault Floyd for his extra upkeep, as the serviceman from the rental company was the *dumbest* man Floyd had ever met, in fact. He'd once left half a sardine sandwich locked under the glass of the LIZARD KING while he went off on a hunting trip. People tempered their complaints at first because the sandwich kept balls from going down the left side. But the stench that week made Floyd's revenue anything but optimal.

And Floyd was suckered on "Optimal Revenue"— another phrase from a catalogue. The key, he'd read, was "proper placement," and he was always dragging the games back and forth in search of that magical configuration. You'd play the GRAND HOTEL on Monday and it would slant to the left; come back Friday and the same machine would be across the room next to the candy machine ("Customers tend to have change left over"), and wedged under the phone, with a whole new set of eccentricities.

I think this all had something to do with Floyd's stint in the military, which seems to affect some people's capacity for reason when it comes to civilian economics.

Still, most of Floyd's catalogues continued to rate pinball a good notch below the main attraction: the Great Enhancer, you recall. Floyd managed to recognize that even if the machines attracted nothing more than an assemblage of delinquent scum, the lucky fellow who lent his floor space to those four-legged bandits would at least reap a percentage of the hard cash gulped by the machines themselves. Floyd wasn't picky.

It just so happened that Floyd's business acumen was peaking at the dawn of the "Family Entertainment" era. Floyd's Drive-In turned, rather abruptly, into a "Family Entertainment Center." He ripped out half the pinball games and replaced them with "Foos' Ball," an uncovered, table-top soccer game which was regularly looted of its plastic balls. Out went Foos' Ball—save for a couple, just so Floyd could say he had them—in came a squad of devices that tested your skill at torpedoing enemy subs, and which was an immediate hit. Proud papas dropped by for lunch and lugged their offspring over to the war zone. You didn't win a free game on these things, you won a rank. Admiral. First Mate. Deck-Swab.

Floyd revived "Win A Cheeseburger."

Obviously, Floyd was just as happy if you sank six submarines and one hamburger as the other way around. He knew what kind of food he was slopping, and he wasn't about to get hurt if you spent your money on the games. Floyd was greedy, but he was patient.

Today patience is a cardinal sin in the fast-food marketplace. Get 'em in and get 'em out; the last thing they want is a goddamn pinball machine slowing things down.

Just to be sure, I asked a few experts. A spokesman for Arthur Treacher's says there's no space for pinball because Treacher "units" are "so functionally arranged." Dunkin' Donuts says, "We are very reluctant to allow any equipment other than what's specified in our package." Burger King, pressed, replies, "Company policy."

The classic rebuff, though, comes from the corporate Wendy. "She" notes, "At Wendy's, operations is the name of the game. We're there to offer quality food service quickly. And for this reason we want to keep our dining rooms clean, and people comfortable, and without the noise and distraction of a pinball machine. We're," she concludes, "not an entertainment center. We're an eating establishment."

Now, I've thought this through. . . . I think they're afraid of attracting riff-raff.

I played my first pinball game in a pizzeria. I was three. There was an electric bowling machine alongside and I have a vague memory of getting stuck in it. From that point on I went with pinball.

For years I had a real Jones. When I was nine and forced into a family camping trip, my father even brought along a plastic, battery-run pinball game as a precaution, but up in the mountains some hillbilly kid observed that the tiny gadget resembled "the thing you put yore foot on when you git new shoes" and then, without malice, stepped right through it.

I could blow three dollars a day on pinball, which lots of people said was foolish. I didn't think so. It just happened to be my vice. I know it didn't make me riff-raff.

A kid named Vern Jefferson used to give me an unbelievably hard time, his argument centering on the "lack of a tangible reward." Now, Jefferson himself used to shell out nearly that amount for pieces of styrofoam which he *burned*.

Jefferson's touchiness probably stemmed from his stunted little brother Bo's being an absolute fool for the game, and constantly shaming the family name through his efforts to support his habit.

Was Bo Jefferson riff-raff? That's a tougher question. I remember when they caught Bo sneaking out the dog door at the hardware store. The chain-and-pipe man had stopped by to do some late sorting, and he held Bo at bay with a blow-torch while someone fetched the owner. After inventory: nothing missing except a half-roll of dimes. Poor Bo

had been hunting for his private El Dorado—the cache of slugs rumored hidden in the storeroom. The dimes were only taken in desperation, he said. I'm sure that's true. I once saw Bo encounter a dollar bill and a dime in the middle of a parking lot and instinctively go for the dime. That's how it was.

Woolworth's was about the only place that tolerated his presence. He had to prop himself on a crate in order to glimpse the action, and, frankly, the sight of Bo tap-dancing in mid-air and bashing at a machine with every extremity seemed to unnerve a lot of people. He was banned (Texans *love* to ban) from Chum's after leaping high in the air to celebrate a match and coming down knee-deep in a shipment of X-ray specs and ventrilo-discs he'd had no business standing on; and from the bowling alley for, I'm pretty sure, breaking a bowling ball. He had crates strategically stashed all over town. A busted melon carrier on the streets of Paris generally meant Bo had been booted from yet another establishment.

Bo had a gimmick for plundering a certain Williams TURF CHAMP whose insides were coated with the equivalent of three entire swine. On a cold day the play-field would congeal, slowing things down to Bo's speed. For a 10, 20¢ investment, he could rack up a good 15 games, which he'd then sell off to another patron at a bulk rate. That got him banned from the rib joint. (Later, Bo tried greasing up the MONKEY TIME at Woolworth's by pouring Mazola oil into the coin slot, an uninspired idea which deserved to fail.)

Bo was finally withdrawn from the pinball circuit after the discovery that he'd been shaking down his schoolmates for their milk money. They came down hard on Bo, and after that I'd see him about twice a year, always wrapped in a military school uniform that made him look like Dondi.

But one of the highlights of my youth was seeing a man drop dead while playing the CITY SLICKER at Chum's. He had five free games to go, and I have a clear memory of Bo Jefferson waiting impatiently for the medics to haul the fellow away so he could get at the machine.

But did that make Bo riff-raff?

Bo, I'm convinced, was lucky to get out of pinball when he did. At least he'll remember it as a forbidden pleasure; he wasn't around to witness the great decline.

I first encountered a three-ball game in a Dallas airport lounge, right next to a Hot Shoppe. The cashier had some story about their being special games for people who didn't have time to play a full game between flights. So I didn't bother keeping my guard up outside the airport. The truth was: A Williams BIG CHIEF could be perfectly healthy in Paris but have a eunuch twin anywhere in Fort Worth. Today, these castrati randomly abound—monuments to the most spiteful whim ever to emerge from the town of Chicago—along with games sporting dead match-mechanisms like withered limbs, that new breed of pinball noise, and a space-age scoring plate. Shit, in 1963, Teddy Lorton ran up 220,000 points on the DEATH VALLEY in Chum's and bought a round of pucker gum for the house; today you get that many just for pushing the Start button.

Floyd's was clearly on the road to ruin when I left Texas. Floyd, whose policy had been to roll out the red carpet for anyone with a dirty dime, was starting to get a bit fussy. There was the odd request for a shirt to be tucked in, and the man who had once informed a mother and her two daughters that they could "suck his dick" if they thought the hamburger buns were stale was putting up cardboard signs advising WATCH YOUR LANGUAGE.

I can't watch my language.

These days my pinball is under control. During a year I'll go on a couple of binges in the same spirit that an ex-junkie will chip occasionally, but the truth is that pinball has turned the same, sad corner that pool did when it became pocket billiards.

So picture this. My mother calls from New Smyrna Beach, Florida, and invites me down for a visit.

Can't, gotta write about pinball.

"There's a huge arcade down here. Can't you write about that?"

I'd made this Florida trip three years straight and she'd never mentioned this place before.

There was a long pause at her end.

"Well . . . you know how you used to get."

Lord, you should've seen this place. It had everything: a luncheonette, war games, Skee-Ball, miniature golf on the roof—and 30 pinball machines. And *regulars.*

That old familiar rush whipped through me when I walked in. My first thought was, "Go easy. Don't kill yourself." I picked out a game called MATA HARI, a game Bo Jefferson could have whipped on his flat feet. A couple of kids, about 14 years old or so, paused to gawk at me and soon were offering hot encouragement in the way of third person commentary.

"He's tearin it up!" This was ideal, you see, to tear it up. Normally I hate for people to talk at me when I'm playing, but I figured these boys might be luminous with local color. I invited them to join me in a couple of games, and whenever it was my turn, they felt obligated to sort of announce the proceedings. One, named Calvin, got so worked up I had to tamp him down a bit. At another point, I gave the machine a sharp poke and the second kid, Rick, turned to Calvin and said, "He hits it."

They watched reverently for a moment. Then Calvin said, "You like hittin it, don't you?"

Once he'd absorbed a tactic he'd work it into his spiel: "Hit it again, there you go, yer tearin it up, hot dog, tear it up, yeah, she's gettin wet—"

On Day Two, Rick and Calvin were practicing "hittin it" when I arrived. They both started shaking like friendly dogs. Rick yanked Calvin away from the MATA HARI, instructing him to "Let the man tear it up."

Calvin seemed pretty subdued, limiting his commentary to an occasional "Un-*real!*" We all tore it up for a while and I earned their respect by tilting the machine four times. I kept trying to find out if any true-spirited players survived in this place. "Come on," I finally asked Rick. "Didn't anybody ever tip over a machine?" Rick shot me a frightened glance.

Day Three. Rick and Calvin friendly as ever, but suddenly *very big* on Foos' Ball. Both were hunched over the MATA HARI when I showed up, but they were actually using it as a table while they wolfed down several hot dogs bought "piping hot" from the Radar-range. (The hot dogs came wrapped in cellophane, which Calvin insisted was edible.) After much prodding, they got me to join them in a game of Foos' Ball. I played goalie halfheartedly for a few minutes, but after the fifth ball got past me I gave the metal goalie a little spin and cursed loudly for Rick's benefit. Rick stiffened slightly and said, "You gonna tip over the machine?"

Calvin said, "Un-*real!*"

On the last day, Rick and Calvin had vanished and I got in a good two hours of uninterrupted play on the MATA HARI before a kid scared hell out of me. It was the spitting image of Young Bo Jefferson, picked up in the backglass. I watched as he skulked toward me, pushing the Re-set button on each machine until he reached mine. I tried ignoring him, but after a lot of neck craning on his part, he caught my eye.

"Yo!" he said. "Borrow a quarter?" I forked it over and he took it with a silent sneer. His skin color went from gray to ivory when he started up a game, a sign of true addiction.

"So," I said cheerily, knowing I'd landed my source at last, "you Florida kids play a lot of pinball?" The kid ignored me and gave the machine a slap. He was starting to get peevish. In the same spirit that you'd pat a wild dog eating a lamb chop, I asked again. His second ball went straight through the machine and the kid rapped the glass sharply with a skull ring.

He turned to me. "Shut up," he said. "Will ya?"

Now, I learned back in Texas that it takes a special kind of desperation to say "Shut up" to the man paying for your game. This kid was definitely on edge, I figured he could be goaded into anything.

He shot off his last ball and locked himself into position. I waited until the ball was at a crucial spot, then pointed to a target: "What happens if you knock that down?" The kid bellowed as he lost sight of the ball, and the game ended. He stood before the machine and trembled; I knew this was it.

I leaned over and whispered, "Tip it over."

He flung himself at the machine. I grinned. Then the kid emitted this sort of flesh-rending sound. The machine was *bolted to the floor.*

I emptied my pockets into the machine while the kid sputtered, shoving in quarter after quarter until the game started spitting them back. *Bolted to the floor.*

"Tear it up," I said, and these were the last three words I spoke in New Smyrna Beach.

Once, I stumbled on a nickel pinball machine. This was on one of my runs to Dallas, in a 9 X 12 restroom of a one-pump gas station owned by a guy named Riley. Directly opposite an exposed toilet. An intact, nickel pinball machine. The only other time I'd seen a nickel game was in a San Antonio diner, where you had to give the counterman a dime and then he'd come over and plug it in for you.

Riley, a sport, offered me a free fill-up if I could beat him at his own machine. After he'd racked up 12,000 pre-inflationary points he got conversational, and asked where I was headed. I told him Dallas. "Yeah?" said Riley. "There was a man in Dallas with a dog that played pinball. Someone I know seen it." I was dubious, but made a mental note to look into it.

A car honked outside and Riley excused himself. "That's my score for three balls," he said. "But if you beat it with five my offer's still good." I played another 20 minutes and didn't come close. Riley eventually returned and watched while I played two more games. Then he started to fidget. He said, "Listen, boy, I got to use the can."

I went on playing.

"Uhh. Sit-down style."

As I left, I heard the unmistakable sound of a pinball machine being dragged across a cement floor.

A few hours later I was battling the GRAND HOTEL at Floyd's when the pinball-playing dog popped into mind. Although I rarely initiated conversation with Floyd, I mentioned Riley's claim.

Floyd snorted with considerable derision. "A dog played pinball, huh?" He licked some mustard off his thumb. His new sound system blared "Holiday On Ice," all strings.

"I seen that dog at the fair last summer, and that dog was a fuckin joke." The *dumbest* dog, in fact, that Floyd had ever seen.

"He couldn't even shoot the ball. He tried doing it with his mouth, but he just slobbered up the machine and his owner had to hit him. *Then,* once the ball's in play, the dog just starts hittin the flippers. No style, just flip flip flip. The only free game *that* dog ever won was on a match."

Personally, I think maybe it was that dog who was responsible for the decline of pinball. Or people just like him.

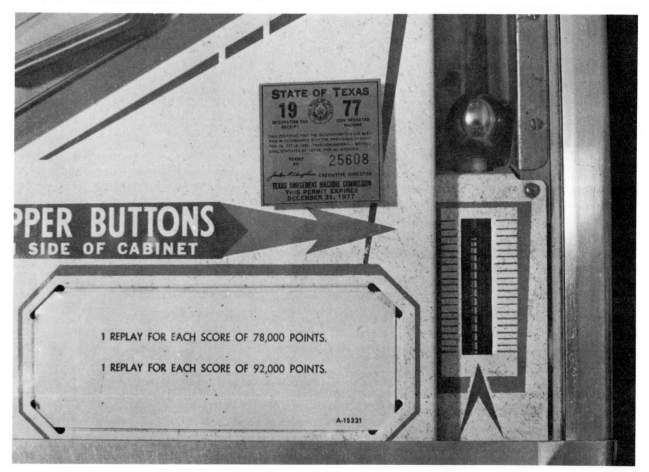

The Compleat Sunset Strip Burger List

All-American Hamburger
Alma Burger
American Burger
Ara Burger
Avocadoburger
Avocado Swiss Cheese Burger
Bacon Burger
BBQ Burger
Beggar Burger
Big Burger
BLT Burger
Blue Cheese Burger
Bob's Big Boy
Buccaneer
Burger Burger
Cado Burger
California Burger
Canadian Bacon Burger
Carl's Famous Star
Casey's Hamburger
Champs-Elysées Burger
Cheese 'n' Mushroom Burger
Chili Burger
Chinese-style Burger
Continental Burger
Cricket Club Burger
Double King Chili Cheeseburger
Dutch Ham Cheeseburger
Egg Burger
Fat Burger
Flamenco Burger
Frank's Fantasy Burger
Fresh Mushroom Burger
Golden Kazoo Burger
Gourmet Burger
Grant Burger
Hawaiian Burger
Health Burger
Heavenly Burger
Hickory Burger
House Burger
Hots Burger
In-and-Out Burger
Irv's Burger
Italian-style Burger
Jeanne's Burger
Jolly Roger Burger
Jumbo Burger
Kamu-ra Burger
King Burger
Knickerbocker Burger
Leonardo Burger
Melting Pot Classic
Mexican Burger
Mushroom Burger

North Woods Inn Hamburger
#20 Bigger Burger
Nut Burger
Old English Cheese Burger
Ordinary Burger
Ortega Burger
Peasant Burger
Persian Burger
Pizza Burger
Portuguese-style Burger
Ranchero Burger
Reuben Burger
Russell Burger
Saloon Cheeseburger

San Franciscan
Sautéed Mushroom Burger
Sourdough Cheeseburger
Spanish-style Burger
Station Burger
Steakburger
Swingerburger
Teriyaki Burger
Texas Burger
'Ton on a Bun'
Welsh Burger
Whitedelight Burger
Zapata Burger

—Brad Korbesmeyer

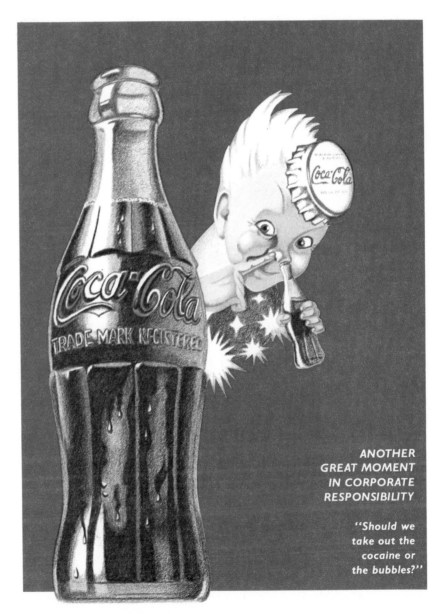

ANOTHER
GREAT MOMENT
IN CORPORATE
RESPONSIBILITY

"Should we
take out the
cocaine or
the bubbles?"

drawing by Tony Fiyalko

NEVER AGAIN ®Ⓤ

And the sons and the daughters come down from the house of themselves, and the apartment-dwellers, and the freeloaders, and Uncle Lou (The Passover Jew),
And the wind of contempt blows against the sea of the good silverware.
And we say: Them again?

For this have we slaved forty hours in this, our own kitchen?
So that the children may pick at the carrots?
So that the meal is without end?
We say: Once again?

But now that the hots may come hot and the colds may come cold.
And the hots, hot. And the colds, cold.
We can finally say: Never again.

For the MacSeder Sack™ Ⓤ has come into the land, and the voice of the dreydl is heard saying: "You will especially like the quality of the goods."
And the Patriarch: "Very reasonable."
And all together now: Never again.

Since when is this a special meal?
For which we make a special deal?
Since: **Never again.**

Never again to the enslavement in the kitchen, and to embarrassing politics, and peculiar foods.
To this we harden our heart and we say:
NEVER AGAIN!

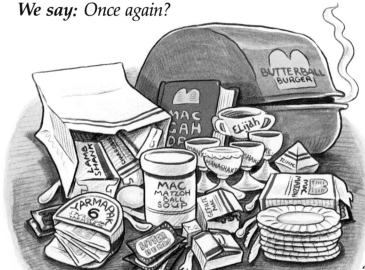

m

MacSEDER GUARANTY MacSEDER SACK™ Ⓡ
"Matzos roasting on the open fire/Old Elijah knockin' at your door"

"Never Again" is a registered Service Mark of MacSeder Guaranty. Not available wholesale anywhere.

drawing by Rick Meyerowitz

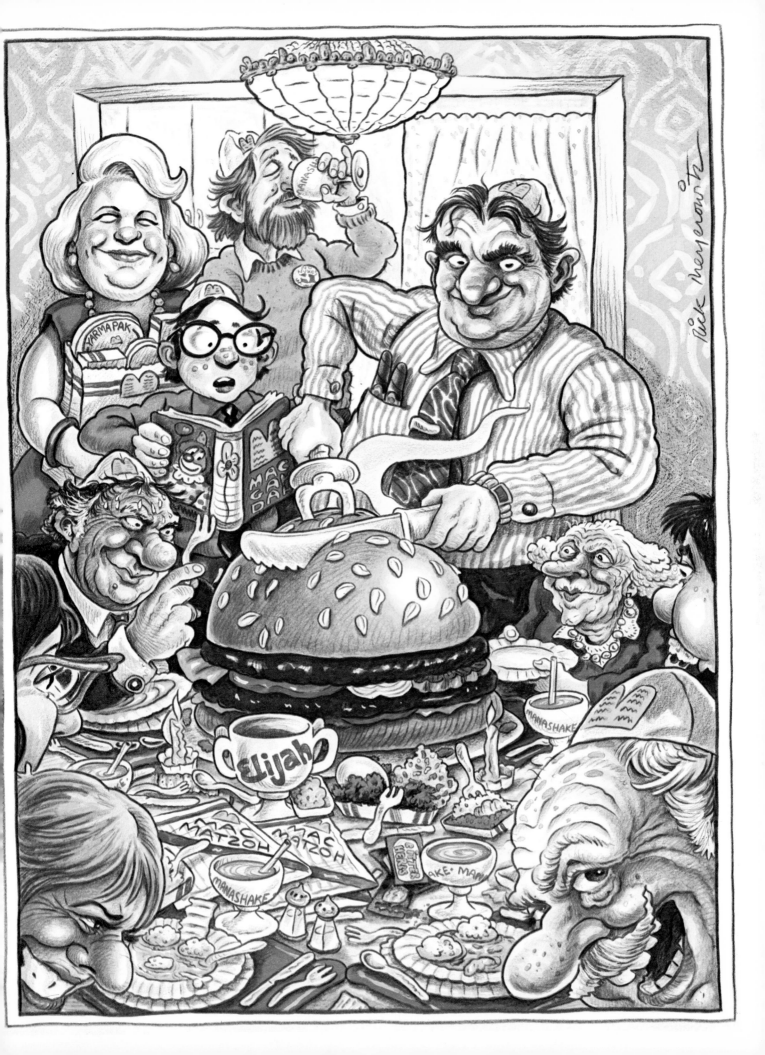

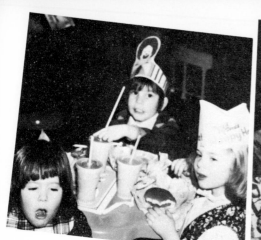
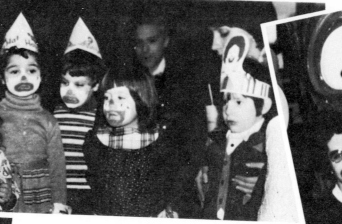

The Birthday Party

by Richard Foreman

Restaurant

I wonder how she's doing. She's all alone in the south.

(Enter with cake "Happy birthday to you
Happy birthday to you
Happy birthday dear—
HAPPY birthday to you"

Wait. (Pause.) There's some mistake

(Pause. Other rises, at other table.)
I think I'm the one that was intended for

(They go.)

Now we can continue our conversation

(Happy Birthday sung through at other table.)

I could drive you south, if you'd like to visit her

Promise one thing

What

Obey the speed limit

O.K.   (Panel rear revealed)
by me.

It's my FORTIETH birthday

You have five more to go.

How do you know what?

45 . . . minus 5

—gives 40. That's how old I am today

I THINK I COULD HELP RESOLVE
THIS ARGUMENT FOR YOU

Asshole

You see, it's my birthday

I don't like being called names like that

—If you belonged to the same sex as me, I'd shove
it up your ass

I want you to apologize to your friend. (All get crowns.)

ALL
Let's have some cake!

(Pause.)
Let's have some cake.

(New people enter: more crowns.)

There was a time, do you understand, when the gods used
to walk the earth

Ah, that's what I'd like.

A God that could have shattered this table

I can go so far as to spill this drink

I can go so far as to throw it

It hits: nothing

My eye. (Pause.) It was-the-sight-that-did that it was the
anticipation of the sight. Slight. It was the sight that
did that

"Here's another" (Mountains, sea)

If I could be on the top of that mountain—

(Arrival.) Here we are, at the famous Boule d'Or
Restaurant

What, would you mind repeating, is their specialty?

MEAT

ALL

Meat!

"Insight. . . . sometimes follows meat"

The END

204

photographs by Stan Siegel

Incident at Stuckey's

CARBONDALE, ILL. Illinois October. The fall came on; it coughed up the last flecks of summer, then moved over everything and the land turned hard, the air cold.

At Stuckey's on Grange Street the birthday party for Kenny Coughlin, four years young, was in full swing. Having polished off his meal, Kenny and his honorable colleagues ($2.00 a head) were ripping the wrapping off his gifts. A terrycloth jogging suit appeared. Kenny's smile was easy and sure. Is anything so fine as a young man into whose face death has not piped its yellow breath?

"You know," wondered a mother, uneasily, until a bystander drifted away.

Meanwhile, at the stainless steel counter gleaming like confetti in the wind and sun, a disturbance was getting up a full head of steam. "Sir, I put your change right there," said a black fry boy.

"Then where is it now?" responded a frustrated customer.

"Don't ask me," came the retort.

"Look," said the contender. "There's a dime here. A dime, and a nickel. Where's the quarter?"

The bearded franchise manager moved into the picture. "Just step aside, sir. You're blocking folks."

"Next," said a uniformed redhead.

"Fine," said the cheated man. "I'm not moving."

"What quarter? What's he talking about, quarter?" said the black fry boy.

"May I examine your purchases?" slithered the manager.

"Next. Miss, next?" said the red-head.

"Do you know who I am?" asked the man, who was someone.

"Set down the napkin holder, sir. Sir?"

Smile, Kenny, in your Incredible Hulk warm-up jacket. There's no such thing as a free lunch. Or justice. As the poet once said, Plus ça change?
—Barney Stone

Battered Wives

DQC from the files of the Bureau of Quality Control

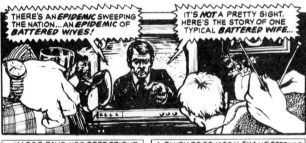

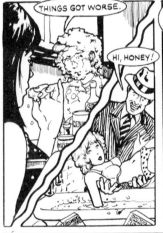

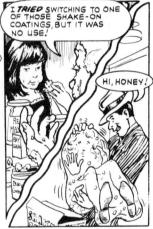

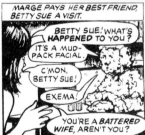

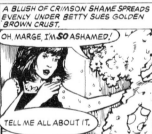

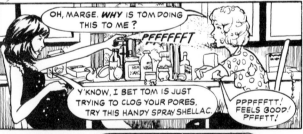

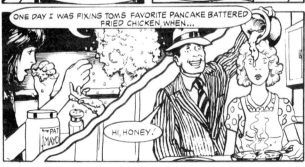

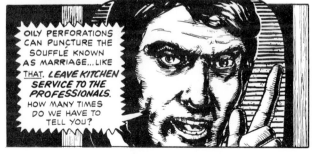

drawing by Bruce Emmett, text by Andrew Zimmerman

Deep Frying

by Tim O'Brien

Agnars Svalbe, a boy of 20, a Seaman Second Class with two full years of service aboard the U.S.S. Tensile— a submarine, now a disabled submarine, actually a *sunken* submarine — had pretty much grown accustomed to a daily diet of C rations. Fact is, Agnars thrived. Even in better times, when the vessel's galley turned out elegant meals of, say, braised veal and fresh buttered parsnips, or perhaps a barbequed side of beef served in the company of lettuce and raw broccoli and a tomato or two, even then, when the larder was full and bellies were plump, yes, even then, Agnars had often skulked away to indulge in a quiet feast of C's. It was a matter of temperament. Agnars simply preferred his food from cans. Why? He didn't rightly know. The cleanliness of vacuum packing, perhaps. Or the delicate—some might say bland—spicings of salt and BHT. Whatever the reasons, Seaman Svalbe was not one to squander those precious underwater hours in self-analysis. All he knew, all he cared to know, was that he liked the sweet taste of peaches in a heavy sugar syrup; he liked the slightly briny odor of turkey loaf as it plopped out of its olive-drab tin; mostly, though, he liked the absolute fidelity of C rations, the absence of surprises, the knowledge that, when a can was opened, he would be granted no more nor less than what he expected. Finally, in his most philosophical moments, he liked C's for their democratic evenhandedness. Officer or EM, captain or yeoman: each received the same product in the same portion from the same far-away kitchen.

Besides, there was no point in complaining.

"Change what can be changed. Accept what cannot."

Agnars said this to Ensign McGeefe.

McGeefe, a rake, winked at Seaman First Class Melinda Long, then scowled at Seaman Second Class Svalbe. "Agnars," he said, "you give me indigestion. Zip up."

And of course Seaman Svalbe blushed.

"I was seeking the sunnyside," he said. "Sir."

"Eat."

Agnars, always a good sailor, obeyed. He ignored McGeefe's little giggle; he ignored Captain Brill's sad gaze; he even ignored Seaman First Class Melinda Long, who, as

ever, was tickling McGeefe's thigh under cover of the table.

In situations of peril, he well knew, people tended to seek comfort in familiarity.

"What really gets me," McGeefe said to Melinda, "is Svalbe's good humor. I mean, *geez.*"

"Yes, sir," said Melinda. "Aye-aye to that."

" 'Accept what cannot, change what can,' " McGeefe mocked. "What crap. If it isn't botulism, it's Svalbe's stupid proverbs."

"He's cute, though."

McGeefe winced. Apparently Seaman Long had given his knee a playful squeeze—her fingers were powerful, she was famous for them.

"Cute!" McGeefe said.

"Well, not really *cute,*" said Seaman Long, "but ... happy-go-lucky-cute, you know?"

"Happy-go-nutty," said McGeefe.

McGeefe grinned at this bit of wit, proudly, and Seaman Melinda Long, much impressed, grinned right back at him, fondly. They were lovers, of course. With her right hand—topside, so to speak—Melinda fed McGeefe a spoonful of canned ham and eggs; with her left, below decks, she inspected the crease on his khaki trousers.

Captain Brill could ignore it no longer.

"Look," he sighed. "Cut the fraternization."

Melinda shrugged. "Aye-aye," she said. "Except it isn't fraternization."

"No? Then what is it?"

"Love," smiled Melinda. "Pre-nuptial affection. Sir, we're *engaged.*"

McGeefe coughed and looked away. Melinda beamed. Captain Brill's eyes wobbled—he was not a well man.

"Engaged, you say?"

"Signed and sealed," Melinda said. "I guess you could say I'm the happiest darn girl in the Navy."

She stroked McGeefe's knee; McGeefe paid close attention to his C rations.

"Engaged," the captain murmured.

"Roger-dodger. Happened just last night. Bingo."

"It stinks."

"Sir?"

The captain gazed woefully across the mess room. "Malodorous," he muttered. "Bad, bad news. Sub sinks, discipline goes to hell. I don't like it."

"Well," said McGeefe, suddenly alert, "I suppose we *could* postpone things. The wedding, I mean."

Seaman Melinda Long glared at him.

"Or maybe not," McGeefe said.

Seaman Svalbe, seated beside the captain, smiled and snatched Melinda's hand: "Well, gosh, congrats all around! I'm pleased as punch. Beauty is in the eye of the beholder."

"You're a doll," said Seaman Long.

No, Melinda was not a pretty woman. She was, however, almost without question, a woman. Who could really blame McGeefe? Under the circumstances, trapped some 900 fathoms beneath the North Atlantic, no hope of rescue, he could've done a sight worse. She had brains. She had brawn, too, but she was certainly no man-eater. Just the reverse. She was affectionate toward the opposite sex, patently affectionate, *physically* affectionate. Hadn't she enlisted in the Navy for that very reason? A socially acceptable alternative to Newark singles' bars? A way of touching plenty of bases plenty fast? Granted, Melinda could sometimes come on a wee bit strong—third runner-up in the sub's wrist-wrestling competition—but at the same time she could also be generous and sweet and even sexy. In her own way.

Though somewhat too muscular, though virtually hipless, though broad-faced and flat-chested and ham-handed, Seaman Melinda Long had those qualities of hardiness and endurance which, in the days of the wild west, were so appealing among pioneer women. Indeed, Melinda *was* a pioneer. The first female ever to serve aboard a Class AA nuclear sub. The first to sail beneath the Arctic icecap. The first to be given responsibility for turning the silver launch key to initiate a firing sequence that would conclude by dispatching twelve warhead-bearing Poseidons on their intercontinental journeys toward Peking, Vladivostok, and points west. Melinda had balls. She took her job seriously. She even practiced. After the accident, when other members of the crew began half-stepping, skating, sulking in their bunks, Melinda was always at her launch station by the crack of dawn—although true dawn, of course, never came. Like an athlete in the off-season, she kept herself mission-ready with a daily regimen of sit-ups and push-ups and knuckle-busters; she was forever squeezing tiny rubber balls as a means of maintaining wrist strength—key-turning power. She was tough and dedicated and chipper. Six months earlier, when the sub sank, she was the first to recognize that here was a chance to blaze a brand-new trail through a man's world: She was the first female sailor to be lost at sea. She did not take this honor lightly.

All told, Ensign McGeefe was a lucky man.

And this is exactly what Agnars told him at the mess table: "Sir," he said, "you're a lucky, lucky man."

"Or else you're pussy-whipped," said Captain Brill. He wagged his head. "Besides, I think shipboard weddings are against the regs. I'm sure gonna check it out."

Melinda shrugged. "I *have* checked."

"And?"

"And it's perfectly legit." Her voice had a truck driver's snap, a movie starlet's teasing lilt. "Look for yourself. Code R-12, Section 23."

"Sounds fishy."

"The regs don't lie, sir."

Captain Brill, a sad and confused man, gazed for a long time at his C ration applesauce. Applesauce: as mushy and sodden as his brains. He felt lost.

"The *regs* say it's legit?"

"Absolutely, sir. In situations like this—cut off from normal command channels—an officer-in-charge, that's you, has the authority to do dang near anything he wants. Including hitchin' folks up."

"Smells rotten as meatloaf," the captain muttered, though without much emotion. "Sounds unNavy."

Melinda pouted. McGeefe looked on with a glimmer of hope. The captain ruminated. Agnars helped out: "Live and let live, that's my theory."

"You *bury* people at sea," said Captain Brill. "*That's* Navy. *That's* SOP."

"So? Just another civil ceremony."

"I don't like it."

"Nothing lavish," Melinda said. "Friends and family. Right, Ensign McGeefe?"

"Jack."

"Ain't that right, Jack?"

"Yeah," McGeefe said, eyes on his C's again, "I guess that's right, baby."

Captain Brill sighed. He pushed his applesauce away, letting Agnars go to work on the leftovers, then, bleary-eyed, he got up and made ready to go.

"One thing for sure," he said. "It isn't like the old days."

"Nothing is," said Melinda.

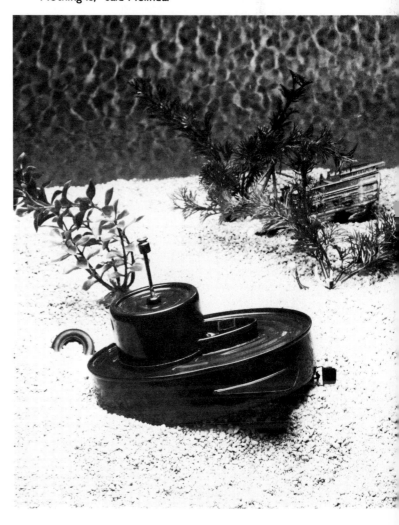

After the captain had retired to his quarters, Melinda and Agnars and McGeefe were able to pursue the matter at greater leisure. Melinda was pleased that the engagement had been brought squarely into the open. McGeefe wasn't so sure. It might've been handled more diplomatically, he thought, and perhaps at a more opportune moment. "Breakfast just isn't the time," he said. "Not these days. Besides, baby, things like this can get ticklish. Can't rush 'em through."

Agnars nodded. "Haste makes waste."

"There it is," said McGeefe.

"An apple a day keeps the doctor away."

Melinda, who had been munching on a tropical chocolate bar, swallowed, peered first at her own hands, then at her formidable belly, then at Seaman Svalbe, then, finally, at Ensign McGeefe.

McGeefe tried to smile.

"Look, Bub," she said, slowly, one word at a time, "don't go yellow on me."

"*Course* not."

"I been good to you. Remember that time in the generator room?"

"Hey, how could I forget? All I'm saying is—"

"I been *darned* good to you, Mac. *Too* good. Didn't even ask for a *ring,* just took you at your crummy *word.*"

McGeefe was flustered. He looked at Agnars for help, then thought better of it.

"Honest," he said, "you've been a sweetheart."

Melinda stared him down. "The point is this: You an' me are officially betrothed, by jiminy, and there's no backin' out. Roger that? Try, an' I'll cream your hairy little—"

Around the mess, sailors were cocking back their hats, listening in.

"Easy, baby," McGeefe said. "No sweat."

"You *had* me."

"Shhhhh."

"You did, dadblast it, top to bottom and back up again, the *works!*"

Weakly, soberly, desperately, McGeefe pledged his allegiance, swore to his honorable intentions, promised her the grandest wedding ever. McGeefe was not a brave man.

"No skippin' town, buster."

"I won't," McGeefe purred.

"*Can't.*"

"That's gospel truth. I can't."

They kissed. Right there, surrounded by 88 chowing-down swabbies, centerstage on the chrome and steel mess room, they kissed and made up. Then, to seal it, Seaman Long gave Ensign McGeefe's nose a sharp, playful, hurtful tweak.

"There's just for starters," she said, meaningfully. "Later on, Jack, I'll show some *real* affection."

Agnars took it all in with the benign smile of a genie.

These were his friends. His best and only friends. True, McGeefe could be a first-class jerk sometimes—most of the time—and, true, Agnars often felt a bit abused by the ensign. But what the heck? He didn't really mind washing McGeefe's undies, or keeping the guy's shoes shined, or rolling his joints for him, or shampooing his hair each Tuesday evening. Friendship, Agnars kept reminding himself, is a matter of give and take. Give and ye shall receive. So even if it sometimes seemed that McGeefe only tolerated him, that was okay by Agnars; toleration was nothing to sneeze at, not by a long shot. Most of the crew, after all, wouldn't even go that far. Except Melinda. Melinda actually seemed to like him. Amazing, boggling, but true. They were buddies. Pals, maties, partners. In fact, up until McGeefe came along, they'd even been bunkmates—not *sleeping* together, not like *that,* just . . . just friends. Close. Thick as thieves, he thought, snug as two bugs in a rug. Agnars thought that way.

"I'm sure you'll be happy," he told them. "Mind if I finish off that pound cake?"

When the U.S.S. *Tensile* sank on the first day of April, some 200 nautical miles off Nova Scotia, there was no real panic. In fact, for the first hour no one knew about it. Not even Captain Brill. "He was caught napping," Agnars said later. "So to speak." The giant sub simply glided down to the seabed, landed softly, and did not move. A mystery. The engine room boys—old hands at the nuclear power game—could find nothing amiss in the ship's circuitry or computer print-outs. The generators kept turning. The lights stayed on. The radios worked. The turbines were ship-shape. The missile systems functioned splendidly. Except for the fact that she wouldn't float, the U.S.S. *Tensile* was in tip-top combat shape.

"Sabotage," some said.

Others said, "Ghosts."

"We been *sunk,*" said most.

Captain Brill, of course, established immediate radio contact with Navy Command HQ in Minnesota.

"Try this," said some of the best minds in submarine technology.

"Try *that,*" said other experts.

"Jesus," said one, "abandon ship."

In the end, after three weeks of tinkering and testing, the Navy informed Captain Brill that the *Tensile* was being removed from the official rolls.

"Removed?" the captain said.

"Deactivated," said a radio-voice from Minnesota. "Decommissioned."

"Yeah, but what about *us?*"

"It's a problem, no question about it." The radio-voice clucked sympathetically. "Thing is, Captain, there's only one way to raise that goldurned submarine."

"So do it."

The radio-voice paused. "No *can* do. I mean, like, we *can* but we *can't*. Follow me?"

Captain Brill sat down.

"See, the way we got it figured is this: You're pinned down by simple weight. A law of physics, right? Too much weight, no float. Otherwise she'd just bob right up to the surface and we'd hook up a line and tow her home, hunky-dory."

Captain Brill, never a man to jump to conclusions, just waited.

"Problem is," the radio-voice said, "you *haven't* bobbed up."

Captain Brill had to agree.

"Too much weight. What I'm saying is, well, we *could* get rid of that extra weight, but we *can't*."

It began to dawn. Slowly at first, then in a quick radioactive flash. Captain Brill nodded.

"Fire the missiles," he said. "Save our hides."

"Exactly it!" The voice from Minnesota crackled with static. "A real war college dilemma, huh? But naturally you see the stopper."

"Moscow."

"There it is," the voice said, soberly. "Right now a launch is pretty much against policy. But, hey. The picture could obviously change."

"Don't count on it, though?"

"Gee," the radio-voice murmured. "I really wouldn't."

Captain Brill considered the options. Eyes tight to his periscope, watching the flood-lit ocean floor, watching the eels and silver-bellied mackerel, sardines and scallops and oysters, flat flounder and chubby tuna, a whole ocean full of food, the captain licked his lips and tried to think clearly. No, he didn't want to blow up Moscow; he was a decent man with humanitarian instincts. On the other hand, he valued his life, and the lives of his crew, and he was determined to do all he could to preserve those lives. He couldn't rule out a launch, not if it came down to it.

A last-ditch alternative.

For now, though, he concentrated on less drastic measures. Oxygen was no problem—the *Tensile* had her own Atmosphere Production System. Power, too, was abundant—30 pounds of plutonium, enough to last a dozen lifetimes. Water? If they ran out of water, they'd just open the hatches and hike home.

Food, that was the issue.

According to the chief commissary steward, the vessel was stocked with sufficient Class A rations to keep them going for maybe two months. Class B's—powdered milk, some moldy beef, surplus coffee and sugar—might tide them over for another month or so. After that, there was only a four-month supply of C rations.

"Then what?" Captain Brill murmured.

The commissary steward shrugged. "Nothin, man. You don't *go* lower than C rations."

In an eloquent, somewhat rambling speech to his crew, Captain Brill explained the predicament. "The world is amuck in greed," he said at one point, "the balance of power is askew, the teeter-totter trembles, the tightrope twangs, we walk with an umbrella in one hand and a cane in the other, swaying, keeling, leaning left to balance right. This vessel—this poor, humbled, sunken ship—remains, for ill or better, a counterbalance to terror. Indeed, laddies, we shall suffer down here. Perhaps we shall perish. But we must remind ourselves, even in the act of starvation, even as we eat our own cuticles, munch our own excrement, that our duty is to the world above. Equilibrium! The U.S.S. *Tensile*, though grounded, still has punch. She remains armed, she remains ready. Believe me, lads, the Chinks and Rooskies will think twice before tangling with her, and with us, and with the good ol' United States Navy. We need to rise above petty greed. We need to see the big picture."

No applause, of course.

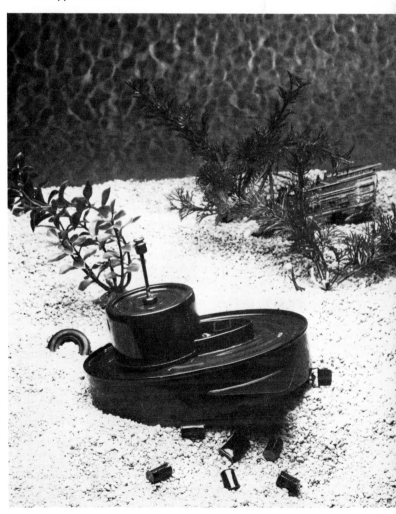

But the captain continued. He outlined rationing procedures; he urged the maintenance of strict combat discipline; he assured the men, and the single woman, that the Navy was doing all in its power to raise the U.S.S. *Tensile*. What harm could a white lie do?

"Buck up, mates," he said. "Be brave. Show me what you're made of. Think *deterrence*. Think *big*. Now man your stations!"

When the speech ended, Agnars and Melinda and McGeefe spent a long time in silence.

Even Seaman Svalbe, ordinarily the most serene of sailors, seemed deeply troubled.

"Gosh," he whispered, "I think we're in over our heads. We're in hot water."

Melinda blinked; McGeefe stalked away.

"No fooling," Agnars said, "I really think we're up the creek without a—you know."

Even with strict rationing, the Class A and Class B victuals lasted only 12 weeks. So for nearly four months now, day upon day, the crew of the U.S.S. *Tensile* had been subsisting entirely on a diet of purified sea water and unpurified C rations. Except for Agnars, who loved C's, and Melinda, who was too engaged in other matters to give a hoot, the crew was edging close to outright rebellion.

The men were suffering.

"I'm *sick*," said the chief petty officer.

"Food poisoning," said the gunnery mate. "C rat DT's."

"Launch the friggin' missiles," the bos'n said.

Agnars, though, was a stabilizing force.

"Come on," he would say, gently, "the chow's not *that* bad. Think of all the starving kids in China."

Captain Brill, after studying the regulations and his own conscience, decided he had no choice but to permit the marriage of Seaman Melinda Long to Ensign Jack McGeefe. Who knows, he thought, maybe a nice festive ceremony would be good for morale.

Melinda was thrilled.

McGeefe was not so thrilled.

The ensign had been having second thoughts. He confided in Agnars.

"Okay, she's the only game in town. But, hell's bells, you know? I'm young, I'm a good-looker, I'm built like a prince. Now, believe me, I don't want to bad-mouth Seaman Long, but, holy cow, the broad *scares* me."

"Pickers can't be choosers," Agnars said.

"But even *so*."

Agnars nodded. He was using his P-38, the standard C ration can opener, to scrape grease from McGeefe's fingernails. Agnars was fond of that P-38; it served as a screw-

driver and icepick and dental floss and hair-trimmer and, in this case, a fingernail file. A hundred different uses. Some folks even claimed the P-38 was worth more than the contents of the cans it was designed to open.

McGeefe inspected his fingernails. "Nice job."

"Thank you, sir."

"Just give 'em a quick file job, nothing fancy."

"Aye-aye."

McGeefe sighed. There were booze splotches in his eyes. "Thing is," he said, "the chick's got her heart set on me. Not that I blame her. But I fear she might try something drastic—I got my own personal safety to consider. She's *tough*. The whole mess is tough."

Agnars clucked.

"So anyhow the upshot is, maybe you'd—you know— talk to her. Explain things. How I'm basically crazy as the Marines about her, I really am, but how I just can't see jumping into a thing like marriage."

"Sure," Agnars said, "I understand."

"You'll do it?"

Agnars shrugged. "Why not? You know what they say."

"What's that?"

"A friend in need—"

McGeefe hustled away.

Aboard the U.S.S. *Tensile*, as on every ship of the sea, there was a sailor who had seen it all, done it all, been through it all, visited every port of call from Hong Kong to Naples, left his initials on the bulkheads of a thousand different vessels, ridden out typhoons and squalls and outright hurricanes, served before the masts of schooners and freighters and canal boats and tugs and destroyers and cruisers and every other make and model of water-plying craft. He was the old-timer. The silent one. The carver of whalebone and the rigger of sails and the fixer of gadgets. Legs bowed, back strong, a knit cap fixed permanently over a bald skull, he was the *Tensile's* salty guru.

Some called him Reb; some called him Little Jim. Everyone, though, called him The Sea Ditty Man.

He never spoke. Never. If asked for advice, he would answer with his eyes or his deeds or his ditties. He had no age. He wrote no letters and received none. He rolled with the sea. He refused bunkmates. He neither took nor gave orders. He held no formal job aboard the *Tensile*, yet, when trouble came, he held every job.

The Sea Ditty Man was a survivor. He had survived Pearl Harbor and Midway, New Guinea and Okinawa, and he would survive the sinking of the U.S.S. *Tensile*. He was a floater, a raftsman, a bobber, a scarred piece of driftwood that somehow always came to shore. Even as food ran short, as C rations caused diarrhea and cramps and stomach ulcers among the other less hardy members of the crew, The Sea Ditty Man seemed to suffer no ill effects; on the contrary, he smiled his secret smile, whittled himself a new pipe, and composed ditties later to be chanted aboard other vessels and in future times of duress.

While his mates moaned, The Sea Ditty Man sang.

*Oh, the **Tensile** sank*
To the deep dark dank,
A missile ship was she.
And her only prayer,
Aye, her final dare
Was to start World War Three.

   Yo-ho-ho
   We gotta blow
   Moscow into the sea.

Oh, the crew ate C's
And they got disease,
They couldn't take no more.
And the only way,
Aye, to save the day
Was to start the final war.

   Yo-ho-ho
   We gotta blow
   Moscow into the sea.

Yes, Agnars was a friend—in word and deed—and, as promised, he presented McGeefe's misgivings to Seaman Melinda Long.

It took place in the sub's launch control center, a gleaming room filled with computer banks and communications gear and security mechanisms and all the other hardware of long-distance warfare. It was not the ideal spot to break bad news.

Patiently, adding a few soothing frills here and there, Agnars delivered Ensign McGeefe's message. Melinda, of course, went ape. She sputtered, tried to speak, banged her fist against the chrome launch console. Tiny bubbles popped between her lips. Her eyeballs did a weird little dance.

Agnars, ever understanding, simply waited.

He watched his best friend swivel in her chair, kick the Code Verification Box, then lunge for a punching bag that dangled from the Fuel Stabilization Gauge. For maybe 15 minutes she worked out on the leather bag, both fists, lickety-split, making it sing. Agnars looked on with combined affection and awe. She was something, this woman: power, speed, agility, concentration, danger. He'd never seen a quicker pair of fists.

Finally she sat down. She wasn't even breathing hard.

"All right," she said, "now listen up."

She wiped her brow, checked the instrument panel, and leaned back.

"Tell ol' Popeye McGeefe *this*. Tell him the wedding's set for Sunday. Either he shows up or he eats plenty o' spinach. Read me, sailor?"

Word for word, Agnars repeated the message back to her.

"Good enough. Two options: Marriage or spinach. An' there *ain't* no spinach."

Melinda was right. No spinach. In fact, very little of anything. According to Captain Brill's latest inventory, the *Tensile* was down to 12 crates of C rations—enough, perhaps, to last another week. The supply list looked like this: 15 cans, pineapple bits; 10 cans, fruit cocktail; 19 cans, peaches; 10 cans, applesauce; 38 cans, pears; 100 cans, "main dishes" (ham and eggs, stewed chicken, beef and potatoes, turkey loaf, pork); 53 pound cakes; assorted tins of crackers and cheese; 100 tropical chocolate bars; and 64 miniature packs of Chiclets.

For a crew of 92, this was not a lot of food.

"What we have to do," Captain Brill told his commissary steward, "is cut the daily ration in half. No fudging it. Bang—right down the middle."

The steward made a note.

"Any questions?"

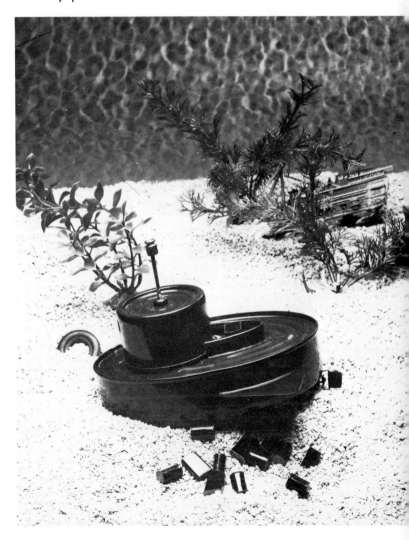

"One," said the steward. "How we gonna handle the mutiny?"

Captain Brill, whose face had weathered like the hull of an old pirate sloop, blinked and tried to put this into focus. "Mutiny?"

"Afraid so." The steward shook his head sadly. "In the first place, C's aren't what you call swell eats, even a *full* ration. I seen silage more appetizing. And here we go cutting it in *half*—the men are gonna be pretty darned upset. Tummies and tempers, both."

"I'm fully aware of that."

"And *then*, sir, we got the banquet to think about."

"Banquet?"

"Yeah, for McGeefe and Long. I was sort of hoping to lay on a decent feed, do it up right. That's my job, I been trained for it."

Captain Brill peered at the man. "Out of the question. Out."

"Aw, but *sir*. The Navy spent six whole weeks teaching me to lay on a genuine banquet. Seems only right we should—"

"Out."

Captain Brill spent many hours at his periscope. In an eerie, almost other-worldly way, he found great pleasure in watching the fish and crustaceans and sea mammals and sharks pursue their daily routines in the cold currents along the ocean floor. He wet his lips. He swallowed. He imagined a seafood platter plump with broiled scrod; a wedge of lemon; a bowl of melted butter; perhaps a frothy stein of beer; certainly a cup of hot fish chowder, heavy on the shrimp. He peered into the periscope, brain tingling with images of Class A victuals. What impressed him most during those long hours of observation was that these sea creatures, many among the most ancient on the planet, appeared to have only one purpose in life, one governing objective, which was to eat. Out there in the elements, politics meant nothing; sociology was extinct; history never happened; math, in the form of trajectories and striking arcs, was purely instinctual; the natural sciences boiled down to what was edible and what was not.

Simple survival—that was the lesson for Captain Brill.

He was a good man. He'd served honorably in the South Pacific and Mediterranean and North Atlantic. He knew the meaning of peril. He knew the pain of sacrifice. Back during the big war, the real war, when subs weren't consigned to any fancy-antsy game of nuclear strategy, no missiles and no warheads—back when you knew your job and you did it and you saw what you were shooting at and you shot cleanly and you were witness to the awful consequences—back then, in these very waters, he had once maneuvered through a whole German wolfpack, crept up on the second biggest battleship in the Kraut arsenal,

lined her up in his sights, then dropped her to the bottom with two torpedoes smack into the boiler room. Bang, down she went. Afterward he'd surfaced to help the U-boats collect survivors and corpses. *That* was war. That was *that* war.

Ah, but things change.

Hour to hour, he watched the pretty fishies. He watched how the big fishies ate the little fishies, and how the big fishies got eaten by even bigger fishies, and how the scavengers gobbled up the scraps, and how, finally, the whole damned ocean seemed to be eating itself.

"Down periscope," he would finally say.

He would sit. He would fold his head in his hands. He would ponder the meanings.

Survival of the fittest.

Wasn't that a lesson?

Eat or be eaten, kill or be killed.

Wasn't that a lesson?

It *had* to be done.

Wasn't that the final lesson?

The Sea Ditty Man, a close observer of men under stress, a veteran of a dozen such disasters, lay face-up on his bunk and sang in his most grizzled voice.

Oh, a valiant man
Was our good captain,
A sturdy chap was he.
With a hero's verve
Aye, plenty o'nerve.
To be or not to be?

Yo-ho-ho
He hated to blow
Moscow into the sea.

But the screw it turned
And our bellies burned
And C's was gettin' low.
The crew was tirin',
Wanted a firin',
But Brill couldn't give the go.

No-no-no
He just couldn't blow
Moscow into the sea.

Yet he had to think
About food an' drink,
The clock was runnin' out.
Discipline flagged,
And tongues they wagged,
Mutiny skulked about.

Yo-ho-ho
He had to blow
Moscow into the sea.

Ensign McGeefe married Seaman Long. All things considered, McGeefe took it pretty well.

"I'm boxed in," he told Agnars a few moments before the ceremony. "No escape hatches, no way out."

"Take it like a man," Agnars said.

"Yeah."

"Necessity—mother of invention."

Actually, it was a splendid wedding. The crew had decorated the sub's mess room with bunting and paper flowers, the bos'n played his whistle, Melinda looked handsome in her blue and white shore uniform, and Captain Brill, although a bit surly, officiated with a properly solemn demeanor. When it was over, the sealing kiss delivered, McGeefe had the look of a badly beaten boxer: humbled and wobbly and puzzled. Melinda, by contrast, was radiant. Agnars had never seen her looking better.

"Hot damn!" she kept saying.

She thumped the captain on the shoulder.

"Hot damn, sir!"

Afterward there was food. The chief commissary steward, who believed in his work, simply hadn't been able to resist the opportunity. He laid out a feast. A no-holds-barred, full-scale, sit-down banquet. Drawing on the last of the C rations, the steward prepared a surprisingly toothsome C stew, a well garnished fruit salad, a pimento-dashed cheese dip, and—for toppers—a tropical chocolate mousse lightly minted with oil of Chiclet.

The men glutted themselves.

"I told you so," Agnars kept repeating, eyes wet with appetite, "I told you C's was Number One stuff, I *told* you."

Even Captain Brill, who'd been feeling sickly of late, dizzy with the enormity of what he soon had to do, even he couldn't resist digging in until he could dig no more. Within 20 minutes the crew had eaten it all: every cracker, every pineapple bit, every morsel of turkey loaf, every tropical chocolate bar. The cupboard was bare.

The captain sighed.

McGeefe mumbled to himself.

Melinda glowed.

The Sea Ditty Man scribbled lyrics at a corner table.

Agnars suggested that the darkest hour is just before dawn.

Oh, yes, it was a long, terrible night for Captain Brill. Through his periscope, he dreamed of reptiles and beady-eating eyes, a world consumed, metabolism, the release of energy, protons and electrons spinning in eternal orbit, fission, fusion, critical mass. He dreamed of haves and have-nots. He dreamed he was dressed in spangled tights; he was a circus lad; he was young and muscled; drums rolled; he stepped into the spotlight, stepped onto the tightrope,

wobbled forward while the crowd held its great collective breath; he danced for his dinner; he tottered high above the worldly arena, leaning left then right, working without a net; sleepwalking, numb, he moved across the tightrope with the precarious humanoid gait of the two-legged; he faltered; he feared; he swayed; his empty belly dropped, his hands clutched vacuums, pretty butterflies came from his lips. Lord, he was hungry. Eyes tight to the periscope, dreaming, watching himself perform high in the yellow spotlight, Captain Brill mulled the alternatives. He did not want to die. He did not want the world to fry. But what can a hungry man do?

During that same long night, in another part of the vessel, Ensign McGeefe lay deep in the arms of Seaman Melinda Long. He was pinned to the mat, his shoulders twitched but then relaxed, he was down for the count. McGeefe sobbed. Melinda stroked his jaw, wiped his eyes. She purred to him. "It's all right," she whispered, "it's all right."

In other parts of the ship, men made out their wills and last testaments; there was some groveling, some anger, a great deal of bitterness. "What's a few Commies?" said some. "It'll happen anyway, why not now?"

Agnars tried to calm them. But for once he was at a

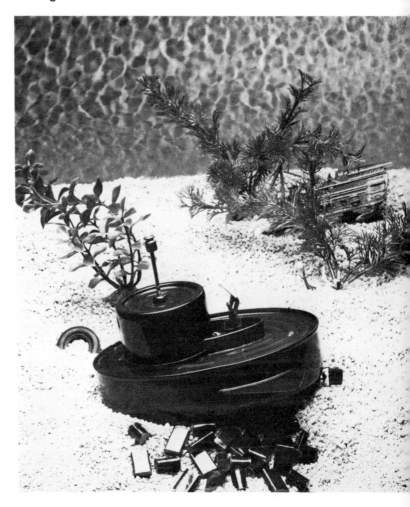

loss for tested vocabulary, he was on his own, and all he could come up with was, "What will be will be." It didn't help much.

"Amen," someone said.

It was a bright, lovely morning. The sky was blue. The water was blue. Blue mixed with blue, and the world was like church. And there was the sun. The sun came gently from the sea and arced east to west as ever, a miracle, and the sea was as vast and motherly as Planet Earth. The world was pacific. A filtered purple light bathed the blue sky and blue sea. There was no wind. Not a breeze, not a whisper. The doldrums settled in and nothing moved, not even the waves; the waves were heat-frozen, the troughs lapped outward to the horizon, one then the next, forever. It was a serenity that took the world's breath away. The simple elements. Evaporation, condensation. The silent whir of physics.

The U.S.S. *Tensile* bobbed to the surface.

She gleamed silver and sleek under the tracking sun. For a long time she simply bobbed, untethered, perhaps unmanned, an artifact of history. Buoyed by the unmoving sea, she drifted to the shores of many continents, never touching, then back to sea, like a messaged bottle that would never be retrieved. She bobbed prettily under the sun. The sun never let her go. The planet no longer spun on her axis, the sun no longer set, and the U.S.S. *Tensile* floated brightly on a sea of sculpted peace.

One day, which was the same day, a hatch opened.

The Sea Ditty Man appeared.

Unsteadily at first, whistling, he stood on the vessel's conning tower. He wore his knit cap, he carried a seabag on his shoulder, he needed a shave. He was an old, old man. He was old, but not without resource.

"Yo-ho-ho," he sang.

He breathed deeply, he smiled and wagged his head, he'd been through all this before. He let the sun warm his face, he thought back on all the other shipwrecks and beachings of his long career, he clucked sadly, knowingly, almost wisely.

At last, with nothing left but legend, The Sea Ditty Man sang.

Oh, the Tensile sank
To the deep dark dank,
A missile ship was she.
And her only prayer,
Aye, her final dare
Was to start World War Three.

   Yo-ho-ho
   We had to blow
   Moscow into the sea.

The Sea Ditty Man inflated a yellow life raft. He stocked it with water and the last of his meat. He threw in his seabag, gave the *Tensile's* gleaming hull a final affectionate tap, wagged his head, hopped aboard, rigged a sail, and began paddling. The Sea Ditty Man did not look back. He had a sailor's superstitions; looking back was bad luck. He looked forward.

Oh, Melinda she
Turned the silver key,
We heard a mighty roar.
But the ship didn't rise,
T'was a pack o' lies,
We was trapped forever more.

   Yo-ho-ho
   We was dumb to blow
   Moscow into the sea.

The Sea Ditty Man set course for Norfolk. He hadn't been to Norfolk in a long time, he wondered if the Old Salt Tavern was still in operation. He grinned. Lord almighty, he'd have some ditties to chant! This time he'd blow their bloody minds. The *ultimate* ditty!

He giggled and paddled faster.

So the lesson here,
One we all hold dear:
Center isn't holdin'.
For the least o' cause,
Aye, the slightest pause,
Bye-bye earthly golden.

   Oh-oh-oh
   T'was sad to blow
   Moscow into the sea.

Yet we had to eat,
We all craved meat,
Survival of the fittest.
An eye for a pie,
Let Poseidon fly,
Because . . .

"Fittest," The Sea Ditty Man muttered. A tough one to rhyme. He removed a bone from his bag and munched on it idly, watching the sea, thinking of Agnars and Melinda and McGeefe and Captain Brill and all the others—*fittest,* this one would take some thought.

Oh, well, he had plenty of time.

Yo-ho-ho
We had to blow
Moscow into the sea.

214

model by Jim Wilson, photographs by Carl Waltzer

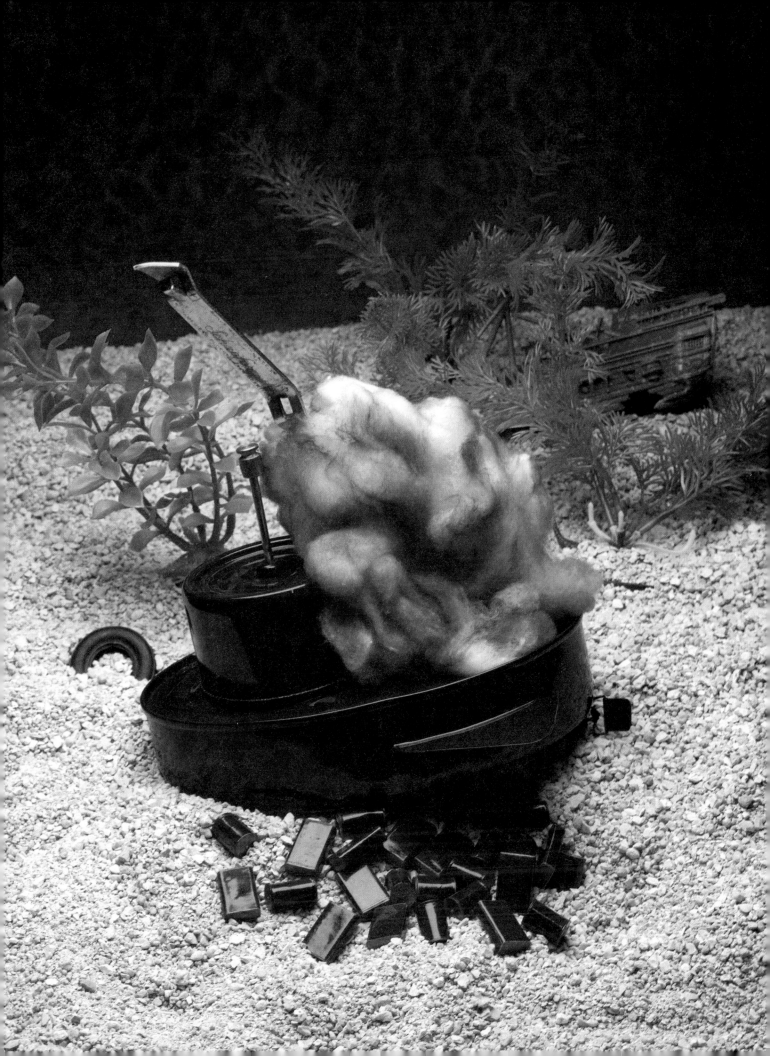

THE NEW CENTURY

The ribbons are off the state! The secret is out of the woodpile. Construction is complete, the food is fresh, our dream is realized—the CENTURY O' PROGRESS is about to open!

This, the largest exposition ever organized, will celebrate America's love affair with Eating:

Cheap

Out &

Pronto

through thousands of expertly designed pavilions, halls, displays, exhibits, pushcarts, stands, tak-u's, My-T-Marts, high school bookstores, booths, street fairs, and stalls.

So, how do I get there?

Don't bother asking directions. For your Fairgoing convenience, the main—and only—entrance is located on the **southern** border of the CO'P (née Illinois, née Land o' Lincoln). Just across the Mississippi River from SE Missouri and SW Kentucky. To reach it, just board our floating Vestibule of Anticipation, that's the Samuel Clemens, the historically impressive Mississippi keelboat whose dedication "The Greatest Food For The Greatest Number" is supported by "pretend-" Doric columns on the main deck. When room for a party of 500 or 600 becomes available inside the Fair, you, your family, and your car, from which you are never separated, will be ferried across to the historically significant former city of Cairo. There you'll be issued a CO'Passport, turtle wax, and Mantra.

Then what? I mean, how do I get around?

In your own auto. And you'll never have to worry about getting lost, or about missing anything. At other fairs, you not only failed to see half the pavilions, you probably didn't see them in thematic order. That's the advantage to our single-lane, one-vehicle-at-a-time Century Highway, which snakes back and forth, back and forth, across the CO'P much like the intestines inside your very body. It assures that you'll visit every exhibit in proper sequence.

And where do I sleep? Like that.

Most visitors will prefer to sleep in the privacy of their car. It's clean and safe—and safer for the car, too. In the morn, you can stop by any of the

ON OUR NEWEST FRONTIER

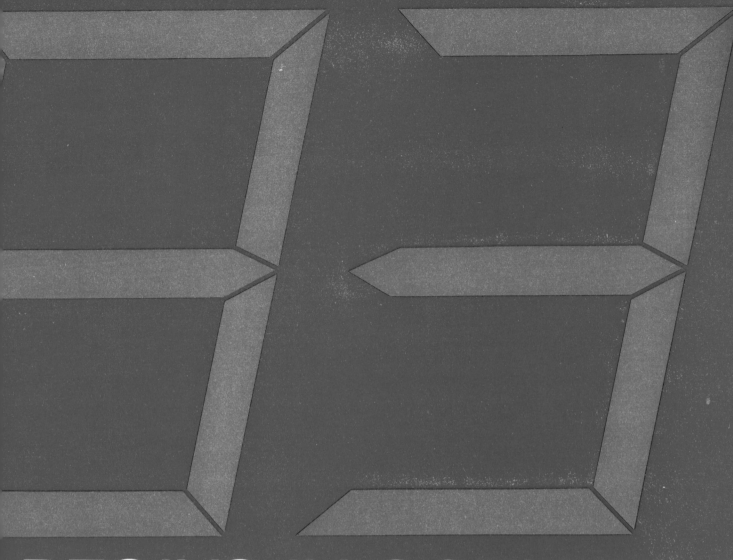

BEGINS IN OCTOBER.

Fair's 136 Showertats containing 399 showertitos® in 7 styles. If you do insist on clean sheets, however, merely present yourself at any of the residence-clusters that are just off the Highway, behind the pavilions, and which have not been designated official staff quarters. <u>These unrestricted residences are NOT paviliarly-associated but ARE part of the CO'P</u>. They have invisible "To Let" signs out front and a collapsible bed awaiting you in the living room. And fellow "bunkies" whom you'll probably spend half the night swapping CO'P adventures with, when it's not your "Watch." So ring any bell. Any time. You're expected!

It sounds like a lot of things to remember.

Sure! Maybe there is a lot to learn. But you'll have help. Upon arrival, you'll receive an official 3264-page, 8½" x 11" guidebook, **FairWays and Means.** It contains all the rules and regs. It will also be revised frequently, and you will be expected to purchase future editions.

I guess it sounds like fun. At that.
Oh, yes.

So when does this amazing Fair open?
October 8, 1983—the 112th anniversary of the first Chicago Fire. And, coincidentally, the third anniversary of ChiFire 2.

Ummm. Has anyone—?
Sure. That <u>is</u> an odd date to select.

Or is it? 1871—most folks digging gold. Chi, a prairie dump, burns to the ground. But a modern metropolis goes up in its place! 1980—Chi's getting a bit sluggish again. Whoosh! Place burns like a bitch. And what do we get? O'Progressland. Rising from the ashes, like a good steak.

OK, OK, I'm ready. What'll it cost me to get in?
Nothing. Nada. Zip. Zero. It's free. We've spent billions to teach people about food, and we don't want anyone missing it because they can't afford a $2 admission.

Think of it as …
Oz on Earth.

THE CENTURY O' PROGRESS.

To Hell with Reese's

by **Roger Rosenblatt**

In recent years it has become fashionable to confess a liking for junk food, primarily because confession is always fashionable; and when one confesses a liking for junk food, after all, how charming and innocent that sounds, as compared—say—with a liking for heroin or for decapitation. He who in public admits preferring Twinkies to mushrooms is greeted with cheers. Others about him fess up at once, each jabbering his own secret love, until images of Devil Dogs, Tastycakes, Yo-Yos, and Mallomars heap in the air like imps purged from the soul. Ah, the amusing baby sin.

Of course, it is a lie. All eager confession of junk food love is a lie, for the confessors are not confessing their essential sin at all, are in fact covering that sin by the false confession of admitting they like sweets. Yet sweetness is no more the essence of junk food than acquisition is the essence of theft. To steal is to show how petty you are; just as to eat junk food does not show how tasteless you are, but rather how cheap.

Now, cheapness is not something people readily admit to, but a lack of willpower is; so it is perfectly okay these days to speak of Twinkies. Twinkies are sort of pretty. Twinkies look like Mo Dean. You will not, however, find many people speaking the same way — as I am about to — of Reese's Peanut Butter Cups, at least you would not have found so 20 years ago. For with Reese's Peanut Butter Cups there can be no doubt that one is confessing something very special indeed, and that he is doing so not in order to avoid hell, but to remain there.

I am free of Reese's now, with all that the idea of freedom implies, so I may talk with some ease. I assure you, when I was at my deepest point of involvement with Reese's, I would have told no one — although in the beginning I made an effort. The beginning occurred in a movie theater on 14th Street in New York, on the long block that stretches between Third Avenue and Fourth. The theater was the Academy of Music, an old New York opera house with piled balconies and chandeliers the size of clouds. By the time of my childhood there were stage shows, the dregs of vaudeville, in the Academy of Music, but no opera. And by the time of my adolescence, the singing had stopped altogether.

The first movie I ever saw was in the Academy of Music — *A Night at the Opera,* fittingly. And I must have seen a hundred other movies there over the years, although at the moment I seem only to remember *House of Wax* and a dozen jungle pictures starring Victor Mature. It wasn't really what you saw in the Academy of Music that left the lasting impression; it was where. That vast, old theater was the darkest theater you can ever imagine. It was, I believe, the darkest place in the world.

So it was appropriate that there, at age 14, and rollicking with "Ah, wilderness!" innocence, I should first taste a Reese's Peanut Butter Cup. I remember clearly where I saw it — at the bottom of the candy case, in the lower right-hand corner. Its square shape was different from the other candies, flatter than Chunky. And the wrapper was orange and yellow, like Halloween. No one else bought one — why? A chocolate cup with peanut butter inside sounded terrific to me. And so it was.

Yet when I asked my friends if they had ever heard of a Reese's Peanut Butter Cup, not one of them had. Moreover, when I described to them what a Reese's consisted of, they inevitably looked horrified, as if I had just told them of something so vile and loathsome it could only be the product of a sick mind, something only a sick mind could enjoy. I began to wonder if I had in fact stumbled upon a forbidden candy, something left by Satan himself, in the lower right-hand corner of the Academy of Music candy case as a trick temptation, like a dime on the sidewalk. As for what so disgusted people upon hearing of Reese's, I am not sure. Perhaps it was the combination of two such fattening elements, or of two elements that might properly be separated into a lunch, instead of being heaved together like a compressed car; or perhaps it was the sweetness with the salt.

All these factors, of course, were precisely those that attracted me to Reese's in the first place, yet it was also clear to me that Reese's had touched upon a special frontier of junk food not previously explored. I knew of people who ate butter plain, and who ate sugar plain, and bacon raw; but they did such things in the privacy of their homes. I suspected that Reese's was like one of those depraved acts gone public. In any event, I was uniformly shunned whenever I dropped the Reese's name, so after a while I kept my affection to myself.

That did not prevent me from returning to the Academy of Music very often, nor from buying Reese's very often — though I always managed to get to the candy case alone, leaving my friends in their seats, and to eat my Reese's as quickly as possible. The trouble with wolfing down a Reese's, however, is that the chocolate and peanut butter become confused. What one wants to do—what I soon learned to do—is to take a great deal of time in the eating, to edge through the jungle of chocolate

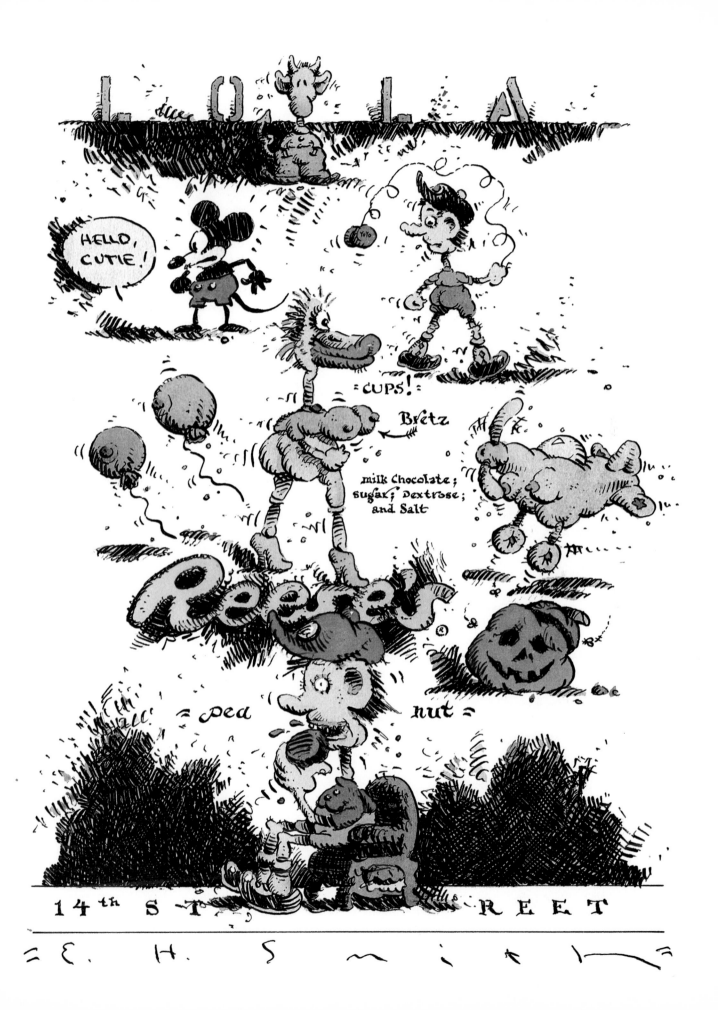

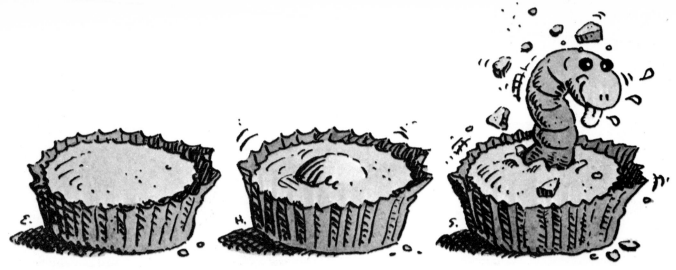

as slowly, as languidly as possible, before plunging into the peanut butter sea.

Soon, needless to say, I started eating Reese's Peanut Butter Cups all by myself, where I would be free of ridicule and scrutiny. And soon, too, I began going to the Academy of Music all by myself, which was unlike me since up till then I much preferred the company of friends. But at the age of 14 one makes decisions one can't control. There were movies I simply wanted to see, and instead of gathering the world about me — for solace and approval — I headed off on my own for the dark Academy.

Where, of course, being alone, I could eat Reese's to the content of my heart and mind, could eat them at any speed I chose. Nor did it take long before I was buying not one Reese's at a time, but two; and then not two, but three. Three was my limit, only because three seemed limitless. To be eating one Reese's, that was bliss. But to be eating one Reese's, and to know that another Reese's awaited, that was heaven. And to know that, and further know that another Reese's awaited afterwards — that was more than bliss or heaven. That was hell.

For as I sat in the pitch black of the old opera house on a Saturday afternoon, usually rainy, gnawing on the forbidden cup, and staring deep into some voodoo dance being performed for Victor Mature, I sensed for the first time in my life, in all its dimensions, the enormous pleasure to be derived from capitulation. Without planning it or knowing it, I had been borne into the heart of darkness. I wondered how dark it could get. I wondered if there was anything on earth more tempting than a Reese's Peanut Butter Cup.

And then I found out.

One afternoon between features, I stood before the candy case, having pointed to the lower right-hand corner, as I had been doing by then for months. My three beauties in hand, I headed back across the huge hallway. The hallway was dark, like the rest of the Academy of Music, dark and musty, smelling of perfume and popcorn. And the carpet was red. It stretched from one end of the hall to the other, and from where I was walking toward Her to where She was walking toward me.

In every life there are what we call "fleeting moments," moments of intelligence or recognition made intense by their brevity. One sees a lovely grove of trees from a car window, and is made forever mellow. One hears a harp in a hotel room, and weeps at the recollection of the music. Or one sees — as I saw then — what must have been the cheapest-looking girl in the history of 14th Street sashaying toward me like Lola of *Damn Yankees*.

She wore a pink halter that was falling off, and shiny black toreador pants that were soldered on, and she walked up very slowly and confidently, and she stopped with her hands on her hips, and she smiled, and she said: "Hello, cutie." And she said it to me.

Now, I was not what you'd call a man of experience. No girl had ever called me "cutie" before, and no girl who looked like that had called me anything. Yet even without experience I knew in that fleeting moment that there was experience standing before me, experience in toreador pants. All I would need do is to say something like "Hi, baby" without giggling or stammering, or even just a simple "Hi," and moments later the two of us would be sitting together in the balcony of the Academy of Music, making out, or worse. Perhaps I didn't have to say anything. Perhaps I could just smile a knowing smile.

But I didn't have a knowing smile. All I had was terror and three Reese's Peanut Butter Cups that were melting with my opportunity.

Then, as it had to, the moment fled. Lola sized me up for what I was, and sashayed away forever, for which I was equally grateful and depressed. Was this hell, after all — the torment of one's own inadequacies? A world of missed opportunities? No. It was knowing as deep down as you could know that you really wanted the opportunities to be missed, that the heart of darkness was you.

After that, my passion for Reese's Peanut Butter Cups gradually diminished; first to an affection, then to a taste, and finally to its present condition, a thing one can take or leave — which, I suppose, is a form of contempt. Today whenever I eat a Reese's, I feel nothing of the evil pleasure I once felt, in part because Reese's have become acceptable, even popular over the tolerant years. But the truer reason for my disaffection is that for me Reese's were involved in a test of civilization, were in fact the test of civilization themselves. Which I passed and failed.

Xmas Dinner

by Mark O'Donnell

Imagine it is Christmastime. Across the nation, cocktail waitresses exchange cartons of cigarettes. Divorced mothers give their married teen-age children sled-sized boxes of supermarket chocolates. Bulletin boards break out in shredded tinfoil bunting and what appear to be the larva of adult-sized candy canes. Magazines fatten with advertisements, like doomed geese on table scraps, and the smell of holiday baking fills the conversation of the tediously nostalgic. The world opens its mouth like a caroling choirboy or a coal chute, waiting for the particularly oral tradition of Christmas to stoke its reticent imagination.

The Xmas routine is man's spiritualized rendition of the midwinter hoarded-nuts bash, a practice dating back millions of years, when our species was more of a tree shrew and suckled its young without the benefit of paperback books. (Note for the beginners: The coy greeting-card shorthand for Christmas is *Xmas,* a cavalier revision that as yet has not been extended to Xgiving or Xoween. By analysis one assumes that Xmas denotes the birthday of Jesus X, presumably an assassinated radical; inasmuch as X symbolizes the unknown quantity, there are sound religious defenses for its use. Besides, some of the most potent icons in Western Christmas culture are X-shaped: the screw-on stand for the Christmas tree; the XXX that comically signifies the labels on liquor bottles; the X through the names of those who failed to give presents last year.)

Anyway, you are imagining Christmastime. Using your fine-tuning knob, imagine it is Christmas morning. Snow can be gently falling, if you like. That runs you extra. Except for scattered discount drugstores with ambitious branch managers, the work-a-day world has been put aside. People everywhere rise early (except for a few drug addicts and Jews) to convene on moccasin-tread in the family room for a photogenic session of Gift Exchange. Hallways thicken with the swish of discarded tissue wrap and the flash of Polaroid cameras. The air dampens with the smell of raisins, licorice, and perking coffee. Ding Dong Sara Lee On High. O for Oral Holy Night. And yet, this often-simulated routine is mere preliminary to the true social-petting-and-grooming that is yet to come, the true participation-through-acquisition that culminates in the splashy domestic production number scientists call Christmas dinner.

Dickens and his imitators (of which he is one) have long extolled the figgy splendors of Christmas dinner, and it is their depiction of the "jolly coachman" holiday that doubtless prompts many to drink to violent excess on the occasion. Although boars' heads, goose, flaming puddings, and interesting tablemates are generally limited to the largess of fiction and coffeeshop placemat pictorials, even its theoretical nature makes Christmas dinner instructive: It is the quintessential illustration of the Real disappointingly aping the Ideal. Basically, Xmas dinner is Xgiving dinner with a holly centerpiece, but even that is optional. The real difference is that at Christmas, no one is hungry. (It is that vague, continuously "stuffed" feeling that makes the day seem endless to some practitioners.) The panoply of platters carried pinkish and steaming from the kitchen, like monstrous newborn babies, are eyed with academic interest only; most of the by-now-wilted wassail have been

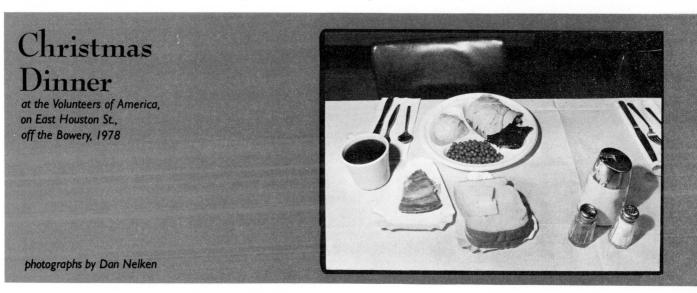

Christmas Dinner

at the Volunteers of America, on East Houston St., off the Bowery, 1978

photographs by Dan Nelken

conceding to pastries and highballs since early in the day, and the meal has no more urgency than a ground-breaking ceremony.

As morning ends, the house burgeons with tiny, non-native grandchildren, busily spilling tumblers of Pepsi on carpeted stairways and pounding on the unused piano with a fervor reserved for the musically ignorant. Distant relatives (though clearly, not distant enough) have accumulated in corners with boilermakers and pre-rehearsed observations on the propensity of others to age and/or fail. Resident teenagers are brooding upstairs in their rooms, or, if they are gregarious, in the rooms of friends, generally over the pathos of being insufficiently misunderstood. Transient teenagers seek each other out and complain about the obligation that forced them to participate in the event. (The ability to be discontent in order to be sociable is the first adult attribute many youngsters acquire.)

The matriarch of the family (the self-designed *sine qua non* of these to-dos) will be insistently unassisted in the kitchen, doing what sentimentalists call "bustling" and psychoanalysts call "guilt induction." The patriarch, who emerges briefly to carve, is not comfortable in this wave of modern humanity; in company he betrays a noble bewilderment comparable to a Navajo chief set upon by tourists. He generally ends up down in the tool room perusing old Yuban cans full of bolts, or out in the back yard cleaning the rabbit cages.

There is a certain delectation in completeness, and all these types are assembled in much the same spirit as the creamed corn and Brussels sprouts they are about to surround. However, before you imagine the gallery sitting down to dinner — and I hope you're imagining enough chairs to go around (this holiday, you'll note, places great demands on the imagination) — remember that no one is expected to be hungry, and consider instead the curiously *visual* function of Christmas food. While we digress perhaps the guests can work up an appetite.

Whatever the merits of "Silent Night," Christmas has always been more of an assault on the eyeballs than on any other sensory apparatus. The eye in December learns to regard red and green as a stimulating rather than garish combination. Fruitcake, surely, and hard candies in the shape of teensy satin pillows or rigid ruffles, demonstrate the appeal of looking at some foods rather than eating them. The arid, crumbly, camel-colored cut-outs that man recognizes as Christmas cookies and sprinkles with a fine confetti of "festive fixin's" — what better illustrates the strange duty of Yule edibles *to be representative art*? Ordinarily, a chocolate chip cookie is just that: a chocolate chip cookie. We don't look at it and say, "Oh, I get it, it's supposed to be the moon, only there are little Nigerian astronauts walking around on it." There is no pressure on it to tell a story. But Christmas cookies must be bells, stars, pine trees, trumpets, or paddle-limbed humanoids. The abundance of the season crams multiple functions into homely objects, giving them the shape if not the tongue of angels. The quasi-traditional Xmas gingerbread house is the most perverse elaboration on the narrative food: a dolly cottage shingled in cookies and heavily marketed by companies who also urge you to give cheese wheels as bon voyage gifts. Here the food lurches into three dimensions, gets even more dry and dusty with not being eaten, and parades about as far from a wholesome life-style for itself as food can get. Its contrivances are meant to titillate the viewer into greater hunger, exploiting a primordial urge to eat one's toys. While being "too nice" to eat, no one minds. Similarly, if people actually *like* candy canes, why are they always around the house, even in midsummer, like currency left over from a foreign vacation? Most families liquidate their candy cane stock by giving it out as Xoween treats. Even a child senses that there must be something wrong with candy canes; otherwise, why would every institution he visits after December 1st give him one *free*?

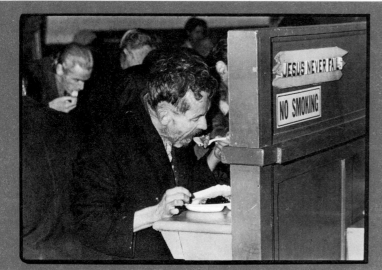

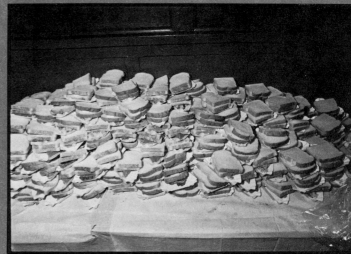

Your imaginary relatives have been cooling their heels long enough, however. Let us free them from the limbo of your mental freeze-frame. A morass of midwinter bounty reclines before them, shinier than trophies and warmer than a hired escort. If any assembled here feels a revulsion akin to that of Tchaikovsky on his wedding night, no one mentions it. The board is groaned over admiringly (Christmas dinner being one of those rare meals that require a gestalt appraisal) and a romantic soul generally observes it's a shame to eat it. Through the courtesy of all available piano stools and phone books, everyone is sitting, except for the matriarch, who daubs at her work like a model railroader. Exhorted to rest, reminded that she has been on her feet all day, she counters with a self-sacrificial chuckle and retires to the kitchen to load gravy boats. This satisfies her scions, and the prayer of grace is prefixed to the meal with the briskness of attaching a postage stamp. There follows a Homeric clatter of silverware, and the Extended Family as we know it begins extending bowls to each other.

Various prestige guests such as yams or miniature corn imply the special nature of the meal, and a shivering cylinder of cranberry reminds the viewer that this is a holiday. Dull-as-dishwater dishes like peas or celery seem radiant, dressed as they are in the seldom-used good china (a sensation comparable to seeing sitcom stars in high-budget costume dramas). Each platter circulates like a celebrity. Everyone constructs little kingdoms on their plates, creating rolling lowlands of vegetables, ridges of potato and stuffing, and a capital city of turkey. Like a Thanksgiving Day parade, or for that matter, like an armored tank procession through Red Square, the ostentation instructs us to be grateful.

Surprisingly, you and yours manage to put it away pretty extensively. The conversation breaks above the stock-exchange hum in enthusiastic, disconnected bursts, and is invariably the progressive assertion that Ma "really outdid herself this year." After solidarity is thus expressed, the assembly begins to fragment: As pie and coffee arrive, the grandchildren have joined the dog under the table or headed up to the attic to play with Dad's old toys; the teens resume their brooding on a full stomach; the distant relatives aggregate in corners, resettling like crows after shotgun fire, for further glutinous consultation on the shortcomings of others. Those who left home at an early age help with the dishes. The partriarch stays at table, since it insures him a little privacy.

In half an hour or so, potato chips and soft drinks are offered and accepted. The resilience of man's stomach is in some ways as magnificent as that of his heart.

Finally, though, heart and stomach are dismissed for the day. Coats, gifts, and children are gathered and counted. Physical exhaustion is interpreted as the glow of intimacy, and relief at having discharged a duty is read as affection. Involuntarily, the cold tick-tock of accomplishment makes mental checkoff marks next to the names of each relation who surfaces within hugging distance. Pledges of undying faith are renewed, and then no one has to see each other for a while. Love can be real without being comfortable.

Imagine the snowfall you imagined earlier has stopped. Car headlights have ceased swooping around the front of the house; the visitors who were visited upon it have gone. A salad of giftwrap and ribbons whispers underfoot. Leftovers are ignominiously crowded into Tupperware quarters. Forgotten new toys commingle under tables with old toys the grandchildren have hauled down from the attic. The day recedes like the tiny dwindling star of a switched-off television screen. Your imaginary house petrifies with silence at that point in the story when the moral is expected, but nothing in the air officializes.

Unplug the tree, put out the lights as if you were putting out the cat. Christmas and its undelivered epiphany darken, as any object would, under the influence of distance or settling night.

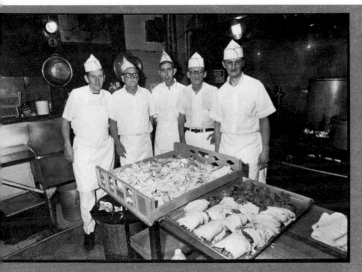

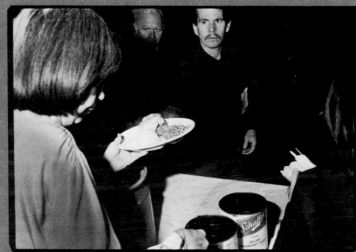

MO: Sir, why aren't you traveling to the Century O' Progress? **CURLY MO:** I don't know. Is it a good idea? **MO:** It's a great idea!

FairWays & Means 2

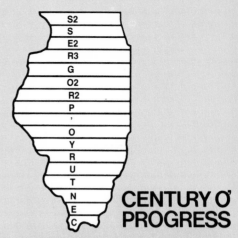

CENTURY O'
PROGRESS

**Official
Souvenir Guide**

**$29.95
Second Edition**

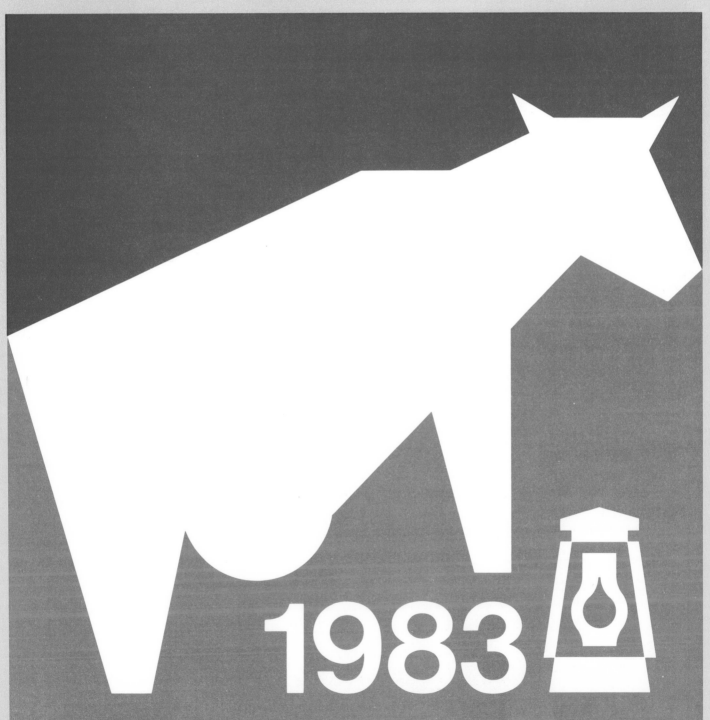

1983

saucers and plates. "Oh yeah?" you'll say.
Ecumenical Dinner. Rabbi Fagin shows young Paddy and Kathleen O'Reilly how food is made kosher. The wise old man enriches the children's brief lives as they enrich the matzoh with their own protein and iron.

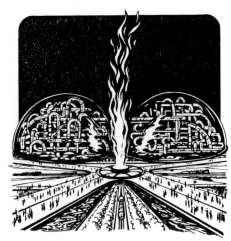

2467E. PILLAR OF FIRE

Think how difficult life would be if we were unable to perform so simple a function as "breaking wind." Hard to believe: But each day the average human digestive system produces more than three (3) million cubic feet of explosive, noxious vapor. If this "gas" is not vented safely, the entire GI track can detonate with a force equivalent to 50 lbs. of TNT. Yet, how quick we are to complain when someone, to use the vernacular, expels gas—little realizing that the alternative is a devastating blast that could rattle windows two miles away. Symbolizing bodily tranquility, then, the Pillar of Fire features an eternal, 25-foot pillar of flame fed entirely by flatus piped to it from the CO'P's 670,000 drive-in toilets. Conceived and

executed by Beauregarde & James, a Wheeler, Ala., architectural firm, the POF by night casts the glow of "150 million Cross power" over the Mississippi Valley, where perhaps it lights the way for new Huck Finns and Tom Sawyers, paddling their way to Cairo, to be free.

Charms

"And the Glow From That Fire Will Surely Light The World." Scientific displays explain how natural intestinal fuel can reduce our reliance on imported oil.

Cook Your Own Goose. Whether it's steak or fowl, at the casual but intimate POFateria you're certain it won't be overcooked or underdone because *you* supply the power. After placing your order, close the door on your booth, set your sphincter for broil, and before you know it you're cooking by the seat of your pants. Enjoy a drink before dinner? Don't forget the bar; it's the ideal place to let go with friends.

That occasional cloud of dust you see on the horizon is not a tornado. It's just a herd of some of the Fair's 25 million head of cattle stampeding someplace. Any visitor to the Century O' Progress may join these gentle creatures, often called the Otters of the Plains because of their playful dispositions, as they scamper about. Occasionally, one of these fellows may die of old age, or from exposure—say, to your fender. Do make sure the poor thing is dead. If it's in agony, won't you take the time to back up over it once again? Then, attach a colorful "Jazz Baby" or wasp-white Old Chi-town Cowcatcher to the front of your vehicle, scoop the brute up, and transport it to the nearest Hospitality Hole, where you will receive our thanks. Do not, of course, attempt to make a meal off the carcass. That's a bad idea. It's not important to know why. But don't let your clothing or any other part of your body come near the former cow. That's only common sense! Sure!

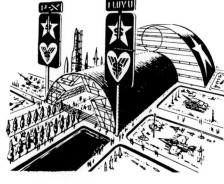

2468E. PX I LOVE YOU

United States Military Cuisine and the brave men who eat it provide the theme for this pavilion, an attractively corrugated Quonset hut housing a wide variety of coded cans containing army-style food. Children can play with the empties out back.

Charms

Tongues of the PX. Your ears will stand at attention as experienced drill sergeants teach you the meaning and pronunciation of mess hall, messkit, and Messerschmitt. You'll learn that the language of war fare is not a pretty thing. But somebody's got to speak it.
"The Long Gray Chow Line." West Point in myth and mirth, a 19-minute, full-color animated movie integrating actual combat footage with zany barside or "campfire" tales of legendary "Good Apples" in their "lowly plebe" days at The Point. Watch—
☆*The volunteer army ridiculed* by Tecumseh "Official" Sherman (W.P. 1840) as he furtively spirits a sack of greasy mutton off to his quarters.
☆*In between walking* "punishment tours" for concealing a classmate's pistol in his footlocker, Jack "I Was Going To Surprise Him With It" "Binglepuss" Pershing (W.P. 1886) spills unauthorized popcorn all over his tactics theme. Watch those paws!
☆*A tiff breaks* out between Doug "Flirty" MacArthur (W.P. 1903) and Jon "His Generation's Binglepuss" Wainwright (W.P. 1906) when the latter is promoted to "Hot Beverage Corporal" without the upperclassman's approval. After Flirty threatens to "bust him down to Cold Beverage Corporal," they settle it over a warm draft beer in the Secret Chapel. "At least it's not warm volunteer beer," says the discreet Flirty.
☆*In a dream* sequence, Anastasio "Say 'Little Chicken'" Somoza (W.P. 1946) imagines leading a platoon of hungry GIs on "egg raids" along the Rhineland. They find a peasant girl with great eggs.
☆*And, finally, what* if Dreyfuss had been a 260-lb. lineman with the Navy game just days away? No difference, says Mimi "K.P." Yapa (W.P. 1980), who stumbled upon evidence that the Jewish lieutenant was actually selling math test answers to the Germans. For her

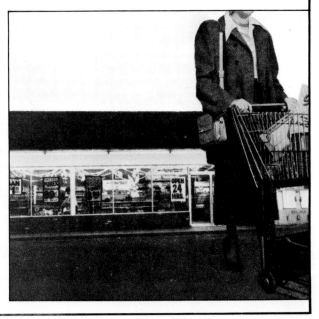

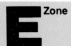

sleuthing, the French government honored K.P. with its coveted Vichy Award.

☆Th-th-th-th-th-th-that's all, Mister!

Tray of the Unknown Dinner. On the bottom engraved in oak leaf can be found a complete roster of things soldiers have never eaten.

Captured Food. Here you can sample kidney pies taken during the War of 1812, Apache corn muffins, and paella from the Spanish-American War. Afterwards, you'll understand why they're called the "spoils of war."

Black Market in Miniature. A re-creation of the famous one outside Fort Bragg, North Carolina. Stroll the childlike cobblestone aisles in single file, perhaps sampling from the squash and corn (in season), nylon stockings, penicillin, whole blood, 14th Century Flemish masterpieces, cream soda, watermelons, chocolate babies, and licorice boys separated from healthy Mamas who were not "complainers." Continuous entertainment is provided about the area.

☆☆☆☆☆☆☆☆☆☆☆☆☆☆☆☆☆

A FairWays FeaTure

Gold Grass Essay: "Animal Pride"
by Amy McQuigley, 12 years old,
Marion County 4-H Club, C-Zone
("It's the Whee Zone")

Once there was a cow who started as a baby calf but grew up by being helped by a little boy who was like its father. And the calf was always hurting itself by getting into trouble or doing something stupid like following the boy into the **kitchen** after he did his chores though it really wasn't the cow's fault because she loved her father who was the little boy. So the cow's father (the little boy) had to punish the cow but she would never learn because she wanted to be with her father so much. And the boy would kick her and heave her down stairs and put her inside the dishwasher and turn it on to Sanitize Cycle and beat her with **kitchen** chairs and things like that and worse. So they kept on having to call the vet to take care of the cow who would keep not feeling well after these things happened to her but the "father" loved the cow and didn't want them to take her away from him so when the vet would come the boy would say how the cow had gotten into accidents and that she had brittle bones and was accident prone or was clumsy so that they wouldn't know she had been punished by her father for being a bad cow and sometimes you could hardly see the marks on her after a while because her hair was pretty dark. They never took the cow away from the little father who wanted to take good care of her until when the 4-H fair happened in town and the father took the cow to the fair where it didn't win any prizes because it limped and one eye didn't work so good so then the boy-father slaughtered the cow and then when they graded it it came out just short of Prime so the boy was happy because he never really liked the cow anyhow. EVEN though the cow really loved HIM.

334 small words
counting introduction: 350 exactly

☆☆☆☆☆☆☆☆☆☆☆☆☆☆☆☆☆☆

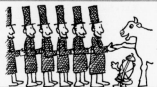
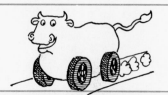
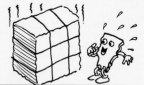
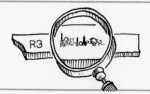
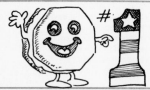
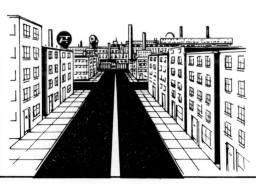

This, and the other 95 Cattlog pages in FairWays 2 should inspire precious memories of your CO'P-Stop when you get back to Idaho, or wherenot—but please note that most of our keepsakes have been designed to enhance your visit while it is in the present tense. That's why we say: When it comes to souvenirs, the Fair's notions are revolutionary. Items may be purchased at souvenir shoppes or participating pavilions.

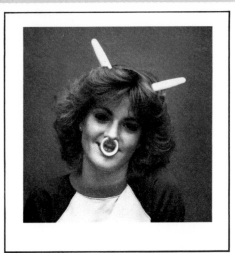

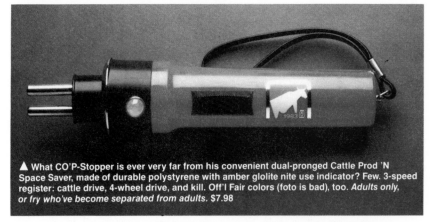

▲ What CO'P-Stopper is ever very far from his convenient dual-pronged Cattle Prod 'N Space Saver, made of durable polystyrene with amber glolite nite use indicator? Few. 3-speed register: cattle drive, 4-wheel drive, and kill. Off'l Fair colors (foto is bad), too. *Adults only, or fry who've become separated from adults.* $7.98

◀ Guess what our little Cowtie Pie, Naomi, has in her hair? Nooooo, and that's not even *funny*. Her Bossy Dress-Up Kit contains **horns** (✔ answer), nose ring, red neck-harness, soft-white adjustable underbelly, and body scars (not shown). **BOSSY DRESS-UP KIT!** $21.95

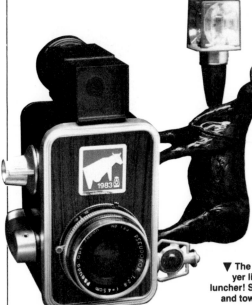

◀ Granger than truth! Forget about making snap decisions when you've got the *authorized* camera of the Fair's Public Relations folk. Handgrip is shaped like their mascot— Media Blitzen! Plus, a flash attachment that really works! $10.95

▼ The *Original* Li'l Abattoir. Turn yer li'l cowpuncher into a cow-luncher! Starter set comes with belt and towel (not shown). Dozens of accessories. And belt is made of huggable horse, of course. [**Of course!**—Ed.]. $35.00

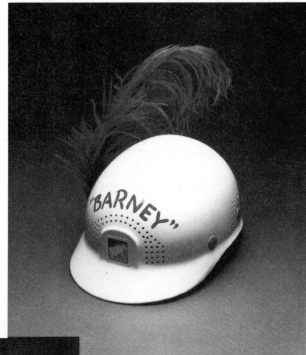

▲ Green-feathered (color is off) meatguy's cap as seen along the Butcher's Block, 14730–15190. St. Patty's Day fun every day o' the year. Made of high-impact polystyrene, in 6 colors, 812 recognized names. $18.49

▼ Lounging toy, souvenir of the Rattrap Hutch. Detailed base. $59.50

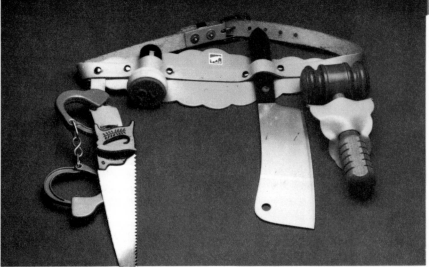

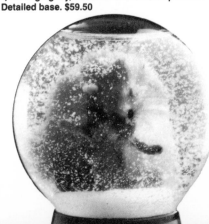

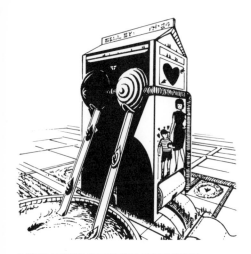

2469E. HOME OF PAPER PRODUCTS

Just across the multilane Panama Common and doglegged around the Mall Des Artistes stands the queerly radiant Home of Paper Products, celebrating "Our Friend, the Mother" at the Fair. *Safe and Sanitary*—in the mind of virtually every Fairgoer that phrase suggests just two things: Paper Products, and the Modern Mom. So the weather-resistant milk carton ("Home"), painstakingly origamied

during a six-month Retreat by relatives and friends of Gus Cinquemani, Carbondale, Ill., is then crowned by two free-standing turretlike globes—one slightly larger than the other. The larger contains 100,000 gallons of chocolaty flavored goodness, while the smaller holds 75,000 gallons of good flavored whiteness. Two corrugated pipes attached to the tower tops convey this treat by viaduct around the Fair. You've probably enjoyed some already. Are you sure you wouldn't like some more?

Charms

Sanitary Arts. When Timmy's cheeseburger falls to the restaurant floor, Mom sanitizes it by wiping the melted cheese with a paper napkin and giving the bun a big kiss. Timmy shows his gratitude by asking for seconds.

Disposable Kitchen Plate Memories. People die and you remember what you were eating. Grandpa. Grandma. The phone rings and Mom turns down the beef bourguignon she's trying out in the new crepe pan. The food is good even if the news isn't.

Hospital Memories. You were grouchy. You'd say, "Mom," you'd say, "how come they divide everything up into sections on the hospital tray?" Like you were some baby. Next day, Mom would sneak you in a chocolate Fridg-Y. She'd wink at you. She'd hide the empty Fridg-Y wrapper in her shirt. Then, after you'd kissed

her, she'd tell you that the Doc said it was all right, because you weren't going home so fast, after all.

Lac Flume. On a 90-second ride, "paper boats" swish dedicated Fairgoers in and out of the good flavored whiteness, and around the outside of the smaller of the two free-standing turretlike globes.

Variety Pack. Three unwed mothers juggle paper plates, then try to act their way out of a paper bag.

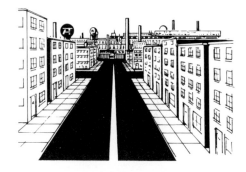

2470E. HISTORIC CARBONDALE

An ancient land with a prodigious future looks to the past in Historic Carbondale, the largest "theme" park in America. Its two-lane traffic, forty churches, raquetball club, absence of imposing pavilions, self-conscious citizenry, and projected retail sales in the $250 million neighborhood suggest insecurity and a cloud, a thin veneer, of smug trade-unionism—in short, Historic Carbondale: America Between the Fairs. A monument to the living past, this near-fully operational, drive-thru historical park was chosen from more than 1,292 proposed sites after it became clear that masses of tasty visitors to local pavilions might result in an overload of the Ante-Breeder, Historic Carbondale's revolutionary, underground nuclear mosquito-abatement appliance (danged Mississippi!). Which could, in turn, produce a seismic shock capable of hitting a fault line running *right under* Milk & Fire, some 145 miles *away*. So picture this, then: Lantern cracks open like a goddamn *walnut* and topples into Cow (Milk), smashing Her bitsy, and now both these babies are going critical on you! Holocaust-efficient? No. Never. Not even to wipe out every 'squita on earth!

☆Please note: 15-minute time limit in Historic Carbondale

Charms

Education. Southern Illinois University has been preserved intact by filling each room and all of its buildings with a low-density, polyurethene foam. Otherwise, schoolchildren still attend classes in edifices of pre-cast concrete faced with marble, slate, flagstone, limestone, gypsum, terrazzo, some with aluminum siding and unalterable hellhole

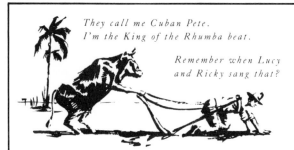
Most of Illinois' 11,688,213 residents were glad for the opportunity to contribute their quarters to the CO'P. In fact, only the Illinois Board of Law Examiners, aided briefly by the last two justices of the Illinois Supreme Court, actually attempted to challenge the placement of the Safeway Impulse Buyorhythma on the Springfield site of their former chambers. The Buyorhythma was forced to open its registers several days late. In the end, however, one and all chipped in on the creation of this truly Eminent Domain.

"Hey, how can I get a pavilion?" visitors tend to wonder after the unexpected pleasures of a Mr. Moody, a White Trash, or an I Don't Think My Career Is Dead Yet. Although the CO'P is mainly a Food Fair, occasionally a maverick is permitted to slip through if he [or she—viz., I Don't Think My Career Is Dead Yet. **And we don't either, Liza.**—ed.] impresses the Fair with his sincerity. Competition is stiff, but if you think you qualify, the man to see is the Hon. Chas. Silverfish "Available" Wu. His office is high atop the Lid Dome.

A FairWays FeaTure

MILK & FIRE

The ancient and modern worlds have no dearth of monumental wonders: The Great Pyramid, the Colossus of Rhodes, Hoover Dam, the Giant Rat of Sumatra. But none of man's works is as awesome or, frankly, as inspiring as MILK & FIRE, the symbol of the Century O'Progress.

A. Located in the temperate **R**-Zone (on the former site of the "rough part" of Springfield, Ill.), MILK stands more than 1000 feet (over 300 hands) high at her big shoulders. She is both a replica of "Dunce," Mrs. O'Leary's cow who started the Great Fire of 1871, and a complicated vision of the grease bath inferno at the U-Spit Steak Pit & Clam Casino that led to ChiFire 2. Dedicated to **"The Greatest Food For The Greatest Number,"** MILK houses some of the roomiest restaurants at the Fair, including the Bell Room, the Top O' the Guernsey, and the Drover Lounge.

B. MILK's untroubled, dusky eyes gaze silently westward to Promontory Point, Utah, where on May 10, 1869, the Union Pacific and Central Pacific Railroads were joined, forming the Transcontinental Railway. Our magnificent cow stands an eternal watch over that hallowed ground, assuring that the Golden Spike, sanctifying the first Irish-Chinese collaboration, and holding our east and west coasts together, shall not be disturbed.

C. A unique mixture of concrete, sand, and Cheez Whiz® have made MILK the largest, hollow poured-concrete structure in human history. Then, meticulous Old World craftsmen surfaced Her with eloquent grades of wood-grained formica—painstakingly intaglioing Colonial maple, Mediterranean walnut, and bleached pine plastic laminate onto Her flanks.

D. The lantern is fuzzy.

E. Some say that MILK's colossal dimensions are just what a **real** cow would look like to a Martian.

F. FIRE—or, "Wohilo"—an enlarged version of the lantern Dunce used to knock over Chicago, contains a 2000-gigawatt atomic reactor, popularly known as "Hamlet's Payload," which supplies much of the Fair's energy at low cost without damaging the environment. (MILK encloses a much, much tinier version: "Lady Macbeth.") The fail-safe design of the core makes an accident theoretically impossible. But if the impossible were to take place, the triple-redundancy of its safeguards system would restrict any catastrophe to an acceptable damage profile.

G. FIRE means Hope. The lantern is a beacon. Only real close friends of the lantern get to call him Fuzzy.

H. "Hey, kids: Steak doesn't come from a horse," says Fuzzy.

I. MILK: Don't worry. He's just a cocktail party witchhunter.

WOHILO: You mean, a sort of McCarthy on-the-rocks?

*Watch for it this fall on **N**-Zone TV!*

J. In the future, after some technical problems are solved, our noble bovine will start living up to Her name....She'll be able to give

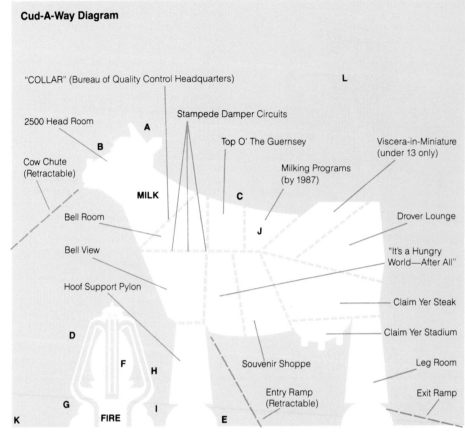

Cud-A-Way Diagram

"COLLAR" (Bureau of Quality Control Headquarters)

2500 Head Room

Cow Chute (Retractable)

Stampede Damper Circuits

Top O' The Guernsey

Viscera-in-Miniature (under 13 only)

Milking Programs (by 1987)

MILK

Bell Room

Bell View

Hoof Support Pylon

Drover Lounge

"It's a Hungry World—After All"

Claim Yer Steak

Claim Yer Stadium

Souvenir Shoppe

Leg Room

Entry Ramp (Retractable)

Exit Ramp

FIRE

A B C D E F G H I J K L

pure, whole milk! As this is written, Her hindquarter muscles are being serrated to allow Her **to actually kneel**—each morning—so a team of specially-trained, champion farmers from the Grange Olympics (**sorry, no Masons**—ed.) can fill their pails with 10,000 gallons of homogenized, pasteurized, low-viscosity Nectar of Hay. The whole thing ought to take maybe 20 minutes!

K. Naturally, before being offered for sale, each drop of Her milk will be carefully inspected to verify that its strontium content is well within proscribed safety limits!

L. Symbols of the Fair's lofty purpose, MILK & FIRE are visible throughout all O'Progressland. MILK has even been spotted as far away as the Will Rogers Actors Home. And WOHILO, it's said, in the Canal Zone. Though that sounds a little fishy.

Some quiet evening during your stay at the Fair, gaze out over the grounds at MILK, our earthbound constellation, rubbing Her enormous torso against the fence of the world (or, "Sky"). On some nights, they say, the glow from Her (baby) atomic furnace casts what looks like shadows of immense herds of cattle stampeding across the sky.

The people go in, the cows go in. The people go out, the cows—?

The longest retractable moving staircase in the world (ENTRY RAMP) sweeps you soundlessly skyward into the BELL VIEW, 450 feet off the ground, where a clean plate-glass window affords a panorama of the surrounding

countryside, notably the thrilling Safeway Buyorhythma and the doughty White Rock Candy Mountain. Closer at hand, contemplate the unavoidable grandeur of the ribbon of cows coursing its way (COW CHUTE) 812 feet off the g-r-o-u-n-d into the 2500 HEAD ROOM—talk about your "pen pals"! Before we tell you why the cows or "cattle" are placed in heavy steel casks and then c-h-u-c-k-e-d or "lowered" into deep, clear, demineralized water where the casks are unscrewed and the "boves" rubbed down by mechanical arms, which they *love*, you won't want to pass up the enchanting, almost tranquilizing spectacle of "IT'S A HUNGRY WORLD—AFTER ALL," in the LaFollette Rotunda, which is about the size of Radio City Music Hall on a good day. Here, simulated tourist buses whisk Fairgoers (or "MILK-men") past rows of ingenuous animated figurines trying to salute—through song, dance, prayer—the starvation and utter hopelessness shackling the lives of those citizens of Ireland or (Big) China still stuck in the "Mother countries." In a final scene, a kneeling MILK-of-the-future is shown providing gallons of milk and side orders of Belgium waffles to the hungry and vanquished. This was all UNICEF's idea. (*By the way*, those tourista buses are amply protected from P.L.O bloodsuckers with bombs in their hand and coo-coo in the hearts!)

The people go out, the cows—?

Coming to it—remember when we said one of those cows had YOUR NAME on it, or at least your initials? Hunky Clancy, head CO'P Dietician, will now do the honors: "Everyone who visits the CENTURY O' PROGRESS will come away with a lifetime of precious memories and, as our gift, a four-week supply of delicious, freshly-slaughtered beef. More surprises: Every creature running with the CO'P herd is only ⅞ the size of an ordinary cow—be forgivin' us, we call 'em LepreCows—because we have selectively bred out all unnecessary or 'tasteless' parts, including the horn, tail, hooves, and Souvenir bones. What remains is just enough meat to feed a family of four for a month! Whoop, there are some cows—girly, girly, girly—now. F-l-a-n-k-i-n-g us. They're on their way down from the cleansing and martinizing facilities in the 2500 HEAD ROOM. Why don't we just lope along with them, Mitch? Or *George,* sorry, that's twice I've done that. And son? Sonny, I wouldn't get too close to that girl, unless your Daddy's put your 'funny' gloves on. Hold 'em up. *Good* soldier! And here's where they led us. Now just slide into this moving comfy chair and you're off on what will surely be a highlight of your entire CO'P-stop: precious MILK's startling anti-climax, CLAIM YER STEAK!

"Entering YER STADIUM, the visitor—you—will note **the 622 torpid 'boves'**[1] milling about on top of a metal plate down in the pit. Soon the plate will be flooded with **two (2) inches of water**[2]. Jutting from your ottoman, meanwhile, at a friendly 45° angle, is a cool cylinder holding dozens of **electrically-charged styrofoam rings**[3], or 'Harpoons.' What you want to do is flip one of these rings, or

---

[1]Maximum occupancy. 622 cows in an enclosed space creates a colorful phenomenon butchers call "Chuck's effect." Plus-623 results in "critical chuck."

[2]For God sake, heed the signs. Don't touch the water. The water means business. You could also be hurt and short-circuit the ride: And what could be worse than sitting around watching 622 cows glow in the dark?

[3]The power-source for both the ride and the rings is our old friend, Lady Macbeth. But don't worry about your own safety, rolling along on your comfy chair. You won't be hurt—you're not g-r-o-u-n-d-e-d.

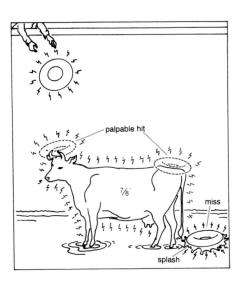

palpable hit

⅞

miss

splash

Harpoons, onto one of these boves, or LepreCows, and that's the way you play our game called CLAIM YER STEAK. You don't have to loop your Harpoon over the cow's horns. You just have to *touch* its body area. Since these gals are now four-hooved **electro-magnets**[4], the Harpoon'll stick like *glue.* Though that's not a word you want to say around cows, is it? Like g-l-u-e!

"Each family gets to throw until they bring one down. As soon as they do, Ranger Chef attendants in flippers and wetsuits race out to 'tag' your beef, branding it with your initials and hometown (for instance: A.F., Natick, Mass.), double-bagging it for easy transport, and slapping the whole thing on a watersled, which speeds off in anticipation of the final step of your Rugged Dream, when you *literally* CLAIM ... YER STEAK!

"In the not-too-distant future," finishes up Hunky Clancy, without the slightest hint of a

---

[4]From cow-catcher to "conductor"—you've come a long way, Bossy!

twinkle in his eye, "you'll find your butchers going much more in the direction of, oh, experimental physics. You know, it's the physicist and the butcher both wears the white apron." Yeah? "Dig. As you wander along here on Butcher's Row—watching them dress your meat, YER STEAK, and listening to the butchers going on about stuff—you'll realize that today's butcher isn't just thinking Cow or Cows but numbers on the order of—" Hey. All *we* want to know is: *Why won't they give us our meat?* "Because ... after dressing, your meat is airlifted to the Abattoirama, the last pavilion at the Fair, where it is hung in our temperature and humidity-controlled aging room, hundreds of feet below the ground. You can call for it after you've settled your CO'P accounts at the Banks of Lake Michigan."

This and that. This whole Fair is this and that.

"Look, buddy, I'm not getting into a whole thing with you. But I'm not trying to fool you. I'm being completely ingenius with you."

☆☆☆☆☆☆☆☆☆☆☆☆☆☆☆☆☆☆☆☆☆☆

Remember the old saw—how cleanliness is next to Godliness, and next to impossible, too? The Fair remembers. That's why each pavilion is outfitted with its own car wash. Because clean cars are "eye fresheners." It's your Fair—keep her that way. "Fair."

There are no dinosaurs at the Century O' Progress. The City of Moline Pavilion came closest to having a dinosaur exhibit, but CO'P Manager Francis Grady said, "No dinosaurs." "Not even the 'Walking Fortress'?" said the City of Moline. "No dinosaurs," said Grady. His foresight has been borne out by recent discoveries that America's precious fossil fuel comes from prehistoric grapes and wafer cookies, as much as from dead big things.

☆☆

Symbiotics

What does a remarkable cow logo and a stunning cow poster of a remarkable and stunning Cow have to do with the state of

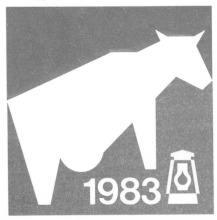

1983

the typographic arts? The answer is, almost everything. They're part of our continued commitment towards a Fair-wide symbol system. Including—and here is the truly amazing part—setting the type for **Fairways 2** in our contemporary COP Cleanskin. Beside which all other faces look hackneyed. COP Cleanskin is our "take" on a non-utilitarian face designed in 1953 by a little Swiss who didn't know anything about this nation's copyright laws. We call our action "reinvigoration." It wasn't easy. The art class who accepted the COP Cleanskin commission missed all their deadlines. That was just plain unprofessional. Then the fonts started blowing up down at the plant. That was just plain sabotage. It's time to begin thinning out the ranks of the Resistance, we think. Men were killed. They died. One last word about COP Cleanskin. You can order it from us for your personal use. The upright is beautiful. The Roman is kooky. COP Cleanskin. Unblemished. Unscarred. Beside which all other faces look acnied.

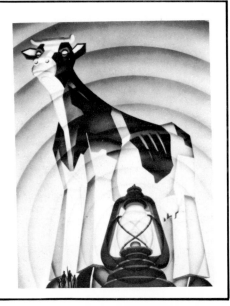

As everyone knows, on May 10, 1869, the Transcontinental Railroad was completed, the Golden Spike was driven, and, in a private transaction, a Chinese man of substance named Hop See "Irrevocable" Wu traded a newborn calf to a craggy-faced Irishman whose eyes danced like a young girl in her first strapless disco gown, Roscoe "Poots" O'Leary. Back in Chi, O'Leary handed the calf over to his wife, The Pooteen.

Of course, that was the cow that kicked over the lantern that burned Chicago that set off the racism... that caused the chain reaction, that is, that built the Century O' Progress!

But, as every theatergoer knows, if you want

THE TRAVELLER'S COMPANION TO THE WORLD'S COLUMBIAN EXPOSITION AT JACKSON PARK

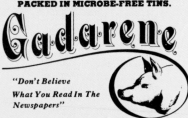
TESTIMONIAL
～ No. 18 ～

I think it high time someone said a good word about the Irish, without accusations that This or That Person was perhaps getting soft on the Green Question. I'm no Green Friend. You boys know that. Those boys burnt our city in '71. There's no rubbing it out, nor wanting to. But all the same, who was it built Our Fair? Not your Palmer House plutocrats, that's sure. They were the ones thought it up. But who went and *built* it? Put their strong backs into it? Was our Irish. See old Jimmy MacGregor throwing his shoulder to that obelisk! Good Jimmy! And thousands more like him. Should a lad be buried alive 'neath a cornerstone of the Fisheries Building, or the Arts Palace, from somewhere came another to take his place! Fancy that. So I think it be high time to re-think our stand on the Green Question. Or at least on worthy Greens. Though I'm no Green Lover and will do what the majority says. **See my booth at the Transportation Building.**

—D. D. P., Esq., Urbana, Ill.

EXTREMELY RAPID CONSUMABLES
by Michael "Jedediah" Stone

All persons engaged in Commerce and the Professions know how consumptive of time and laden with inconvenience is the noon repast to those who would rather apply themselves to the Science of Wealth.

Many Entrepreneurs have sought to magnify their Functionability by abstaining entirely from the luncheon. This manner of gastronomical imprudence is invariably repaid by attacks of ulcers, Palsy, Acrimonious Discharges, Flush Mouth, the Dreaded Indurations and a host of ulterior complaints numerous as they are pitiful.

But hurrah! A Remedy has been at last proclaimed. During ceremonies at the Midway Hall of Cathartic and Digestive Arts at our World's Columbian Exposition, a variegated array of Extremely Rapid Consumables was demonstrated to the Public.

One dozen young men of commodious proportions ingested these Appetitans in jiffy-time, thereafter declaring themselves fully satiated and revivified for an afternoon of Enterprise.

Each consumable is certified tasty, easy to digest and enriched with Substances known to promote Good Health. Most salutary of all, they may be eaten with dispatch at one's Place of Business, sparing the time and expense of repairing to a commercial restaurant.

As these Groceries leave one hand free, rendering dining utensils archaic, it is possible to continue with one's affairs while standing erect or even standing.

These comestibles are manufactured to the highest degree of excellence on the most Modern culinary engines by teams of dedicated young girls and boys. These Victualists, as they are proud to call themselves, may soon supplant the haughty Head Waiter and the insufferable maître d'hôtel as purveyors of the Nation's nutriment.

These Victualists—Ambitious Toilers!—respond immediately to commands of the most exacting gourmand and ask no gratuity, but only a fair wage.

The Speedy Viands depicted here are typical of the vast assortment offered for Sale, all of which lay claim to the following advantages. Each weighs less than two pounds and is small

---

THE SALIVATOR

This meal is constructed of a Baked Potato and a succulent bolus of Ground Beef held together by a handsome bun, of which there are several styles, some for ladies, some for men. The top is excavated to permit the application of condiments, and the base has been entunneled to allow drainage of same. Each sandwich is protected by a solid oak container with brass fittings and a double action lock. Manufactured by Concordia Eateries of Aliquippa, Pa.

THE BAG O' CORN

Sometimes the palate's desires cannot be sated by sandwiches, which is when a Side Order of a Bag O' Corn will delight both Tongue and Tummy. Freshly shucked kernels are coated in a Curative Trout Sauce and supplied in a Clutch Bag for which you will find many uses. This is the successor to the widely acclaimed Chest O' Broccoli. From Gotham Tastesmiths, Inc., City of Industriousness, N.Y.

THE SCALAPINO

This elegant sandwich would look completely at home resting on the mantelpiece of the finest home. It embodies an International blending of German Sausage and Latin delicacies, and is seasoned with a generous dollop of Hemp. Its producer, Ovia Foodarium, Norwalk, Conn., advises that it is "A Complete Meal in Every Bite—Everything But the Soup."

THE MONTGOLFIER

This glacial conformation, the perfect conclusion to any meal, can be had in three flavors: Vanilla, Chocolate and Glycerine. The ice cream is constructed according to the most exacting specifications, then imprinted with truly Aesthetic Contourations by newly patented devices that interlock each scoop, allowing them to be piled Ten High without fear of Toppling. Even the most vibrational eater will not be failed. Available from the Anthracnote Frappery Co., Swansea, Mass.

to clap at the curtain call, you've got to sit through the play. The "Greenos" and, sometimes, "heathren Chinee" were callously treated for many years across the U.S.A., all because of one mistake.

This theme was fearfully avoided by Irish writers of the period, such as the one below, whose presence in the '93 Guide testifies to a relaxing climate. Still, the Illy-Irish had seen too many of their kind routed from their beds and forced to hop the Underground Railway for Boston. Their early interest in convenience foods was no accident, and neither is this excerpt's place in **FairWays**.

—Ed.

AND MIDWAY PLAISANCE, CHICAGO, ILLINOIS, U S A, EIGHTEEN HUNDRED & NINETY THREE

enough to be concealed in a Gentleman's pocket.

Also, each Manufacturer warrants the durability of his Wares. They are pledged to remain free from Decay and Effluvium for up to ten months after their Date of Purchase.

On no account will these provisions emit offensive Vapors or take on discordant Hues, no matter if they are stored in Heated, Tropical, Toasty or Damp environs.

Plus several eminent Physicians report that the regular intake of Extremely Rapid Consumables restores deranged organs to their proper function and nutriates the blood so that the Body feels refreshed and invigorated.

Those who are chronically fenestrated, suffer from rectal expectoration or are subject to fits of phlegmatic incontinence because they are incapable of producing sufficient quantities of ammoniated bile, have been observed to benefit most splendidly from an exclusive diet of Rapid.

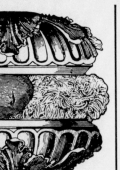

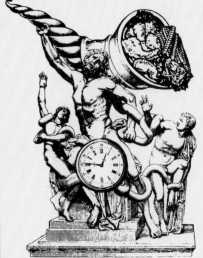

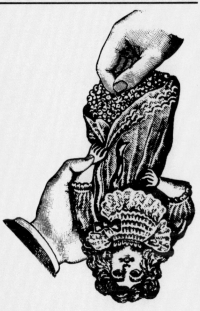

| THE SALIVATOR | THE SCALAPINO |
| THE BAG O' CORN | THE MONTGOLFIER |

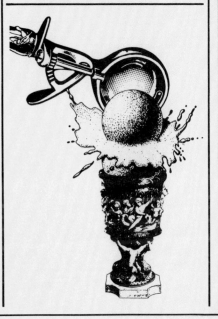

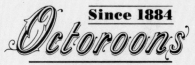
TESTIMONIAL
~ No. 19 ~

This Great Fair—what can be said by a small-town newspaper owner and decidedly amateur scribbler that has not been said already? This Great Fair, Great White City—beacon of American Enterprise, colossus of Chicago's exalted mission. The Great Fair heralds the future—just a scant seven years away. And a crusty, wizened old owner and publisher, off to sample those Extremely Rapid Consumables he has just paened, finds the happy strength to write

Begone Charon! Nasty Shade
I'll have no truck with Father Time,
'Long's I get ten pennies for every dime!
—*M. "J." S., Carbondale, Ill.*

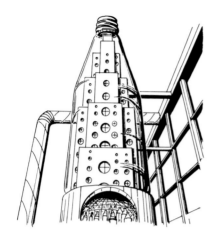

0001Y. CANDOR OF THE LEMON LIME-LITES

☞ *Focal Exhibit*

Business was way down. The lemon-lime manufacturers got together because it was in their best interests. Lemon-lime drinks are still good. But the bloom's been off the rose since the late '60's. It was probably those kids burning down buildings. People were just more zestful then. If this doesn't work, God knows what will. This cooperation and spirit of mutuality got them named a FOCAL EXHIBIT.

Charms

Grand Design. Someone was always "uncomfortable" with the idea for this, or for that. So you end up with a cardboard traffic cop out front—"arresting the eye," said Fresca, childishly. The cop (or "CO'P," more cleverness) is reciting (how? who cares?):

> Flow forth again o lemon-lime in flowing
>   flows from fountains
>   Where teeming soda jerks once teemed
> And gush again from far-flung Vendos when
>   the innocent child brings forth the
>   requisite coin
> And stream again in green-gold sparkle from
>   the green unquiet bottles
> O'ermastering, lo, my soul with thy scent
>   and tang.

Somehow the Wink people got control after this.

Bigfoot. No one quite knows how the Wink people got control, but a theory is that Fresca was getting preoccupied with the press junket, and Mountain Dew, something about the stock, and you can never count on Seven-Up in situations like this, so there was the opening. Wink had a paperback from an airport drugstore and it told them *roughly* how to find Bigfoot. Which they promptly did, picking a "probable" sighting in Manitoba and zeroing in, and impressing just everyone, even Seven-Up, who allowed it was "shameless." And they're pretty sure it *is* Bigfoot. There may be a couple of "fudgy" things at this pavilion, but this Bigfoot seems a sure shot, more or less. Though Wink may be hedging a bit, as this FairWays goes to press, with their insistence on thanking Mountain Dew for pointing out the airport drugstore, and Fresca for coming through on the nets and spikes.

Feeding Bigfoot, Or: Forty Winks. Now this is pretty good. You've got your Bigfoot, and he's being force-fed Wink until he passes out. That's strong. And if they'd had a couple more weeks it probably would've been unforgettable. Even Seven-Up started coming around, churning out the P.R.: "He may not always look happy, but that's just his way of saying 'thanks.'" Everyone was mortified.

Lime-Lites. Mountain Dew was pretty ticked off at the theatrical productions, "Up With Wink!" and "The People, Wink," and mustered Fresca for support, but let's face it, no one's lining up for these shows, though they're not half bad. No Broadway, but is Broadway Broadway, anymore? Seven-Up was a big booster of the shows and said none of the

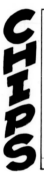

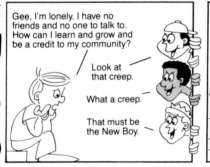

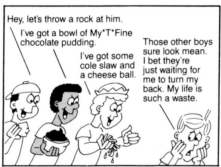

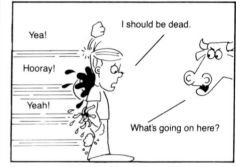

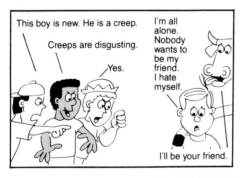

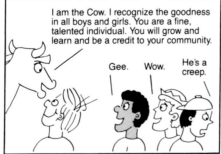

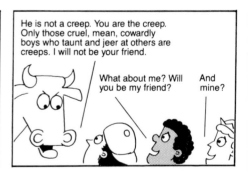

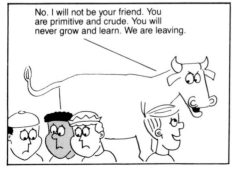

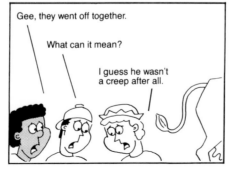

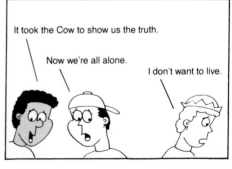

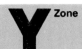

Colas had anything like them, but then Seven-Up started writing the publicity again and you've got to keep Seven-Up away from the publicity. "Just whose stringent standards are we using here?" sniffed a very condescending Mountain Dew when they got a load of the ads: "How Far May A Man Throw His Thoughts?" There was nothing about sparkling limey tingle. "And no savage attacks on Colas," said Fresca. "They're murdering us and we're not pounding back."

Fry Lime-Lites. Will lemon-lime bounce back? Or will Cola stay on top? Watch them set the Probability Table with a sparkling can of Wink.

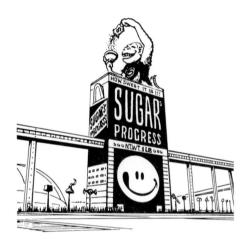

0002Y. SUGAR'S PROGRESS

Sugar begins his Journey as an ape stuck in the Morass of Molasses. As he makes his Way he becomes Fairer and quicker running. By the end of the first leg of his journey, he is Unspotted and entirely refined. Not content with his Personal redemption, he seeks that of other foodstuffs. He subdues the bitter Caffeinated Drink and makes him acceptable to Palate.

Let's not go worrying about having to use our cattle prods in self-defense, shall we? Prods are dispersal tools only. All rumors are in error. There was, and is, no "Shame of the S2-Zone"! All cows are kept under control by 40K H_z (cps) tone generators buried in the 300-foot high and "matching" 300-foot deep Illinois retaining walls. Now that's o'progress for you!

A homemaker from the U-Zone ("it's the You-Zone!") writes, "The guests were strolling up the front walk. Then, oh-oh. A leg had snapped off the couch! Immediately, the chest of Belgium waffles was in my hands: I pulled forth a few, propped up the couch leg, answered the ringing doorbell—and none of my company was the wiser! Dogs don't eat them like furniture, either." Furniture propper-uppers? Now that's ingenuous!

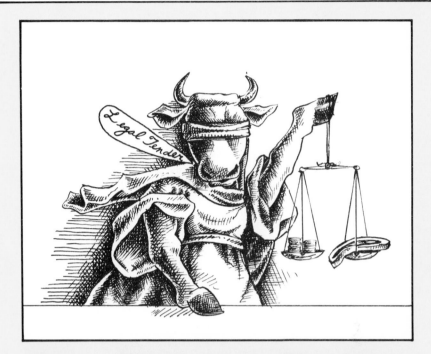

The Butcher Scales of Justice.

Little children—little fry—are having a dispute. Who settles it?

A Judge. Good ole Mom, probably.

Bigger fry are having a dispute. Now what? Mom's probably dead, or she can't even feed herself. Who settles it?

A Judge.

But this time there's no intimacy. Just a cold courtroom and some ratty-robed party hack who only wants to move on to the next case on his docket. Which rhymes with throw-away-de-key-an'-lock-it. Which is just the sort of snap decision such Guardians are always handing down. That's why—these days—too many of our system's "sore losers" are becoming "freak winners." Like America's a lottery or something. Is that Fair?

"Nooooo!" cries Bossy O's. You know us ... our gleaming green Astro-Cud (really, ordinary grass) roofs sprout in every one of the Century O' Progress' 17 Zones,* offering a single fixed meal to eager Fairtrotters, except Fridays, when there is a Fishball Alternative.

So every Wednesday, from now until the Fair shuts its borders, we'll earmark 25% of all our daily receipts for a special fund to REFORM THE JUDICIAL SYSTEM.

With your help, we'll give the judiciary just what it needs!

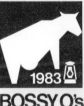

BOSSY O's

*Also known as LADY BOSSY'S in the '-, **P**-, and **R2**-Zones, due to a minor trademark infringement issue held over from the early days of the Fair. The Supreme Court should hear the appeal of *Cinquemani v. Illinois*, 106 F. Supp. 2d 1292 (SD Ill., 1981); aff'd sub nom *Century O'Progress v. Cinquemani*, 1 F. 3d 755 (7th Cir. 1983); cert. granted, 324 U.S. 995 (1983), before this Guide goes into a 3rd big printing! Watch for a name change in your Zone. We regret the inconvenience.

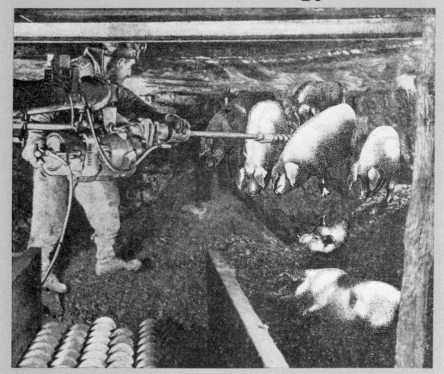
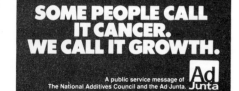
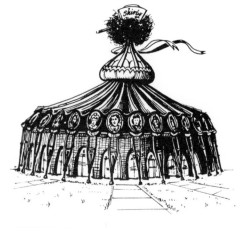

0003Y. FRANK BUCK III's CRIPPLED WAITRESSES

Frank (BRING 'EM BACK IN WORKING ORDER/ "No Fault") Buck III has made his greatest haul. From the snug Catholic working class epicenter of Old Illinois; from Decatur, from Blue Mound, from Forsyth, Mt. Pulaski, and Lovington— "The Beads," to local wags— Buck III has assembled an exotic line of crippled waitresses, many shorty-legged, many buck-and-wing, at least one 40-year Clubber, Sister Mole, and several badly scarred bull hostesses. Toughies all! "No cheapy shots," promises Buck. "No funny dressers. I don't just go for funny." The theme of this most sensational Buxtravaganza is "the unsung people who serve us our food (or direct us to it)." And: "How if we could see these people, it wouldn't be so funny." Still, Buck's paying these tragic figures good money—so he guarantees the Fairgoer "always a complete show," or he'll know the reason why. He points to his world-famous credo as proof of good faith: *If something happens to some of my merchandise, let's split the difference.* Buck himself designed the pavilion as a "short" version of the Library of Congress. Its legend shimmers out front: NO IDEALISM. The words stand tall.

☆*All tips will be pooled. (Policy change.)*

Charms

Cause and Defect. Seminars, photo opportunities, cavalcades, and Monkey-Sees for the fry. These very special ladies of the CO'P may make you laugh, or may make you cry, but you will never forget:

☆*Shirley Locky, the* one-armed waitress who carries meals in her teeth. Don't be afraid, Mom—just stop sending her back for more napkins!

☆*Craggy—make* that crabby—patootsed crippled crones slipping on loose floorboards? Buck's brought back plenty of floorboards: He fashioned them into a "pretend" space capsule and the hurty-girlies sit around *inside.* Take all the photos you want. But watch those braces!

☆*Holloway's (formerly Floyd's)* Hideaway yielded Betty "The Young Dumpster" Trell— and wait'll you hear how she got her name. "She's my Young Dumpster," says Buck. "My bird of paradise."

Inner Peace. In the pavilion's 78-seat

lunchroom, the specimens tell you their life stories while serving up *any sort* of food or beverage you want, within reason. Specialties of the *maison*? Belgem waffles, of course, and lindy torties. And "Just" Jill, who has never spilled a cuppa—despite losing *both* her monkey glands in a threshing combine accident during the high-point of her adolescence. "It's a funny story how that happened," laughs Jill. And Frank Buck III is sure you'll agree.

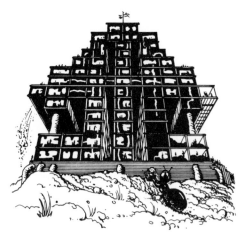

0004Y. FARMITAT '83

How to provide the Fair's future workers, or the workers at future Fairs, with humanistic housing that meets functional, technical, environmental, and budgetary parameters was the conundrum facing the Century O' Progress. Its solution was the "Person Wall" of Farmitat '83 *(latifundium formicarum 'LXXXIII)*. Although Farmitat, with its 27 linked "colony units," features many traditional construction techniques—gardens, patios, catacombs, earthworks, and entry hatches—it also introduces an exciting innovation of utter genus: continual burrowing. In their spare time, the worker-residents will actually claw out their own chambers and hallways. Thus each individual can decide the dimensions of her living quarters for herself—the sole proviso being that no room shall be more than 2 meters long, 1.5 meters wide, and 2 meters high. This element of choice reflects both the Fair's continuing commitment to participatory democracy and its determination to meet the residential needs of a burgeoning workforce.

Charms

Engineering Feets. Continual burrowing demanded the invention of a new kind of matrix: Formics. When coated with saliva—milked regularly from the gums of Farmitat's inhabitants—the surface of this soil-like substance turns as hard as concrete, thus enabling the walls to be cast as soon as they are formed! Another emblem of the driving genus of modern man!

SUPPORT THE KNEADIEST!

A FairWays FeaTure

Opening Day

Fairs have measured histories. A wastrel blows his brains across the Midway, and it becomes a chapter in the '93 Fair. '33—a spendthrift gets locked in a Time Capsule—ditto. Like the way a giant bee crisped in the light fixture is still too frightening to go near and becomes part of your life.

May 1, 1893—Chris Columbus had no idea what he was finding, much less what he was doing, so a blind minister was chosen to half-open Chicago's World's Columbian Exposition. "Everyone says this Fair is a sight for sore eyes," said the metaphor, cracking wise. "But my eyes don't even hurt." When the booing started, President Cleveland was told to press an electric key in a purple plush box. "When you touch this magic key, Mr. President," said the sightless sacerdote, "the ponderous machinery will start!"

May 27, 1933—The whole idea was: that they'd harness a tiny beam from a "remote star," Arcturus (means: Wood Alcohol), 240 trillion miles away, and slap it on a photo cell, and then relay it by telegraph wires to the Great Metropolis, and then somebody at A Century of Progress throws a switch (probably a President)—this was the whole general idea.

October 8, 1983—To the oohs and the ahs of an expectant world, the President became the first human being to officially harness the awesome power of Appetite. And where else, but at the Century O' Progress? There, at the President's say-so, a massive, specially-constructed ("one-shot") Entry Gate, erected on the shore of the former Cairo, Illinois (now point-man of the dainty **C**-Zone), and wrought from *raw protein*(!), was *deluged* with a flood of gastric juices piped from the stomachs of famished Fairgoers—honored dignitaries and sports heroes—who had starved themselves for three full days on the purposefully becalmed Vestibule of Anticipation in the middle of the mighty Mississippi. [**That may be the longest sentence in your FairWays. Anyone disagree?**—ed.] *Minutes* before the catheters were inserted, the V-of-A deck was saturated with the odor of toasted buns in order to stimulate the flow of gastric juices. Just *seconds* after the first wave hit, the Gate was entirely digested. As the newly disgorged crowd swarmed over its remains, many lost the leather heels and soles of their shoes to the still active puddle. This bubbling, ferocious bath of enzymes brought home to bystanders' senses what their reason and taste could not accept: the Century O' Progress was open for business!

☆☆

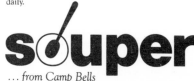

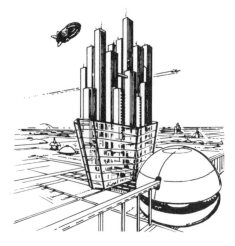

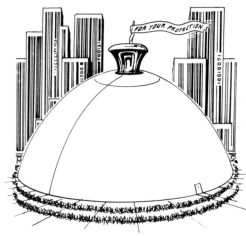

(Beyond, plum void by law.) Who said you can't fit round pegs into square holes? Not the sons of Luther Burbank, that's who not! Using patented genetic techniques (whispering to the pollen by the light of the crescent moon, gibbering at the stamen during the new), the boys have created out of plumb the world's first fully comfortable fruit. Wow!

Sodiomothizer. The fry will hop and pop to the latest in BigBan' sounds on the floor of the Salad Bar Experience. The "crooner" is none other than Lot's Wife! (Don't worry, Dad. It's only some guy—or gal—in a costume.) Between "heats," while "Lot's Wife" freshens up backstage, a long-nosed, cigar-chewing, "salty" fellow talks about how he became "her" portion-control *agent*. Dance and Learn! The CO'P to a Tasty T!

0005Y. PAVILION OF METERED MEALS

Since the dawn of time, when our prehistoric ancestors spent days hunting a mastodon only to find that it was more than could be consumed in one meal, mankind has been beset with the problem of portion control. Refrigeration, stews, and doggy bags were, in their day, inventive solutions to excess, but it was not until the discovery of portion-controlled meals that this burdensome abundance was eliminated altogether. Designed by noted architect I.M. Pei, who once built the Kennedy Center in his sleep, the Metered Meal Pavilion is a tribute to the work of A. Thomas Flud. In 1971, Flud shattered all Newtonian meal principles with his decision that $H = ms^2G$, that is, that hunger equals the mean diameter of the mouth times that of the stomach, squared, times gravity. Flud built a prototype bag of fries that could reduce an appetite to within 1% of satiation. Thus, with a savage slash of genius, second helpings were cut by more than 60%.

Charms

Not Quite a Wrap. Murals convey some of 603 ingenuous shapes Flud devised before hitting on the tastiest configurations that fit snugly the mouth. Sometimes a man fails for 44 years and then—bang—succeeds. It happens. Bang.
Standard Plum. Weight: 58.4 gms. Length: 5 cms. Shape: Ellipso-cubical. Color: buff. Maximum permissible deviation: .01%.

*Yep, Louie. Yep, Muggsy. Oh, you kid-me-not: Those are Salvation Army Warriors and Warrioresses operating the hootch houses, horse rooms, and hoopy parlors of Prohibitionland, on the former site of Joliet, up at the tippy-top, the very cowlick of the G-Zone ("Not the Free-Zone, But Close"). Huh! But this is the **New** Salvation Army, whose tenet "You can catch more flies with shimmery, kind of, rainbow colors than with a very sharp pith" was initially promulgated in May of '81, after the Miracle of the Bank Auditors. Still, some things never change, and much of the SA's energy goes into managing the five soup kitchens left over in old J-Town from the '33 Fair, A Century of Progress, which are that Father Fair's only legacy to the CO'P. Of course, nothing remains of the 1893 Columbian Exposition, our Fair's Granddaddy—and doesn't that just figure? They tell you how much they do for you, how much they do for you ... and they don't do a goddamn thing! It's a shame so little lingers from the Fair's glorious relatives, but perhaps the ghosts of those bygone buildings would be comforted to know that o'progress was just around the corner. The soup kitchens now glitter as clean and modern capuccino houses.*

Everybody knows that God spelled backwards is dog; but did you know that Dieu spelled backwards is ineffable?

0006Y. LID DOME

Ingenuously situated in the CO'P's businesslike "Nothing of Interest" section, the Lid Dome shelters a small band charged with carrying out the day-to-day administrative duties of the Fair. Beyond that, this pavilion, which isn't really a pavilion, provides CO'P-hoppers with a much-needed respite from their Zonal Sprees. A parachutist could see that the Li'l Lid is clearly a jewelbox of cast iron and rolled steel, which some have compared to a mermaid rising trembling and shaken from the sea, with something in her mouth. But viewed from the comfort and relative safety of your car, why, you'll realize that not a darn thing is going on here! Paperwork, maybe; just none of the usual romp and riot synonymous with the Fair (Our Living Cartoon, it's been called). Dr. Fleming's original penicillin bread ("I Choose A Profession," 1929) is sometimes exhibited here. But not now. Nothing here now. Don't bother stopping by. Just give the Lid a friendly wave and head over to the next pavilion. When the penicillin bread comes back, we'll tell you.

Charms

None.

One of the better stories coming out of Re-Ad Camp 4 ("Peoria") had a new arrival saying, "What's the diff between a quarterback and a quart o' bourbon?" and a Ranger Chef "Librarian" answering, "You silly drunken journalist." And that was the new man's ex-profession, all right!

✿✿✿✿✿✿✿✿✿✿✿✿✿✿✿✿✿✿✿✿✿✿✿

TESTIMONIAL 364:
Wanda Dupree, Bennington '82

FW&M: What was that again?
Dupree: Food is more than something we eat—it's something we buy. But it takes months, sometimes years of work by large groups of attractive, college-educated people you'll never meet just to deliver one order of french fries. Thanks for asking, Barney.

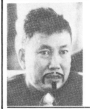

Whatever destiny draws the Dutch to Pennsylvania or a dog to his favorite hydrant also unites the Irish, the Chinese, and wieldy foods.

The Irish and Chinese persecutions in the wake of the Great Fire had generally aborted by the 1930's. (These irrational persecutions had been like having some pretty thing—hair shining like the back side of a table knife—say, "Sorry. Only with doctors.") Irish Santas were once again asking wee ones, "Have ye been good, have ye?" from the sanctity of a Confession box!

The gentle, gossamer-seeming paintings of Charlie "Traffic" Wu on these pages were displayed in the Comestible Group at A Century of Progress (1933).

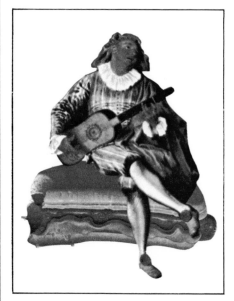

Their preoccupation with Irish concerns is both unusual (for its time) and, to some, not a little distasteful. Still, their uncanny ability to foresee the future surely merits a second glance. (Butter Design Sculpture Gallery, O-Zone, "It's the Vo-de-O-do Zone!")

Misplaced during World War II, this series of stellar Chinartistry was recovered by the CO'P amidst a batch of missing Nazi art treasures. Tragically, however, the Fascists had removed all the marbles.

—Ed.

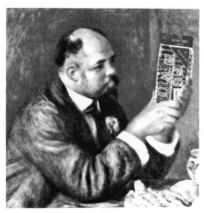

(above) BACK THEM UP: A.L. ALL-STARS!

(left) Detail from cover of The Practical MidWay, 1933-34, illustrates the "I WILL IF YOU WILL" spirit of modern Chicago

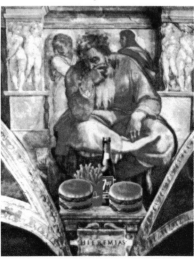

(above) SMALL FRIES TO BISHOP THREE

(below) MELTING ADVERSITY (The Future Shines With The Light Of 1,000 Spare Dimes)

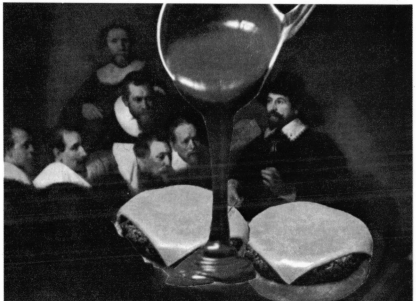

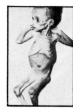 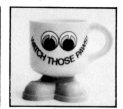
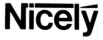

TESTIMONIAL No. 600
Barney Stone

Barney Stone, Assistant Public Relations Director for the CO'P, singlehandedly edited **FairWays 2** *with some help from the Wallechinsky O'Reilly's, and has a fascinating tale to tell. Hard to four-stomach, Barn did not immediately hitch his plow to the Cow. In his own words, his was "an Odyssey through an American digestive tract." We found Barney in his centrally air-conditioned suite inside the Hall of Free Speech, already assembling material for* **FairWays 3.** *Though visibly stirred by some of the new features, he doesn't want to drop the veil too soon. "I won't tell you what I'm doing with these baby pictures," he said. But busy Barney leaned back in his vibrat-o-chair, crossed his legs, picked up a pen and smiled, and agreed to give us His Story.*

FW&M: Hello.
Stone: Hello.
FW&M: Test.
Stone: Oh, I thought—sorry.
FW&M: You thought I was starting.
Stone: I'll just pour myself a pot of black coffee and pick up a pen.
FW&M: Suppose we begin with Dr. Gus Cinquemani, and how you two became a sort of team.
Stone: I knew we'd get to that, sooner or later. Waffle?
FW&M: Thanks. How you two became Ministers Plenipotentiary of Death, so to speak.
Stone: I wish I was older. You know? I was just thinking that. Or younger.
FW&M: Don't play with that. It's on.
Stone: You sure? These things, sometimes they seem like they're working, but they're not working. Spinning and everything.
FW&M: What're you handing me—oh, it's a roadmap of the route you and Dr. Cinquemani took to the fateful Bossy O's! We'll try to reprint that for the FairWayfarers. But using the old nomenclature—names of cities—gets pretty confusing these days. I don't know.
Stone: Maybe if we just print "Not A Map" all over it.
FW&M: Maybe.
Stone: Hotly. Because if we don't *show* it, then I've got to *tell* it, and that's *boring.*
FW&M: We'll leave it for the art guys.

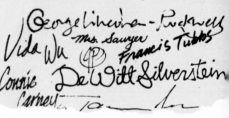

Stone: I walked into the Bossy O's and next thing I knew, Buzz Burdy was dead. They called him Buzz. Probably 'cause he never did anyone any harm.
FW&M: Back it up a little. How'd you first make the acquaintance of Cinquemani?
Stone: You're a regular badger. I used to be a badger.
FW&M: Listen, where can I spit this out?
Stone: What is it? A WAFFLE? Are you *crazy?* They'll come down on us like *Huns!* My *God:*....

The Sony TC-55 Cassette-Corder is inadvertently swatted off the brown table.

Stone: Put that away now.
FW&M: Ha. Some folks like 'em burnt.
Stone: Not burnt! *Well done!*
FW&M: Uhh—
Stone: Yeah, yeah, yeah. Cinquemani. "I swallowed hard." Did you get that? This isn't easy for me. I swallowed hard.
FW&M: This is an interview.
Stone: It can be a "Creative Interview." But... I guess that's why I'm Barney Stone. Room really holds the smoke, doesn't it?
FW&M: Coughs.
Stone: I was a reporter-columnist on the Carbondale *Atom.* Four generations of Stones lived and worked in Carbondale, worked for the *Atom.* Well, only the last two generations actually had to work *for* the paper—my grandfather and great-grandfather owned it, but they both mismanaged it so bad my Dad and me ended up as working stiffs working shifts on our own birthright.
FW&M: That must of hurt.
Stone: My Dad, maybe, was bitter. I never got to ask him.
FW&M: He died when you were very young, then?
Stone: No, I was twenty-seven. I just never thought of asking him. Listen, are we gonna stick to the outline, or what?
FW&M: Talk about your great-grandfather, Mike Stone.
Stone: Mike "Jedediah" Stone. Moved to Carbondale in winter, 1871, after the Great Chicago Fire which, historical hindquarters show us, left so much good in its wake. Modern Chicago. The Hog-Butcher of the Heartland. Porkopolis. A Chicago glowing like the Christmas Tree at Rockefeller Center. But poor Mike had to miss it—the Irish pogroms were starting.
FW&M: Surely the blackest mark on the history of Illinois.
Stone: *Northern* Illinois.
FW&M: He took the name "Jedediah" to "pass."
Stone: Like so many of his co-racialists, even in the "Free City" of Carbondale. He founded the *Atom,* and thus four generations of Stones slaved dutifully at her bosom... until that day, just over a year ago, when my editor hinted that there was "trouble in Paradise."
FW&M: How come?
Stone: I refused to sign his Loyalty Editorial.
FW&M: You're kidding.

Cow of Gold

On the plains of our Illinois, far from the Babylons of the nation's extremities, a new and rejuvenating force has reared its noble mantle.

Like a prairie wind of the people, it has shaken the Tree of Life of the Republic, sending the wormy and anti-agrarian apples crashing to the ground in confusion and disarray.

We know that force as Bossy—the Century O'Progress, i.e.—and like a zephyr She is spreading the clean and rejuvenating scent of the barnyard and disspelling the noisome odors of industrial stench and the eau de cologne of Wall Street merchant-princes in their white buttondown shirts and carrying their imitation leather attache cases, so it seems.

Now comes the nonce of the husbandman! And the citizens of Historic Carbondale have in the vanguard been!

Ignore the carping and sinister voices, breathing the accents of corrupted coastlines, even if they be local, urging resistance to Bossy. Button down your hatches! Raise more pavilions and less hell!

Mankind shall not be criticized upon its Cow of Gold!

[signatures: George Lihewbra-Pvckwell, Vida Wu, Mrs. Sawyer, Francis Tubbs, Connie, DeWitt Silverstein, Carney, etc.]

FW&M: What's wrong with that?
Stone: That's the way I was. Lincohen—the editor—threatened to fire me on the spot: All this surface noise about how nobody read my column, anyway.
FW&M: That's all it was, surface noise.
Stone: And how I wasn't conversing with the English language!
FW&M: Just a *bit* disingenious of him.
Stone: I'll say. I'd written this column chewing out the Fair, that's what had everybody in flames.
FW&M: The CO'P?!
Stone: I had this fixation, you know, that the Fair wasn't going to be careful enough about private property. It was like this oral nuisance suit. But Lincohen says to me, "You're getting a reputation as a knocker." So I come right back at him: I says, "I don't care if I get a reputation as a knocker." That's the sort of loudmouth I was.
FW&M: Incredible. You know it's incredible, don't you?
Stone: I guess. So there was this guy, Dr. Gus Cinquemani, and he was probably about 42 years old, and he had this cockamaimy idea about Mayor Daley's being dead. I shut him right down. Because Daley's alive, right? Then my Fair column runs and here comes Cinquemani again. "Forget Daley," he says. "You were right. I was wrong. It's the Fair we want. Let's get the Fair." "Hey, baby," I says. "The phone is crying for its cradle," and threw him back. He still wouldn't let up on me. Then the heat started down at the *Atom,* and my reporter's instincts lit up like a mobile home torched by Johnny Gas. I called Cinquemani and told him I wanted to get to the bottom of this CO'P. "The Fair *is* the bottom," he rebuffed. "No," I crashed back. "The bottom was Dresden, 1945. I read it in a book." Then a long pause, for tension. "Everything else is jello-with-fruit."

This Week of November 18, 1983 at the Century O' Progress

Sunday	Monday	Tuesday
7:30 FLINTY, FLAVORFUL FLORIDA FEN "Apaches Poisoning the Water." Stirring slice of Americana is enacted with dramatic results. Porpoise Pool.	**8:15** HUNCO HOSTEL Test marketing: Incredible Hulk Children's Enemas. Complimentary refreshments.	**8:00** Fish Toss 10 and younger only AROMARAMA
10:00 CHEF CENTER Lecture: "Well Done But Never A Thank You"	**11:15** Jell-O Pouring Ceremony BALINESE CAFETERIA	**9:00** "Fifth Column": continuous live action. It's hoeing, planting, and road-building day at the GREEN, GREEN FOURTH ESTATE
1:00 FRANK BUCK III's CRIPPLED WAITRESSES Symposium: Do crippled waitresses get better tips? Or do they lose them, for shoddy service? Hmmm.	**12:00** Grand O'pening: BOSSY O'S (#1) T-Zone Soon to be a Fair-Wide Franchise! Today only: the Riceball/Potatoball Alternatives are on us!	**10:30** TRIBUTE TO VEGETABLES Karen Anne's birthday. She'd just be getting up around this time, if she was home with a cold. Little ice cream cups, $1.
2:30 GOLIATHS OF THE KITCHEN Event 36. Steroid Test: Pumping Chow.	**1:15–1:35, 1:40** Jell-O Congealing Ceremony BALINESE CAFETERIA	**2:00** FOODS FOR FREEDOM The 7 Original Astronauts (Glenn, Shepherd, Grissom—go on, just try naming them) assemble "telephones" using empty Tang cans and dental floss. MISTER DONUT SCHOOL OF APPLIED SCIENCE
5:30–8:30 4 Sisters Happy Hour WELLESLEY CLUB $2 door charge. Piano bar.	**3:30** A team of visiting dermatologists will graft a chicken skin onto a turkey roll. MISTER DONUT SCHOOL OF APPLIED SCIENCE	
8:30 MR. MOODY "Il Brodieatore" Benefit $50. Black tie preferred. Cash bar.	**9:00** MICROWAVE MALL Son et lumière spectacle: "Radiation Doesn't Kill People, People Kill People"	**4:14** DRAWING BOARD We get some sort of fuzzy, sort of images you can make out on the PicturePhone. Then we smack it one.
COW NAMED: Fair officials announce that, following a grueling eight-month search, they have chosen a brown and white Jersey cow to replace the late CO'P mascot. After carefully considering all suggestions for a name, she was branded Bossy in a private ceremony.	*THIS WEEK'S CEREAL: Count Chokula®. We know, we know. But they're a whole lot better now.*	**8:00** HISTORIC CARBONDALE Closing ceremonies: Belgium Waffle Week Dedication: Tasty Bel-Jam Waffle Month. Saluki Stadium.

Stone: All the way out to the Bossy O's, it was me and Cinquemani, going back and forth on the Fair. The Doc kept trying to unpin my "Press" badge and substitute this button he says all the guys opposing the Fair are wearing. "First," I tell him, "nobody touches me. Second of all, you take away my 'Press' card it's like a young girl, ripe like an Illinois morn, looking down the dawn of the morn-after"—am I being precise?

FW&M: Sure. No problem.

Stone: You know?

FW&M: Sure. I'm with you.

Stone: She's lost her ... ███ Forgive the French.

FW&M: I think that ought to make it past the boys upstairs.

FACSIMILE

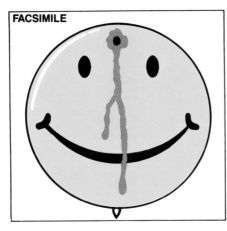

Stone: Pretty cheesy button?

FW&M: In-credible!

Stone: Now look at this lining—this is one of ours—hmm?

FW&M: No comparison.

Stone: Feel. *That* protects your clothing.

FW&M: I can feel how it doesn't scrape the fabric or anything.

Stone: Now hit it. I want you to hit it.

FACSIMILE

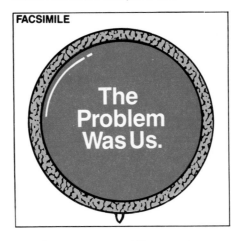

The Problem Was Us.

FW&M: Okay, so you and Cinquemani are driving along.

Stone: Right. And the roads are jammed, just jammed. It's three weeks into the Fair, after all. But Cinquemani's gotta bellyache about it, it's a beep and a bop and a boop—but what I see is people working together, letting their houses be bulldozed for pavilions, then hanging around to *put up* the pavilions. Look at history. Did the Indians do that? I tell the Doc, "You know, Doc, I think the Eighties is going to be a 'Me Last' decade. I think it's time to heal all the wounds." I got real excited and couldn't wait to get back at my typewriter. I had myself a story. I'd show them who the knocker was. This was "The New Automation"—man doing the work of machines—Messiah Populism—and I'd have it before the newsweeklies. And I kept saying, I remember this clearly, I kept saying, "What's so bad about all *this*?" That whole personal property thing of mine was going right out the window.

FW&M: Chews. And then?

Stone: Cinquemani hauls out a Geiger counter—and with it, this story how the meat

---

they're using at Bossy O's is radioactive, for God sake, and how he's going to prove it to me, but then *I've* got to rush right out and put it in the paper. I gave *him* the old hoo-hah laugh, you can be sure.

FW&M: Of course he claimed to have evidence.

Stone: Don't they always? I asked, and he nodded like a junkie. Here's his proof: He says, They've been stockpiling meat for the Grand O'Pening, right?

FW&M: Yeah?

Stone: Well, he says, at night the whole freezer glows in the dark.

FW&M: Boy.

Stone: Yeah. You know? So I says to him, "My friend"—facing him down with my eyes.

FW&M: I love it.

Stone: "My friend ... you better have a second source."

FW&M: Tell the readers what that means.

Stone: That's "reporter." It means: Two people have to say the same thing, within—oh—six months of each other.

FW&M: Did you just hear something?

Stone: Only the boy leaving off the waffles.

FW&M: Hungrily. My God, my *God*, I haven't had a chance to, I couldn't *possibly*—!

Stone: Emember-ray he-tay ape-tay ecorder-ray, K-Oay?

FW&M: What—what did Cinquemani do?

Stone: He was livid. He said, Wasn't seeing for myself proof enough? "Look," I said. "The First Amendment may be a shield, but it's nobody's Cross."

FW&M: So Cinquemani was angry because you were insisting on an additional demonstration, at *another* Bossy O's—only there weren't any other Bossy O's, then.

Stone: And it had to be a *second* Geiger counter, too. I don't miss a trick.

FW&M: Little knowing that in less than a year there'd be 1,252 Bossy O' franchises throughout Greater O'Progressland!

Stone: With more on the way. Plus, a lot of folks aren't aware that Bossy O's also produces the syrup we empty on our Fair-mous Belgium waffles.

FW&M: Maybe they should be made aware. Listen, there's no way you could eat half of this, could you?

Stone: By the time we hit the Bossy O's, all I wanted was a good burger, which seemed to upset Cinquemani, but before he starts going crazy with his Geiger counter I flipped him my Polaroid. "You owe me," I said. "Take a photo for my story. Frame it nice, and try to get in the old bat." This is my talking then.

FW&M: Of course. So that's how the famous picture came to be taken?

Stone: Yeah. And the Doc's smile flashed like a "Don't Walk" sign. A thing like that is hard to forget. "If I take your picture," he said, "and it's all blurry: Will you believe that's from the radioactivity?"

FW&M: I bet you just threw your strong hands in the air!

Stone: Strode right up to the counter, too. Fixed the counterman with a red stare and mouthed, "Big Boss,® with a complimentary Potatoball Alternative."

FW&M: But that counterman was the manager, Buzz Burdy.

Stone: Soundlessly. Yes. Yes.

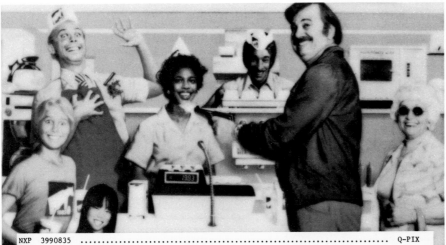

NXP 3990835 .... Q-PIX

WATCH THE BURDY DIE!

T-ZONE ("HAVE A SPREE ZONE"): RECENTLY UNEMPLOYED JOURNALIST <u>BARNEY STONE</u> ASSASSINATES <u>BUZZ</u>
<u>BURDY</u> AT LAST WEEK'S O'PENING OF BOSSY O'S. L. TO R., MORGAN AND JENNY WU OGLETHORPE, ATHENS,
GA.; THE TRAGIC BURDY, MANAGER; WANDA DUPREE, FRY GIRLY; NICHOLAS SCALESE, HOT OIL BOY; THE
IRREPRESSIBLE STONE; AND ANNA HERZOG, VENICE, CA. THE PHOTO IS BLURRY BECAUSE EVERYONE MOVED
WHEN THE SHOT RANG OUT IN THE T-ZONE.

NX-4-5-6   EUR-1-2   CREDIT LINE (BQC PHOTO) 11/19/83

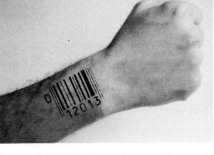

Stone: … And it's the Ambassador Hotel, all over again, that's all I could think. American society is a walk through a **kitchen**: dripping red once-living meat, now carved up at twelve bucks a head, and if you make it through the main course, there's an Arab psycho waiting in the corner. When a messenger from the darker side of America arises, that's all she wrote….

FW&M: Easy.

Stone: Okay.

FW&M: That's the way it *was*—for America, and for Barney Stone. You had foul yellow breath. Now the Fair is here. Periodontal treatments.

Stone: I see what you're hiding there.

FW&M: Oh, it got shoved under these papers, didn't it?

The tape jams.

FW&M: Cinquemani escaped?

Stone: In the confusion. Too bad. But we'll meet again. There'll be no next time for Cinquemani.

FW&M: And you killed Burdy … because?

Stone: A misunderstanding. I paid for my meal. They handed me a lottery ticket. I thought it entitled me to some money back. They disagreed, things got out of hand. Maybe I should have read it more closely.

FW&M: So the Bureau of Quality Control sent you to a ReAdjustment or "Re-Ad" Camp. No. 4, "Peoria."

Stone: Correct.

FW&M: Were you a wreck, going in?

Stone: I think I was pretty much of a wreck, going in. Yes.

FW&M: But you came out—

Stone: Assistant Director of P.R. Editor-in-chief of **FairWays**.

FW&M: How would you explain the change?

Stone: Change?

FW&M: Panicky. Please, the transformation.

Stone: Things went along, and I went along with them.

FW&M: Nice one.

Stone: I went in with an open mind, which is always important. Some Campers objected to the iron-on ID's we were asked to wear. But maybe that's just because they made us buy the T-shirt.

FW&M: Could you put them on beachballs and stuff? Okay, then that was just being childish. We've reprinted one of the attractive patches above. Chews.

Stone: But I think what really turned it around for me was the Bel-Jam Waffle billboard I could see from my register at the kitchen supply house. I'd already had my Two Slogans approved.

> ***If You've Got the Guns,***
> ***We've Got the Dream***
> ***If You've Got the Guns,***
> ***We've Got the Butter***

as well as the first of my Two Rules

> ***Seek the Center, Hit the Middle***

and I was anxious to come up with the second and get out of Camp and right back into the Fair and begin *contributing*.

FW&M: I can't blame you.

Stone: I was stumped, though, until I began to consider, you know, really *regard* that familiar waffle billboard.

FW&M: With the old man throwing the waffles to the swans?

Stone: No. The baby with its cheeks all puffed out with waffles and its tiny hands all covered with combinations of whipped cream, powdered sugar, and fresh strawberries.

FW&M: Oh, the famous one.

Stone: And reaching out to touch that famous painting?

> ***You'll Gobble 'Em Right Up—***
> ***But Watch Those Paws!***

That always hands me a little laffito!

FW&M: Swallows.

Stone: Anyhow, there it was. That was it, that was my #2 rule! I mean, I'm not saying I stole—

FW&M: No one's saying it.

Stone: After all, my version can't hold a white-waxen candle to "Watch Those Paws":

> ***Don't Put Your Hands***
> ***Where They Don't Belong***

It was how my version spoke to me, bold and many-limbed, how it forced me to examine the *very nature* of the Creative Journalist. All this crabbing and probing—why? For what? Had I despised my grand- and great-grandfathers so much, because they busted my Dad and me down till we ended up as working stiffs working shifts on our own birthright?

FW&M: No! That *happened*?

Stone: One bum with a taste for dice, the other for fancy cheeses—yet when he died, they went all through his house and couldn't find a single fancy cheese!

FW&M: Or a receipt for the cheeses.

Stone: Right. Still, I had driven myself to excel, on their account.

FW&M: And you *had* excelled.

Stone: But to what end? You know?

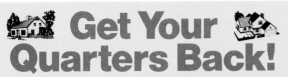

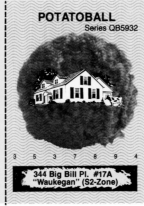

FW&M: I know.

Stone: I was but one of many voices, each singing in a separate key. We journalists think that's admirable. BUT YOU CAN'T HEAR ANY OF THE G-DAMN WORDS! They all run together!

FW&M: Sprinting to the window like a man possessed and half his age.

Stone: Look there. What do you see? And there?

FW&M: Newsboys! There, too. And isn't that a newsboy?

Stone: And listen to their voices. If this window opened you'd hear them singing, "FairWays. /And Means./$29.95./Including 640 color pages./Many with gold!"

FW&M: Many voices, *one key!* And *that* key—

Stone: Is the CO'P.

FW&M: In-credible.

Stone: Funny: But the less questions asked, the more answers found.

FW&M: That is funny. And this is probably a good place to stop.

Stone: Let's celebrate with a heaping plate of waffles.

FW&M: Barney…

Stone: I've never seen anyone with your thirst for waffles!

FW&M: Barn—I haven't even finished my first … oh. Ohhh,I get—

Stone: Shhh. I'll just pile 'em on. Mmm.

FW&M: Mmmmmm. Yum.

Stone: Coughs. Mm—

FW&M: Coughs. Coughs.

Stone: Cough.

FW&M: …all stinkums … Cough

Stone: Cough

FW&M: Cou

STOP.

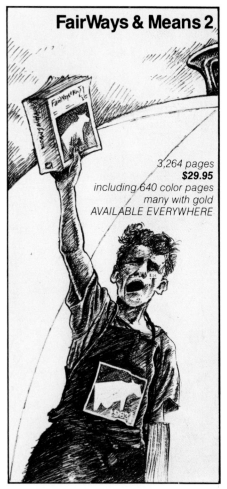

FairWays & Means 2

3,264 pages
$29.95
including 640 color pages
many with gold
AVAILABLE EVERYWHERE

A FairWays FeaTure

**Barney Stone's
—The Great Collaborator's—
5 Past Lives**

Barney Stone has "unconscious memories" of these past reincarnations of himself. He doesn't know we're running this.

1. A "mastodon specialist" at the Caves of Altamira in Northern Spain.
2. Scuola di Tintoretto.
3. A very big *padrone* of Emile Zola. "Go back for thirds, Emil," M. Le Barney would say.
4. Silent partner with Ben Hecht on *The Front Page* (1931).

 Ben: You big stew-bum!
 Barney: You big banana-head!
 Ben: Write it down.

5. Mr. Behind-the-Scenes on *South Pacific* (1949).

 Rodgers: Dum-dum-dum-dum …
 Piano: Dum-dum-dum-dum-Doom-doom-doom-doom
 Rodgers: I c-a-a-a-n't, dum-dum—dum.
 Hammerstein II: Dum?
 Rodgers: Dum-DOOOM.
 Piano *and* Rodgers: Dumdumdumdydumdumdum I'm gonnna clean—
 Barn: Wash.
 Piano and Rodgers (nodding): I'm gonna *wash* that man right. …
 Hammerstein: You're invaluable, Barney.

 —D.W.W.O'R., exclusive for the
 FairWays & Means

☆ ☆ ☆ ☆ ☆ ☆ ☆ ☆ ☆ ☆ ☆ ☆ ☆ ☆ ☆ ☆ ☆ ☆ ☆ ☆

Futurologists beware! Even the General Motors Corp. is fallible. Their Futurama at the '77 Fair in nearby Lincoln, Neb., booted a few predictions, including: toilet paper with Bing Crosby's picture on it (he died); a dolphin Pope; Clay Felker would make a go of Esquire; return of the Jungle novel; funny little squares with colors on them; a flying saucer found frozen under a polar icecap; you should ask your friends for advice; 4-year-old whores prowling the halls at Chrysler Corp.; sonic booms and other "bugs" ironed out of the PicturePhone; white collar crime blown all out of proportion; women in incredible sailing costumes; and a Fourth Reich. However, GM did predict that an entire midwestern state would be host to a World's Fair devoted exclusively to food. How about that? Though most folks figured they meant Nebraska. Or, say, Kansas. Nostradamus, look to your laurels!

*Towering 800 feet above the **P**-Zone stands "Napkin," the world's tallest 58,002-ply soft sculpture. Conceived by Claes Oldenburg, it is estimated that this monument to dinnertime decorum could wipe the face of every man, woman, and child in North America without being laundered.*

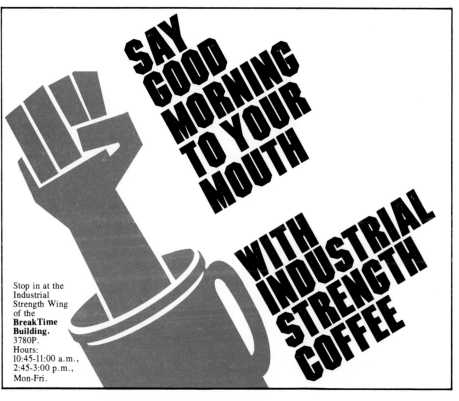

SAY GOOD MORNING TO YOUR MOUTH

WITH INDUSTRIAL STRENGTH COFFEE

Stop in at the Industrial Strength Wing of the **BreakTime Building.** 3780P. Hours: 10:45-11:00 a.m., 2:45-3:00 p.m., Mon-Fri.

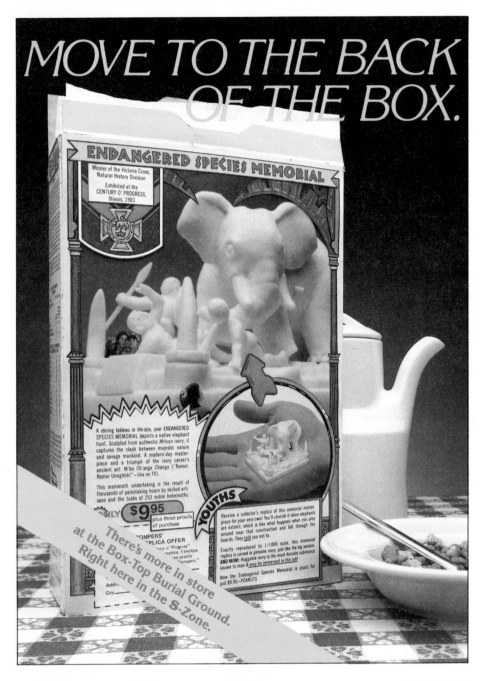

MOVE TO THE BACK OF THE BOX.

(on the box)

ENDANGERED SPECIES MEMORIAL

Winner of the Victoria Cross,
Natural History Division

Exhibited at the
CENTURY O' PROGRESS,
Illinois, 1983

A stirring tableau in life-size, your ENDANGERED SPECIES MEMORIAL depicts a native elephant hunt. Sculpted from authentic African ivory, it captures the clash between majestic nature and savage mankind. A modern-day masterpiece and a triumph of the ivory carver's ancient art: M'bo Ch'anga Changa ("Ramar, Ramar Unnghhh!"—like on TV).

This mammoth undertaking is the result of thousands of painstaking hours by skilled artisans and the tusks of 253 noble behemoths.

$9.95 plus three proofs of purchase

ROMPERS'
REPLICA OFFER
...

Receive a collector's replica of this memorial masterpiece for your very own! You'll cherish it when elephants are extinct, which is like what happens when you play around near that construction and fall through the boards. They told you not to.

Exactly reproduced to 1/1000 scale, this memorial replica is carved in genuine ivory, just like the big version. AND MOM: Huggable ivory is the most durable substance known to man & may be immersed in the tub!

Now the Endangered Species Memorial is yours for just $9.95—PEANUTS

YOUTHS

There's more in store at the Box-Top Burial Ground. Right here in the S-Zone.

and it feels good, no matter what she says. Do it. Do it.

Fabulous Picturephones. We'll get this working. Just give us a moment.

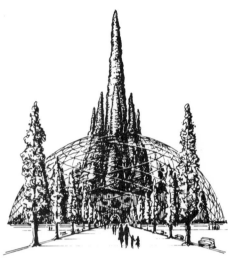

1026S. THE CATHEDRAL OF CURDS

How many wander through life hungering for that perfect, spreadable food, and how few find it? How tragic it is to see pilgrims journey from one restaurant to another, ordering here, taking out there, without ever achieving a sense of fulfillment. The Cathedral of Curds offers these searchers hope and comfort, a place where they can lay their burdens down and re-dedicate their lives to Cheeses. As you pass through the Cathedral, take a few moments to reflect on the meaning of the words inscribed above the altar: "I am the Life and the Whey." Many Fair visitors have found that even a brief meditation reaffirms their taste in the one true Gouda, the Father of Edam.

Charms

Cover Story. This exhibit features what may well be the world's most efficient piece of cheese. A hybrid curd of spreadable cream cheese and stretchable mozzarella, at first it was no bigger than a pat of margarine. Now it covers an area of more than two acres. A miracle you won't want to miss!

A Different Vein. Did you know that if the blue veins of a ripe, one-pound Roquefort were turned into a single thread it would circle your dairy counter over 75,000 times? To demonstrate just how much that is, the acolytes of The Cathedral of Curds have woven those veins into the world's second largest freestanding geodesic dome!

Philly. First a prize racehorse disappears, then a swamp of rare beige Velveeta with chives appears on the spot where, some say, she fell off the side of the world—implying some coincidence between the two events. Isolated instances of spontaneous veneration were paid—but there may not even have *been* such a racehorse. Hourly roundtable (but not *too* round) discussions are led by Monsignor F. X. Saltimbocca, who can also find a Jack of Clubs up your nose.

Garden of the Eternal Shelf-Life. In 1977 the

John Gordon family of Virden, Illinois, went for a picnic in their new Chevy wagon. Six years later John decided to trade in the old Chevy. While tidying it up, he found a cheese-n-cracker package left over from that picnic, wedged in the backseat. As you might expect, the crackers had long since disintegrated. But, astoundingly, the cheese retained the same smiling golden color of six years before! Why don't you and your family let John tell you all about it in the Garden of the Eternal Shelf-Life? The Chevy, the cheese (in its original package), and John's family are on display from 9–6 every day.

Pool of Runny Brie. Leave your small fry here to float a B-B-Belgian waffle boat while you pay homage. They can also eat Lindsey torten, which go nice with the brie.

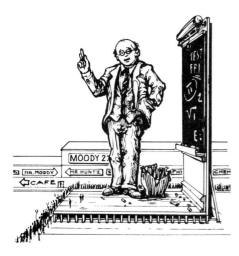

1027S. MR. MOODY

I would like to revise and extend my remarks on Mr. Moody. Readers of **FairWays 1** will recall that I took Mr. Moody to task for his phony "open book" exams and for giving **preference to athletes.** The answers were not in the Chem book. You could turn and turn and they were not in there. Also the turning and turning of the other students in search of God knows what kind of "Eureka" was distracting. And when I would turn to them and say, "You will have to stop turning those pages so fast as my concentration is now affected," they would reply, "You must understand I am only trying to get into a good college." This is your Moody legacy, then. I hated your sharkskin jacket. "Francis Bacon this," you'd say. And your Periodic Table of Elements, yanking it down with a k-*whipppp!* Each week I picked a new lucky atomic number. How come you never asked my lucky elements? How about zinc? **Zinc, Moody!** If I'd been on a team, sure. But Mr. Moo-dee never noticed what he wrought. I bought seven guinea pigs. I named them after my friends, and me, then sat back and waited for them to die. When several months passed and they were still jolly, I opened the window behind their cage. They began to die of the cold, big dead guinea pigs. And one with my name on it. Do you know what it's like praying your friends go first? Moo? And You, when you

saw me filling out the applications, picking one up and saying, "Friend," I hated that, "You'll never get into 'Vard. Your Chem average is a-wayyyyy down!" "Brown would be all right," I said. "Or one of the Potted Ivy. Amherst." You *walked away.* I hated expensive private school. My sentences ended in pain, rather than periods.

Charms

Room of Mr. Huntz. Department Chairman. Must've been Moody's friend. Kept him on year after year. I hated him too.

"Il Brodieatore." This was too a good idea, Dr. Boster! The all-Romance-language opera version of *The Prime of Miss Jean Brodie.* Moody told you I couldn't waste time on extracurricular activities, didn't he? Didn't he?

Extra Credit. What Marty Gogelbeck earned by playing a flashy, much overpraised forward. He's a doctor now. Big basketball star, Moody.

Toss-Up. They let Donny Gieringer out of wrestling because his mother said, "He's not going to be a wrestler." Of course his Chem grades suffered.

I'll Admit It. One day I came to class resolved to kill you, but I had trouble getting through the metal detector. Dioramas recall this.

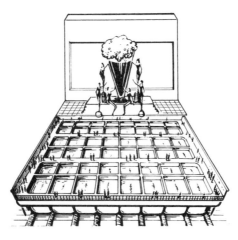

1028S. ICE-COLD AMAZONS

Clad in abbreviated bathing or "Dip"® suits, 44 years of winners (1935-1976, 1981-1983) of the Miss Rheingold contest are individually entombed in solid cakes of crystal-clear ice weighing up to 1400 pounds and change! The girls aren't waiting for some Prince Charming to melt them down. They're here to swap drinking stories—via intercom—clear up those really *nettling* problems of tavern etiquette (Do I *have* to read that stuff on the wall?), and to act as authorities on how long meat keeps in a freezer. Only one ice maiden is missing, 1982's Monica Ginger, who is kept busy these days working for the Fair as wife to the Honorable Jerry Riley, General Counsel to the CO'P. Her spot is symbolically filled by Mrs. Dolores Cinquemani of Carbondale, Ill., who dozes in a state of perpetual suspended animation from which she is permitted only occasionally to awake for blood tests, like in that movie.

Time Vault

De frost is on de do'r
De do'r mus' be lebe op'n
Do de milk sour?
Not if Time be but a hour.
Tho' you kin t'row it down de sink
Eternity mus' also drink.
    —folk wattle

Despite all we have learned of ancient civilizations, there is much we shall never know about them. We may be able to admire the exquisite craftsmanship of Egyptian jewelers or be awed by an Aristotle, but we will never be able to pull back the doily Time has drawn over their lunches.

To assure that our descendants are not denied the culinary legacy of our times, CO'P Ranger Chefs are now busy preparing a Picnic for Posterity. 5000 years from now, perhaps around lunchtime, a band of antiquarians will pry open the Time Vault to be buried on October 8, 1984, beneath the pitcher's mound of the former Wrigley's Field (today: Sermons From Gum, **S2**-Zone).

To aid in selecting its contents, CO'P staffers queried passing Fairgoers.

"I think, a brick. You know, those ice cream bricks?" was the most common answer.

When these responses proved too time-consuming, the Ranger Chefs developed their own solution: filling the Time Vault with a cross-section of the finest mixed nuts available in Greater O'Progressland! Which include: Brazil nuts, fancy nuts, lichees, and unusual white pistachios. *Plus,* the Vault's contents are guaranteed to contain not more than 50% peanuts.

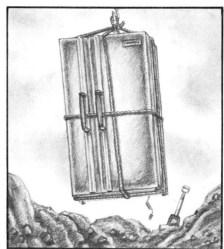

It's bedtime for Bonzo on October 8, 1984, when the Time Vault is rocked into its 5000 year sleep!

Instructions for locating the Time Vault have been printed on leaflets and disseminated to libraries and hospitals throughout the Free World. Each of these handsome pamphlets offers two double-beef hamburgers for the price of one to the person who retrieves the Vault's embarrassment of riches.

This offer is valid only for the year 6984.
☆☆☆☆☆☆☆☆☆☆☆☆☆☆☆☆☆☆☆☆☆☆

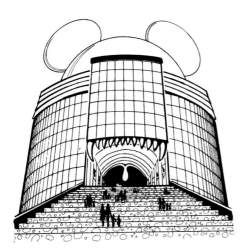

1032S. RATTRAP HUTCH

The Hutch isn't just a better rattrap, it's the best. Fairgoers will want to savor its eye-catching design in Hi-Tech83, combining the latest in modular convenience with the pleasing antique grace of mansard trim. The translucent bubble-domed roof—following a Romanesque curve of least resistance—adds a dynamic contrapuntal undertone of mercy to the otherwise blunt tantalum-carborundum rage. Then it *really* gets going.

Charms

Rats! Trapped Again! Fully automatic, the collapsible grid entrance traps the unwary visitor in a colorful wire mesh wall of reinforced steel prongs. Descending at random intervals, pinning but not penetrating (in much the same manner as helpless rodents of antiquity were immobilized but not destroyed), this Web-o-Steel creates an exciting sense of doom, raising blood pressure, body awareness, and defense mechanisms in preparation for the amusing experience ahead.

Next. Prodded gently, the Fairgoer scurries along a mirror-lit passageway illumined from above by 105,000 twinkle lights arranged in symbolic disarray to limn the 1867 skyline of Bombay, the year we purchased Alaska. Visitors are encouraged to locate on this mosaic images of such meaningful advances in rodent control as the broom and the ball peen hammer, and to inspect the modDay milk chocolate sculpture, "Madonna Deserting a Sinking Ship," which was the centerpiece in the Vatican's POT LUCK crate, though the towels were nice, too! By the way, although the chocolate is sweat-resistant, watch those paws!

Rats! Again! Visitors will want to finish their incarceration experience with a 5-day (mand.) confinement in the Holding Area. They should note the carefully simulated claw-scratch texture of walls and floor. The rich, metallic tints incorporated into the glass roof add a minor touch of decorator elegance to an otherwise purely functional design.

Time Tunnelvision. At 3 P.M. daily in the Holding Area, ex-city planner Robert "The Profit" Moses, President of the 1964 New York World's Fair, will discuss rodent control in Flushing Meadow, if he's up. His Fair solution:

Isolate all the rats by building major traffic arteries away from their shelters, effectively boxing them in. Mr. Moses may choose to title his lecture "Is Extermination Genocide?" though a slight disquisitional detour on whether knowledge is power and, if so, who shall be the knowledge broker? is always possible. On July 4, Mr. Moses will also receive a Brotherhood Flask from both surviving members of the Interfaith Council who can still remember what that stuff was that Fiorello LaGuardia used to put on his hair.

> *Renowned for its choice nubbly asphalt, the Tuskawawee Drive-In Parking Lot constitutes what one critic calls "The Crown Jewel of the Fair." Yet this "bangle" was almost lost to mankind forever. In 1982, the National Park Service decided to turn the giant Alabama lot into a nature preserve. Public outcry led to a "Save the Tuska" committee chaired by Jacqueline Onassis Deng (née Teng). Soon millions of citizens were wearing O, THANKS A LOT buttons and T-shirts. But the outlook remained uncertain until the resources of the CO'P were enlisted. Only a few cynics couldn't believe their eyes when the entire Tuskawawee was air-lifted intact by a phalanx of rotary engines and incorporated into the former Rt. 57 traffic circle. The rolling, nubbly expanse of the Tuskawawee had found a new and better home!*

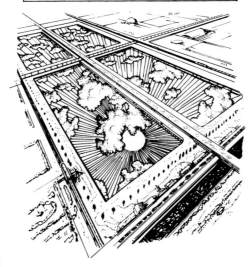

1033S. INSURANCE POOL

Because an unprecedented number and variety of priceless treasures have been gathered for the Fair, an unprecedented means had to be found to guarantee their security. The solution? The Reflecting Insurance Pool. Its 500-foot depth, 600-acre surface, and polluted fluids make it the perfectly secure receptacle for the Fair's jewels of the first water. Of course, that means what you see in the pavilions are actually ⅞ scale replicas of the originals! Interestingly enough, the exquisite workmanship of two reproductions—the crystalized fruit cups of the Balinese cafeteria, and the hanging garden of fetal pigs—made them so valuable they were subsequently deep-sixed and the originals salvaged for exhibition.

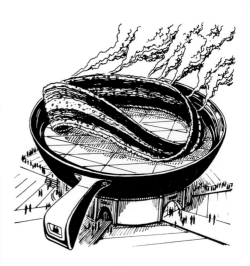

1034S. GREEN, GREEN FOURTH ESTATE

What's grown on the Fourth Estate? Nothing. And everything. Nothing is fomented, that's for sure. And everything—every scrap of info demanded or required by Fairgoers or interested America—is produced right here in the Hall of Free Speech. On the grounds of the Fourth Estate. And sold in the Marketplace of Ideas.

Charms

Format. We went and built the Hall in the shape of a Moebius Sizzlean® Strip. That's because the Sizzlean® part reminds us that, although most presspeople are swine, their by-products can be useful to us all. While the "Moebius" part reminds us that these strips appear to have two sides but in reality have only one. In the same way, although there appears to be two sides to every issue, your side and my side, in reality there's only one side: Our side, the Truth.

Night Dusk. A synthetic beige polyester cloud hovers almost aromatically over the Sizzlean® Strip, perpetually blacking out the tiny Hall of Free Speech, smallest at the Fair. The cloud symbolizes an epigram of the journalist—that "shadow of doubt" that hangs over all but the most carefully managed news. It also contains a Press Club (counter service only) serving waffles prepared in the Belgian tradition, and, directly inside, Copy, a seemingly endless stream of stale, cardboard cups of coffee moving along a conveyor belt under mock deadline pressure. The fry can pitch chocolate cigarettes at their half-empty recesses, provided expressly for this purpose.

Blue Pencil. Both ride and reason, a funny chair bounces you up and down while a computer lets you answer such questions as "Is this going to get the paper in dutch with the airlines?," just the way a real reporter does. The Blue Pencil prevents you from taking any unnecessary risks.

Backgrounder. It's noon. Roaring noon. And there's Herbie Tufo with his press releases, hand-outs, and lists of photo opportunities, sharing them with visiting fourth-esaters on their two-week permits. If it's a *real* hard news day, watch Herbie dig into the Fair's bread-and-butter issues with both barrels. He'll say, "Look, I've got a simple statement to read and then no questions. Please—can I have it settled down? I have a job to do, too, you know." Big old bear—Herbie Tufo!

–30–. Naturally, several journalists—29, exactly—have surpassed the usual media ruck, according to a poll conducted by the CO'P and filled out by *top* journalism professors during their recreation period. Honored in this exhibit include: columnist Kelly ("Call Me Ms.") Green of the Milwaukee *Says,* J. Kevin Clull of *Mr. Iowa,* Pokey Wambsganss of the Beaver (Or.) *Tales 'N Advocate,* and Christopher ("Hi, Guy!") Bathe of *Yachting.* Also: the stirring Wax Dummy of the Unknown Journalist ... #30. It could be you or your children.

Beefing It Up. From time to time, famous writers (such as Hemingway or Stephen Crane) honor newspapers with their presence before moving on to their career. Holographs of a herd of pure-bred cattle wandering aimlessly through a City Room get this point across.

Ingenuously Getting It In. The fall came on; it coughed up the last flecks of summer, then moved over everything and the land turned hard, the air cold.

–40–. It is noted that those who get ahead fast in journalism generally know somebody, but *that it is never too late to be great.* Public relations is not such a bad place to end up. You *can* make an omelette without breaking eggs.

> Some people keep wondering, "Who started the Fair?" That's like asking, Who was behind the oil crisis? Who killed Kennedy?

☆ ☆ ☆ ☆ ☆ ☆ ☆ ☆ ☆ ☆ ☆ ☆ ☆ ☆ ☆ ☆ ☆ ☆

*A Fairways Fea*T*ure*

DON'T FORGET: You earn your CO'P Exit Vita by passing a short exam at the Banks of Lake Michigan, on your way out. So start boning up today. Those FAILING to secure a PASSING grade may be asked to re-visit certain key Zones before re-applying to the Banks. There's no reason to FAIL, though many DO. The answers to these sample questions [below], as well as to the ones on the REAL THING, may be found right here in the pages of FAIRWAYS & MEANS. Happy hunting.

E-Z Secular
569. The main reason for saying grace before meals is to keep God from poisoning your food.
☐ True
☐ False

Stricter
917. Jack is musically-oriented. He keeps his dial tuned to WCO'P. Roy has a drinking problem. Samantha is a lawyer. She admits she has a lot to learn from Mr. Smart, her boss. "I can't believe I'm finally a lawyer," Samantha says. "And getting paid for it!" Question: *Why hasn't anything been done about Roy's drinking?*
  a. Because he's a journalist and they're all drunk so nobody notices.
  b. They sent him out on a story and he was just bombed so he *completely* changed the facts but they thought that was *funny,* so they ran it.
  c. If he was a lawyer the Senior Partners would all get together and say, "Let's get Roy the best help money can buy," but journalists do not help their own.
  d. When a famous doctor *did* try getting some "pertinent facts" out of Roy, Roy just made them up.

© 1983 OBTS, Outward Bound Testing Service
☆ ☆ ☆ ☆ ☆ ☆ ☆ ☆ ☆ ☆ ☆ ☆ ☆ ☆ ☆ ☆ ☆ ☆

The spot price for all leftovers, crumbs, table scraps, and organic detritus purchased by the CO'P's 17 wasp-waisted Food RRRRecyc Centers is set by supply and demand, inventory levels, spoilage, and other factors affecting the meal aftermarket. We ask that you place the remains of every meal in the plastic bags provided for that purpose—first removing crust from enriched buns and separating desserts from entrees—and that you don't, please, ask to be paid more than the posted price for previously-owned foodstuffs. If the RRRRecyc-ers kowtowed to the manners of the marketplace, it would be impossible for them to continue offering reconditioned soups and fruit juices at below wholesale prices. (Besides, a certain Colonel K. has lived "quite flagrantly" off RRRRecycle Security during his six-month stay at the Fair, thank you very much.) Remember, that "OK Used Lunch" sticker on the tray is your assurance of complete nutrition at low cost.

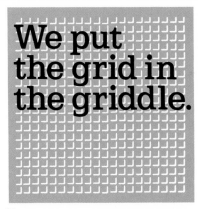
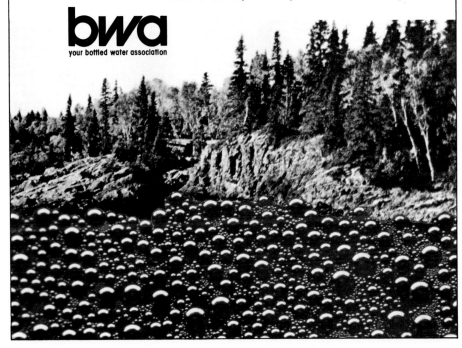

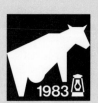

FairWays & Means 2

"The Greatest Food for the Greatest Number"

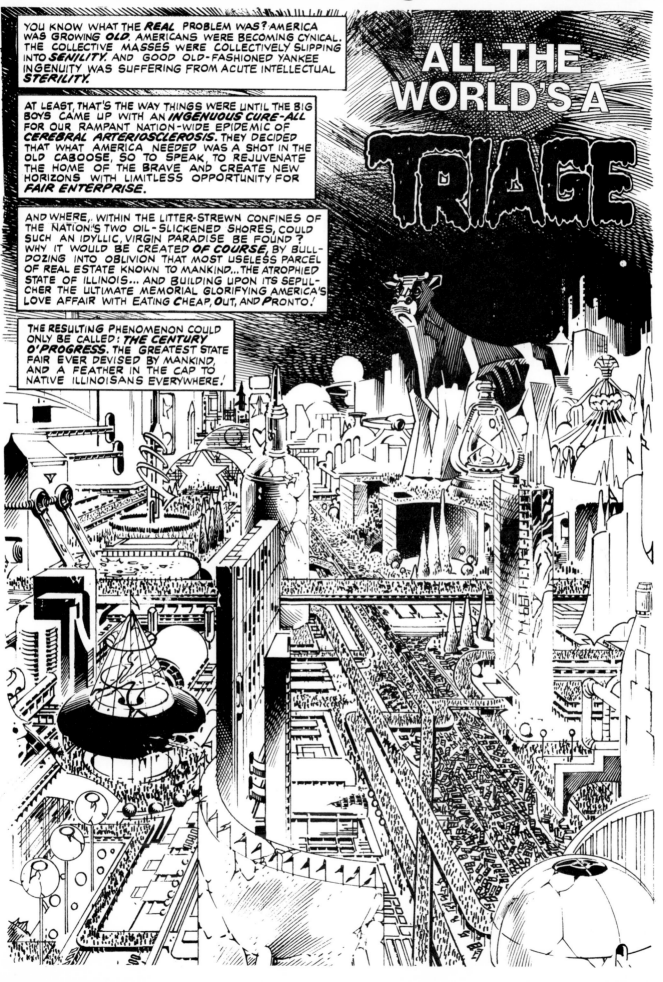

YOU KNOW WHAT THE *REAL* PROBLEM WAS? AMERICA WAS GROWING *OLD*. AMERICANS WERE BECOMING CYNICAL. THE COLLECTIVE MASSES WERE COLLECTIVELY SLIPPING INTO *SENILITY*. AND GOOD OLD-FASHIONED YANKEE INGENUITY WAS SUFFERING FROM ACUTE INTELLECTUAL *STERILITY*.

AT LEAST, THAT'S THE WAY THINGS WERE UNTIL THE BIG BOYS CAME UP WITH AN *INGENUOUS CURE-ALL* FOR OUR RAMPANT NATION-WIDE EPIDEMIC OF *CEREBRAL ARTERIOSCLEROSIS*. THEY DECIDED THAT WHAT AMERICA NEEDED WAS A SHOT IN THE OLD CABOOSE, SO TO SPEAK, TO REJUVENATE THE HOME OF THE BRAVE AND CREATE NEW HORIZONS WITH LIMITLESS OPPORTUNITY FOR *FAIR ENTERPRISE*.

AND WHERE, WITHIN THE LITTER-STREWN CONFINES OF THE NATION'S TWO OIL-SLICKENED SHORES, COULD SUCH AN IDYLLIC, VIRGIN PARADISE BE FOUND? WHY IT WOULD BE CREATED *OF COURSE*, BY BULL-DOZING INTO OBLIVION THAT MOST USELESS PARCEL OF REAL ESTATE KNOWN TO MANKIND...THE ATROPHIED STATE OF ILLINOIS... AND BUILDING UPON ITS SEPUL-CHER THE ULTIMATE MEMORIAL GLORIFYING AMERICA'S LOVE AFFAIR WITH EATING *CHEAP, OUT*, AND *PRONTO*!

THE RESULTING PHENOMENON COULD ONLY BE CALLED: *THE CENTURY O'PROGRESS*. THE GREATEST STATE FAIR EVER DEVISED BY MANKIND, AND A FEATHER IN THE CAP TO NATIVE ILLINOISANS EVERYWHERE!

ALL THE WORLD'S A TRIAGE

AND OH, WHAT A MARVELOUS SPECTACLE IT WAS! WITH ITS ENDLESS MILES OF UNIQUE PLASTICIZED EATERIES AND ITS SERPENTINE ONE-WAY SINGLE-LANE EXPRESSWAY, SNAKING THROUGH THE FAIRGROUNDS LIKE AN *INCONTROLLABLE INTESTINAL SPASM*—AND ASSURING VISITORS OF SEEING EVERY EXHIBIT IN PROPER THEMATIC ORDER.

FROM OPENING DAY BACK IN OCTOBER OF '83 WHEN THE FIRST EXCITABLE CROWDS STREAKED INTO THE FAIRGROUNDS, PAST THE 300-FOOT *HIGH* RETAINING WALL DESIGNED TO KEEP OUT UNDESIRABLES, *HAPPY FACES* HAD THRONGED THE FAIRWAYS, MUNCHING THEIR WAY INTO STOLID EUPHORIC ECSTASY.

THUS, THE CO'P. THE PRIMAL PRIDE OF THE EMERGENT 80'S. THE MESSIANIC MACHINATION THAT GOT AMERICA BACK ON ITS FEET AGAIN. IT WAS WHAT EARTH *WOULD* HAVE BEEN HAD THAT PUSHY BITCH EVE NOT FORCED SOUR APPLES UPON AN UNSUSPECTING ADAM, EFFECTUALLY INDUCING A 2,000,000 YEAR EPIDEMIC OF *GENETIC DIARRHEA.*

AND YET, JUST AS WITH THAT FIRST PENURIOUS POISONING, ALL IT TOOK WERE A FEW BAD APPLES TO SOUR PARADISE FOR THE REST OF US AS WELL.

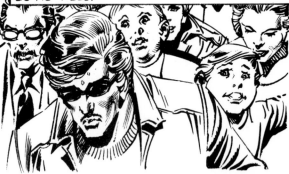

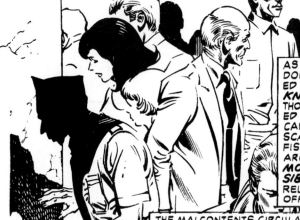

AS IT ALWAYS DOES, IT STARTED WITH THE *KNOCKERS,* THOSE DISGRUNTLED FEW WHO CAN BRING SCAVENGER FISH SWIMMING AROUND *THE MOST RESPONSIBLE* PUBLIC RELATIONS OFFICIAL.

THE MALCONTENTS CIRCULATED RUMORS THAT THE MATCHING 300-FOOT *DEEP* RETAINING WALL HAD BEEN CONSTRUCTED TO KEEP FOLKS FROM BURROWING *OUT.* AND THAT NO ONE WAS PASSING THE EXIT EXAM—NO ONE WAS LEAVING!

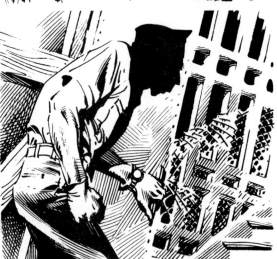

WELL, WHY ANYONE WOULD WANT TO RETURN TO THE HOSTILITY OF THE OUTSIDE WORLD WHEN EDEN COULD BE ETERNALLY THEIRS, WAS A MYSTERY TO ME.

BUT—AS A SIDEBAR TO THAT—I, TOO, HAD ONCE BEEN ONE OF THE MALEVOLENT MALIGNERS.

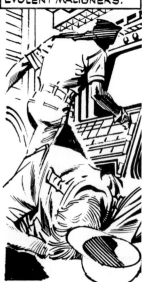

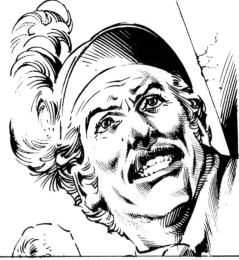

ME? OH, I ALMOST FORGOT. I'M *BARNEY STONE,* EDITOR OF THE FRIEND'S GUIDEBOOK, ASS'T DIRECTOR OF PUBLIC RELATIONS, AND CHIEF NEMESIS TO THE VILE UNDERGROUND PREVARICATORS WHO HAVE VOWED TO *DESTROY* THE CO'P!

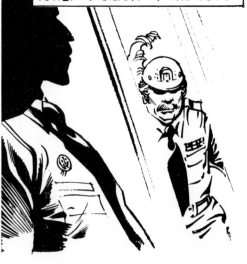

YES. WAY BACK IN MY FORMER REINCARNATION AS A COLUMNIST ON THE HISTORICAL CARBONDALE *ATOM,* I HARBORED SOME AWFULLY KINKY IDEAS OF MY OWN ABOUT *OUR GREAT FRIEND,* THE GREAT FAIR. NOW, YOU MIGHT SAY, I WAS THE GREAT FRIEND'S *BEST FRIEND.*

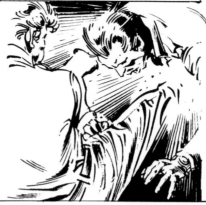

I WAS ABLE TO RECOGNIZE THE BAD DOCTOR ON SIGHT. IN FACT, THOUGH I BLUSH TO ADMIT IT, WHEN I FIRST MET CINQUEMANI I COULD'VE TAKEN HIM WITHOUT A TUSSLE.

MY CURRENT USAGE OF PAST TENSE SINGULAR WAS BROUGHT ABOUT BY MY *FINAL ENCOUNTER* WITH THE *LEADER* OF THE ANTI-FAIR UNDERGROUND HIMSELF! HIS NAME? *DR. GUS CINQUEMANI*, AN ANIMAL VET- AND CHIEF PETTY KNOCKER.

I'D BLOWN MY SHOT, THAT WAS ABOUT THE ONLY BLIGHT ON MY RECORD, TOO. BUT THAT'S ANOTHER STORY.

WHEN I HEARD HE'D BEEN *SKULKING* AROUND THE *R-ZONE,* I SPED RIGHT OVER THERE ON ONE OF THE SECRET BACK ROADS KNOWN ONLY TO TRUSTED PERSONNEL. IT WAS TIME TO PUT THIS BABY ON ICE FOR KEEPS.

BINGO. THERE HE WAS, LIKE A SLAVERING MAGGOT, CREEPING ABOUT THE NOBLE MILK & FIRE MONUMENT— AND BOSSY THE COW AND HER ETERNAL FLAME WERE *DUAL NUCLEAR REACTORS,* WHICH, IF SABOTAGED WITH THE PROPER DEGREE OF EXPERTISE, COULD NUKE OUR GREAT FRIEND RIGHT OUTTA THIS WORLD!

WHICH IS HOW I CAME TO BE STARING DOWN THE YELLOW-BREATHED JAWS OF DEATH WHILE CINQUEMANI THE DERANGED BOUNDED TOWARDS ME WITH THE ADJUSTABLE NUB OF HIS CATTLE PROD SWITCHED TOWARDS *KILL!*

I COULD HAVE BEEN JUST ANOTHER FORGOTTEN OBIT BURIED IN THE BACK PAGES OF NEWSPAPER HEAVEN! INSTEAD I THREW THREE OF BOSSY'S FOUR RETRACTABLE LEG LEVERS— INSTANTLY CAUSING THE MAMMOTH MONUMENT TO *GENUFLECT* WITH A TRIO OF ITS APPENDAGES, WHILE THE FOURTH REMAINED RIGID— SENDING THE WARPED CINQUEMANI HURTLING OFF HIS FEET!

YET THE DIABOLICAL DEVIATE MUST HAVE PLANNED IT ALL! HE KNEW I'D THROW THOSE SWITCHES. HE KNEW, TOO, THAT HIS OWN INALTERABLE MOMENTUM IN COLLIDING WITH THE BEAST'S INNER WORKINGS WOULD BE FORCE ENOUGH TO SEND IT *TOPPLING* INTO THE GREAT LANTERN...

...WHICH IN TURN WAS THE *PRECISE MOTION* REQUIRED FOR THE MONUMENT'S *DUAL NUCLEAR CORE* TO MELT DOWN, EXPANDING THE WATER TABLE, WHICH HAD *ONLY MOMENTS BEFORE* RESTED SO SERENELY BENEATH WHAT WAS ONCE THE GREAT CENTURY O' PROGRESS!

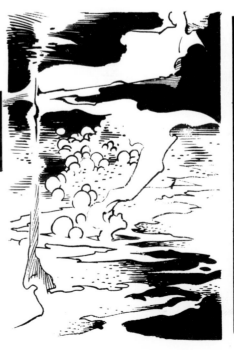

THE COW HAD DONE IT AGAIN! KICKED OVER THE LANTERN. HISTORY HAD REPRINTED ITSELF!

THE KNOCKERS HAD TRIUMPHED. THE CENTURY O' SHOT OFF LIKE AN EXCITABLE PORN STAR, AND TOOK UP A STATIONARY GLOBAL ORBIT SOMEWHERE ABOVE THE STRATOSPHERE OF SOUTHERN TANZANIA!

AND ME? WELL ...FOR ALL THE PAIN AND SORROW, ALL THE LONG HOURS AT MY DESK, I'D DO IT ALL OVER AGAIN, TOMORROW. EVERYTHING. *JUST SO LONG AS NO ONE GOT HURT!*

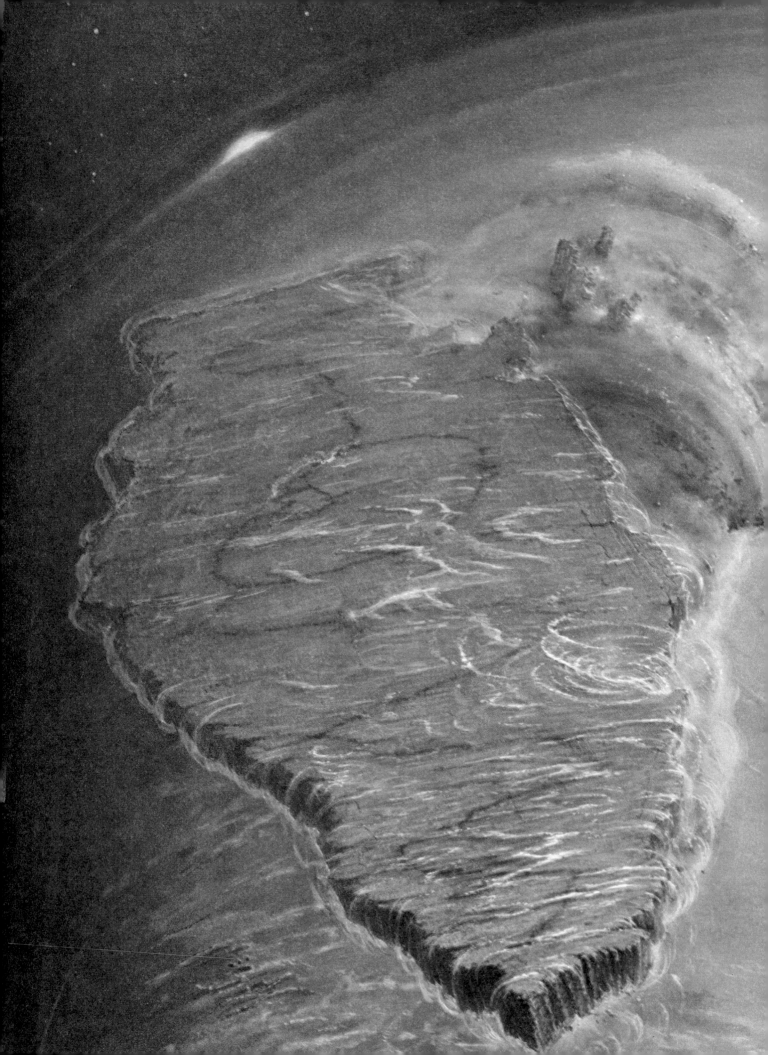